ly

III Patient

Third edition

NS/12

Monitoring the Critically Ill Patient

Third edition

Philip Jevon
RN, BSc(Hons), PGCE, ENB 124
Resuscitation Officer/Clinical Skills Lead
Honorary Clinical Lecturer
Manor Hospital
Walsall
UK

AND

Beverley Ewens
RN, BSc(Hons), PGCE, ENB 100, PG Cert Management
Studies, DPSN, PG Dip Critical Care,
Lecturer, School of Nursing and Midwifery,
Edith Cowan University,
Perth
Western Australia

CONSULTING EDITOR

Jagtar Singh Pooni
BSc(Hons), MRCP(UK), FRCA
Consultant in Anaesthesia and Intensive Care Medicine
New Cross Hospital
Wolverhampton
UK

⊛WILEY-BLACKWELL

A John Wiley & Sons, Ltd., Publication

This edition first published 2012 © 2012 Blackwell Publishing Ltd

Blackwell Publishing was acquired by John Wiley & Sons in February 2007. Blackwell's publishing program has been merged with Wiley's global Scientific, Technical and Medical business to form Wiley-Blackwell.

Registered office: John Wiley & Sons, Ltd, The Atrium, Southern Gate, Chichester, West Sussex, PO19 8SQ, UK

Editorial offices: 9600 Garsington Road, Oxford, OX4 2DQ, UK
The Atrium, Southern Gate, Chichester, West Sussex, PO19 8SQ, UK
2121 State Avenue, Ames, Iowa 50014-8300, USA

For details of our global editorial offices, for customer services and for information about how to apply for permission to reuse the copyright material in this book please see our website at www.wiley.com/wiley-blackwell.

Library of Congress Cataloging-in-Publication Data

Jevon, Philip.
  Monitoring the critically ill patient / Philip Jevon and Beverley Ewens ; consulting editor, Jagtar Singh Pooni. – 3rd ed.
      p. ; cm.
  Includes bibliographical references and index.
  ISBN 978-1-4443-3747-1 (pbk. : alk. paper)
  I. Ewens, Beverley. II. Title.
  [DNLM: 1. Intensive Care–methods.   2. Monitoring, Physiologic–methods.   3. Critical Illness. WX 218]
  LC classification not assigned
  616.02'8–dc23
                                                                    2011034244

A catalogue record for this book is available from the British Library.

Wiley also publishes its books in a variety of electronic formats. Some content that appears in print may not be available in electronic books.

Set in 9/11 pt Palatino by Toppan Best-set Premedia Limited
Printed and bound in Malaysia by Vivar Printing Sdn Bhd

[1 2012]

Contents

Foreword

In the current healthcare environment, there is increased emphasis placed on the early recognition and treatment of the acute and critically ill patient. There is certainly good reason for this, with approximately 80% patients who have a cardiac arrest audited in hospital displaying adverse signs prior to collapse. It is the responsibility of every nurse to be able to effectively monitor patients and understand the significance of what the observations are communicating to them regarding the patient's condition, and what appropriate action needs to be taken. Nurses need to understand that fast and appropriate action can save lives.

This third edition builds on the success of the first two editions. The content has been completely revised to reflect current guidelines and practice. Five new chapters have been added (blood transfusion, infection, critically ill child, blood transfusion and pregnancy) making this a comprehensive guide to monitoring the critically ill patient. This book remains a valuable guide for healthcare staff.

I congratulate the authors on their achievement and I would particularly recommend this book to nurses working in critical care, high dependency care, coronary care, theatres, A & E and the acute ward environment, especially in the ever growing Acute Cardiac, Medical and Surgical Assessment areas.

Jacqui Daly (Mrs)
RN, BSc (Hons), ENB 124,998, 927 and N-14.
Matron and Specialist Practitioner in Cardiology

Preface

When we developed the first edition of this textbook in 2002, it was with high hopes that there would be at least one more edition and, despite no longer sharing the same continent, here we are with the third.

The book has undergone a complete revision with this edition, including the addition of many new chapters as well as extensive updating of existing ones. To ensure that this edition provides the reader with contemporaneous material, an integral component of each chapter is the inclusion of best available evidence, the most current trends in clinical practice and the latest recommendations from statutory and advisory bodies. As we both continue to work within, and be enthused by, critical care nursing, we are uniquely placed to witness and contribute to developments in practice at first hand.

This text is intended to be an aid to the novice critical care or ward nurse in a culture of accelerating ward acuity, as they embrace the challenges that this varied and stimulating specialty offers. It may also serve as a revision tool for the more experienced critical care nurse, keen to update on unfamiliar aspects of monitoring, included in this book.

The worldwide movement targeting improvements in patient outcomes, through the promotion of early identification of the patient at risk, has experienced no higher profile than it does today. It has been evident in the literature for many years that simple strategies, including accurate and appropriate monitoring, interpretation of resulting data, appropriate and timely patient management, in tandem with escalation of care where necessary, is the key to early identification of the deteriorating patient. We hope that this text not only provides readers with the knowledge and skills to contribute to this process but also entices them to explore further.

This book is dedicated to all the critical care patients for whom we have had the privilege to care, past, present and in the future.

Bev Ewens and Phil Jevon
June 2011

Contributors

Jayne Breakwell, RN, Child Dip HE, Paediatirc Sister, Paediatric Assessment Unit, Manor Hospital, Walsall Healthcare NHS Trust, Walsall, West Midlands, UK

Mandeep Dhanda,BSc (Hons), HPC registered Biomedical Scientist, Transfusion Practitioner, Blood Transfusion Department, Manor Hospital, Walsall Healthcare NHS Trust, Walsall, West Midlands, UK

Dan Higgins RGN, ENB998, ENB100, Senior Charge Nurse, Critical Care, University Hospitals Birmingham NHS Foundation Trust, Birmingham and Director, Healthcare Education & Skills Training (HEST).

Recognition and Management of the Deteriorating Patient

LEARNING OBJECTIVES

At the end of this chapter the reader will be able to:

☐ discuss the importance of prevention of in-hospital adverse events
☐ identify the clinical signs of impending or established deterioration
☐ discuss the role of outreach and medical emergency teams
☐ discuss the importance of education and training in relation to the deteriorating patient.

INTRODUCTION

Critically ill patients are not necessarily located within intensive care or high dependency units (ICU and HDU), but are frequently managed within ward areas. There is irrefutable evidence to confirm that early identification and timely management of the deteriorating patient, may negate the need for transfer to these units and ultimately improve outcomes (Jones et al. 2007; NICE 2007). The literature states that, antecedents to deterioration are present in up to 80% of patients before an adverse event, cardiac arrest, unplanned ICU admission or death occurs (Kause et al. 2004). This is postulated to be because of both the inability to either recognise deterioration, and/or to act on it promptly and appropriately, compounded by existing poor communication channels (Schein et al. 1990; Franklin and Matthew 1994). Nurses, by definition, are at the forefront of monitoring and recognising

Monitoring the Critically Ill Patient, Third Edition.
Philip Jevon, Beverley Ewens.
© 2012 Blackwell Publishing Ltd. Published 2012 by Blackwell Publishing Ltd.

...eriorating patients which, in turn, relies on appropriate monitoring and accurate interpretation of findings, accompanied by timely action. If patients are permitted to progress without prompt and appropriate management, adverse events will occur with associated poor survival rates.

The aim of this chapter is to understand the recognition and management of the deteriorating patient.

PREVENTION OF IN-HOSPITAL ADVERSE EVENTS

In-hospital adverse events have been defined as an unintended injury or complication resulting in prolonged length of stay, disability or death, not attributed to the patient's underlying disease process alone but by their health-care management (Baba-Akbari Sari et al. 2006; de Vries et al. 2007). The causes of this have been classified into three subthemes (NPSA 2007):

1. Failure to measure basic observations of vital signs
2. Lack of recognition of the importance of worsening vital signs
3. Delay in responding to deteriorating vital signs

The prevalence of adverse events has been estimated at between 3% and 17% of all hospital admissions, with resulting high human and financial costs (Baba-Akbari Sari et al. 2006). The most serious adverse events classified are unplanned admission to an ICU, cardiac arrest or death, 50% of which are estimated to be preventable (de Vries et al. 2007).

Survival to discharge from in-hospital cardiopulmonary arrest

In the UK, overall less than 20% of patients who have an in-hospital cardiopulmonary arrest survive to discharge (Meaney et al. 2010). These survival rates are also dependent upon the location and time of day at which they occur (Herlitz et al. 2002; Peberdy et al. 2008). Most of these survivors will have received prompt and effective defibrillation for a monitored and witnessed ventricular fibrillation (VF) arrest (Fig. 1.1) or pulseless ventricular tachycardia (VT), caused by primary myocardial ischaemia (Resuscitation Council UK 2010). Survival to discharge in these patients is very good, even as high as 37%) (Meaney et al. 2010).

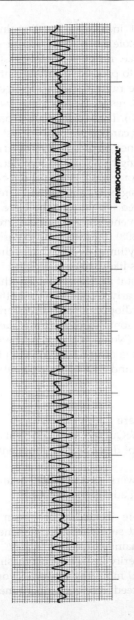

Fig. 1.1 Ventricular fibrillation (coarse).

3

Unfortunately, most in-hospital cardiopulmonary arrests are caused by either asystole (39%) (Fig. 1.2) or pulseless electrical activity (PEA) (37%) (i.e. no pulse, but an ECG trace that would normally be expected to produce a cardiac output, (Fig. 1.3) Both of these non-shockable rhythms are associated with a very poor outcome (12% and 11% respectively – Meaney et al. 2010; Resuscitation Council UK 2010). These arrests are usually not sudden nor are they unpredictable: cardiopulmonary arrest usually presents as a final step in a sequence of progressive deterioration of the presenting illness, involving hypoxia and hypotension (Resuscitation Council UK 2010). In some studies it has been alleged that patients with abnormal vital signs before cardiac arrest have improved survival rates, compared with those who have normal vital signs, thus indicating the preventability of cardiac arrests (Skrifvars et al. 2006; Peberdy et al. 2008). Patients who experience cardiac arrest with non-shockable rhythms have a reduced chance of survival, so a vital approach that is likely to be successful is prevention of the cardiopulmonary arrest if at all possible. For this prevention strategy to be successful, early recognition and effective treatment of patients at risk of cardiopulmonary arrest are paramount. This strategy may prevent some cardiac arrests, deaths and unanticipated ICU admissions (Nolan et al. 2005). The statistics are irrefutable in that antecedents are present in 79% of cardiopulmonary arrests, 55% of deaths and 54% of unanticipated ICU admissions (Kause et al. 2004).

Suboptimal critical care
In a seminal study (McQuillan et al. 1998), it was demonstrated that the management of deteriorating inpatients in the UK is frequently suboptimal.

Two external reviewers assessed the quality of care in 100 consecutive unplanned admissions to ICU:

- Twenty patients were deemed to have been well managed and 54 to have received suboptimal management, with disagreement about the remainder.
- Case mix and severity of illness were similar between the groups, but the ICU mortality rate was worse in those whom both reviewers agreed received suboptimal care before ICU

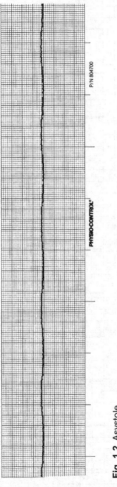

Fig. 1.2 Asystole.

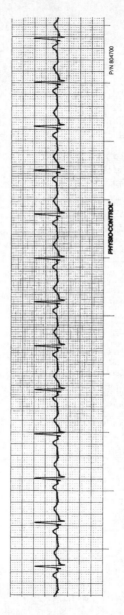

Fig. 1.3 Pulseless electrical activity (PEA)/sinus rhythm.

admission (48% compared with 25% in the well-managed group).

- Admission to ICU was considered late in 37 patients in the suboptimal group. Overall, a minimum of 4.5% and a maximum of 41% of admissions were considered potentially avoidable.
- Suboptimal care contributed to morbidity or mortality in most instances.
- The main causes of suboptimal care were considered to be failure of organisation, lack of knowledge, failure to appreciate clinical urgency, lack of supervision and failure to seek advice. Junior staff frequently fail to recognise deterioration and appreciate the severity of illness and, when therapeutic interventions are implemented, these have often been delayed or are inappropriate. The management of deteriorating patients is a significant problem, particularly at night and at weekends, when responsibility for these patients usually falls to the on-call team whose main focus is on a rising tide of new admissions (Baudoin and Evans 2002).

Despite gaining criticism for alleged methodological weakness, this groundbreaking study was the catalyst for many other reviews and studies pertaining to the management of the deteriorating patient and the recognition of clinical antecedents.

Even more disturbingly, earlier studies of events leading to 'unexpected' in-hospital cardiac arrest indicate that many patients have clearly recorded evidence of marked physiological deterioration before the event, without appropriate action being taken in many cases (Schein, et al. 1990; Franklin and Matthew 1994).

Deficiencies in critical care management frequently involve simple aspects of care, e.g. failure to recognise and effectively treat abnormalities of the patient's airway, breathing and circulation, incorrect use of oxygen therapy, failure to monitor the patient, failure to ask for help from senior colleagues, ineffective communication, lack of teamwork and failure to use treatment limitation plans (McQuillan et al. 1998; Hodgetts et al. 2002).

The ward nurse is uniquely positioned to recognise that the patient is starting to deteriorate and to call for appropriate help (Adam and Osborne 2005). However, recognition of the deteriorating patient remains inadequate (Beaumont et al. 2008; Odell et al.

2009). Strategies to prevent in-hospital adverse events are based on certain elements: the early identification of the deteriorating patient, escalation of care, timely and appropriate management, and the early transfer to critical care areas as appropriate.

Guidelines have been produced to enable organisations and individual clinicians to design, implement and evaluate a strategy to identify and manage the deteriorating patient to improve outcomes.

Best practice – measurement and documentation of observation

The accurate measurement of physiological observations is essential in detecting the deteriorating patient and reducing adverse events.

- All patients in acute care settings should have observations performed
- All patients should have observations performed on admission (NICE 2007)
- Observations should comprise as a minimum:
  - *Respiratory rate*
  - *Oxygen saturation*
  - *Heart rate*
  - *Blood pressure*
  - *Temperature*
  - *Level of consciousness* (NICE 2007; ACSQHC 2010)
- **Frequency of observations should be consistent with the condition of the patient, but at least once every 8 hours and documented in the monitoring plan**
- Observation charts should display observations in graphic format

---

Best practice

Escalation process should:

- be a formal documented escalation process that should be available and applicable to all patients at all times of the day
- support and authorise the clinician to escalate care until a satisfactory response is achieved
- be tailored to the organisation's characteristics and available resources
- allow for a graded response according to the degree of physiological abnormality, e.g. increase in frequency of observations, interventions

by ward staff, review by medical team, summoning urgent assistance, transfer to a higher level of care
- specify the levels of abnormality for which care should be escalated, for whom the care is escalated, who else to contact when care is escalated, timeframes for requested response and back-up options for obtaining a response if this fails
- consider the needs of patients with advance directives

(ACSQHC 2010)

CLINICAL SIGNS OF DETERIORATION

The clinical signs of deterioration and critical illness are usually similar regardless of the underlying cause, because they reflect compromise of the respiratory, cardiovascular and neurological systems (Nolan et al. 2005). These clinical signs are commonly:

- tachypnoea/breathlessness
- hypotension
- altered conscious level (e.g. lethargy, confusion, restlessness or falling level of consciousness). (Kause et al. 2004)

Tachypnoea, a particularly important indicator of an at-risk patient (Goldhill et al. 1999), is the most common abnormality found in critical illness (Goldhill et al. 2004). In an early study it was identified that a raised respiratory rate (>27/min) occurred in 54% of patients in the 72 hours preceding cardiac arrest, most of which occurred 72 hours before the event (Fieselmann et al. 1993).

TRACK-AND-TRIGGER SYSTEMS

Most hospitals in the UK now use some form of track-and-trigger system, e.g. early warning scoring system (EWS), to identify deteriorating patients, and are an important component of risk management strategies (Donahue and Endacott 2010). There is a lack of rigorous evidence to support any single track-and-trigger system above the others, but it is important that organisations introduce a tool based on best evidence surrounding reliability, validity, specificity and sensitivity, and on local requirements (Gao et al. 2007). It has been recommended that some type of physiological track and trigger system should be used to monitor all adult patients in acute hospital settings (NICE 2007).

EARLY WARNING SCORING SYSTEMS

The recommendations from *Comprehensive Critical Care* (Department of Health 2000) were the widespread implementation of EWS systems and outreach services. The EWS systems have been developed as a tool to enable ward staff to combine their regular observations to produce a physiological score (Sharpley and Holden 2004). They are based on the premise that there is a common physiological pathway of deterioration in the critically ill patient, which can be detected by simple ward-based observations (Goldhill 2001).

The most commonly used scoring system is an aggregated system wherein a weighted score is attached to a combination of blood pressure, pulse, respiratory rate, oxygen saturations, temperature, urine output and simplified level of consciousness (AVPU) (Fig. 1.4). A trigger response is activated when the patient reaches a certain score and the designated escalation process is triggered. Nursing and other healthcare staff must then alert the designated expert help following local protocols. Escalation policies are put in place whereby a failure to improve (or to receive prompt help) results in the immediate contact of more senior members (including consultant staff) (Baudouin and Evans 2002). Clear guidelines should be drawn up to guide the nurse in when escalation is necessary and whom to contact for help (Fig. 1.5).

Each hospital should instigate a track-and-trigger system that allows rapid detection of the signs of early clinical deterioration

- **A**lert
- **R**esponds to **v**oice
- **R**esponds to **p**ain
- **U**nconscious

(Resuscitation Council UK 2011)

Fig. 1.4 Level of consciousness.

JOONDALUP
HEALTH CAMPUS

ADULT OBSERVATION CHART
EARLY WARNING SYSTEM (EWS)

URN: ....
Surname: ....
Forename: ....
Gender: .... D.O.B. ....

Ward:.................... | 0 | 1 | 2 | MET |

DATE		
TIME		

TEMPERATURE X
>38.5° / 38° / 37.5° / 37° / 36.5° / 36° / 35.5° / 35° / <35°

SYSTOLIC B/P ONLY V
>200 / 190 / 180 / 170 / 160 / 150 / 140 / 130 / 120 / 110 / 100 / 90 / <90

BP

PULSE ●
≥140 / 130 / 120 / 110 / 100 / 90 / 80 / 70 / 60 / 50 / 40 / <40

RR / MIN ●
>35 / 30 / 20 / <8

SpO₂%
95 / 90 / <90

OXYGEN / MODE L/min eg. RA HV, NRM

PAIN SCORE 0-10
ALERT ● A
RESPONDS TO VOICE ● V
RESPONDS TO PAIN ● P
UNRESPONSIVE ● U

EARLY WARNING SYSTEM SCORE

TEMPERATURE SCORE	
SYSTOLIC BP SCORE	
PULSE SCORE	
RR SCORE	
SpO₂% SCORE	
AVPU SCORE	
EWS TOTAL SCORE	
NURSE INITLAL	

| TOTAL SCORE 1 – 3 INFORM SHIFT COORDINATOR AND REPEAT OBSERVATIONS IN ONE HOUR | TOTAL SCORE 4 – 6 MEDICAL REVIEW WITHIN 30 MINUTES AND IF AFTER HOURS, NFORM CNC | TOTAL SCORE ≥ 7 OR 1 PARAMETER IN RED BOX MET CALL | ALTERED EWS ☐ |

Fig. 1.5 Early warning system (EWS) algorithm, Joondalup Health Campus. (Reproduced by kind permission of Fiona Legg and Beverley Ewens.)

and an early and appropriate response (NCEPOD 2005). These track-and-trigger systems should be robust, cover all in-patients and be linked to a response team that is appropriately skilled to assess and manage the clinical problems (NCEPOD 2005).

The main advantages of EWS systems are as follows (Gwinnutt 2008):

- Simplicity: only the basic monitoring equipment is required (usually readily available on acute wards)
- Reproducibility between different observers
- Applicability to multiprofessional team
- Minimal staff training required.

The early recognition and treatment of the deteriorating patient can minimise the occurrence of adverse events and reduce the level of intervention that a patient may have otherwise needed (ACSQHC 2010). However, these clinical signs of deterioration are often subtle and can go unnoticed. It is therefore essential that tools and systems, based on best evidence and designed for individual organisations, be developed, put in place and evaluated, and available to help the practitioner identify signs of deterioration. Ultimately this may prevent adverse events and improve patient outcomes. However, over-reliance on a scoring system to identify the deteriorating patient should be used as an adjunct to clinical judgement not as a replacement for it.

The efficacy of a variety of EWS tools designed to enable practitioners to identify the deteriorating patient has undergone extensive evaluation and discussion in the literature. However, the reliability and validity of these varying systems are lacking and further work to validate them is recommended (Gao et al. 2007).

Best practice – Early warning scores (EWS)

EWS systems should be based on the best available evidence.
  EWS should reflect validity, reliability, specificity and sensitivity:

- EWS should be designed to reflect subtle changes in condition
- EWS chart should be straightforward to use and unambiguous in its design

- Implementation should be planned and coordinated
- Extensive education strategy is needed before implementation
- Specific escalation policy should be attached to the EWS, e.g. whom to call and when
- EWS calling criteria can be adjusted for specific patients, e.g. chronic disease
- Ongoing audit of EWS charts should be undertaken to assess completeness and accuracy
- Ongoing review of specific incidents where calling criteria were not adhered to
- There should be on-going education of staff and auditing of tool
- EWS systems should be designed for the organisation's requirements and resources
- EWS systems should be used as an adjunct to clinical decision making not as a replacement for.

ROLE OF RAPID RESPONSE TEAMS: OUTREACH AND MEDICAL EMERGENCY TEAMS

Critical care outreach teams

All acute trusts should have critical care outreach teams (CCOTs) in some format (NCEPOD 2005). It has become evident over the last decade that, due to escalating patient acuity, decreasing nursing numbers and skill mix initiatives, there has been an increasing need for critical care skills external to the critical care unit and the need for a formal CCOT available 24 hours a day, seven days a week has been acknowledged (NCEPOD 2005; Wolfe 2008). The seminal report – Comprehensive Critical Care (Department of Health 2000) – recommended the development of CCOTs in all acute trusts as a component of complete reorganisation of critical care services across the UK. These services have been established in accordance with the 'intensive care without walls' philosophy as one aspect of the critical care service outlined in *Comprehensive Critical Care*. The composition of this service will vary from hospital to hospital but it should comprise individuals with the skills and ability to recognise and manage the problems and complexity of critical illness (NCEPOD 2005). The composition of CCOTs has evolved to be senior ICU nurses and/or physiotherapy and medical staff. It is recommended that CCOTs should not replace the role of traditional medical teams in the care of inpatients, but should be seen as complementary to them (NCEPOD 2005). The role of CCOTs can be variable and based on local needs, but fundamentally comprise (DoH 2007):

- Supporting hospital education programmes and initiatives by sharing critical care skills
- Monitoring and auditing the management of at-risk ward patients and working with ward staff to improve processes
- Providing expert skills to critically ill patients in ward areas
- Expediting admission of the critically ill patient to critical care areas and providing safe transfer
- Contributing to the early rehabilitation of patients, recently stepped down from critical care areas
- Delivering a follow-up service for ICU survivors after hospital discharge
- Delivering safe critical care practice to patients being kept in ward areas until a critical care bed is available
- Assisting in the identification of patients, for whom critical care services would be futile
- Undertaking evaluation and education of track and trigger systems and rapid response teams.

Best practice – critical care outreach teams

- Clear operational guidelines of the service
- Structured work practices
- Ownership by senior hospital managers and clinicians
- Clear lines of communication and accountability throughout the organisation
- Strong links with other teams to share practice and disseminate ideas
- Identify and address training needs in ward areas
- Act as a resource and support for ward staff

Despite widespread acceptance and intuitive belief in the benefit of outreach teams, there is an overall lack of evidence to support their use (Holder and Cuthbertson 2005; Gao et al. 2007). However, recent evidence does allude to the benefit of CCOT follow-up visits to ward patients after ICU discharge and the associated potential reduction in mortality and hospital length of stay (Harrison et al. 2010).

Medical emergency teams

Medical emergency teams (MET) is an example of a rapid response system which have been introduced in many hospitals to identify, review and treat at-risk patients during the early phase of their deterioration (Jones et al. 2007). The MET model has replaced the more reactive cardiac arrest teams, wherever they have been implemented. The MET responds not only to patients in cardiopulmonary arrest, but also to those with acute physiological deterioration, usually in response to a recognised single system trigger (Jones et al. 2007). MET was first developed in Australia in the 1990s in response to the evidence that delays in treatment could result in preventable deaths (Jones, et al. 2007; Schmid-Mazzoccoli et al. 2008). They are now commonplace in Australia (Cuthbertson 2007). The MET system is an example of a system designed to provide pre-emptive management of the patient at risk.

METs rely on calling criteria (Table 1.1) whereby the team will automatically be alerted. They will then attend, assess and treat the patient as required with the explicit aim of preventing deterioration. There is conflicting evidence that indicates that MET is associated with longer-term survival in some patient groups undergoing major surgical procedures (Jones et al. 2007). However, activation of a MET relies on the system's users and, despite MET being well established in many health-care systems, delayed responses by staff have been reported in the literature (Galhotra et al. 2007; Calzavacca et al. 2008). Members of the MET may include:

- experienced ICU nurse
- anaesthetist
- physician.

Best practice – Medical emergency team (MET)

- Calling criteria should be evidence based
- Staff must be aware of the MET calling criteria
- MET calling criteria should be visible in all wards and departments
- Staff should carry individual copies of MET calling criteria
- A designated leader coordinates MET calls, e.g. medical registrar
- Regular education sessions to update staff

Continued

- MET education sessions on all staff orientation programmes
- Audit of all MET calls to identify trends and deficiencies
- Audit of cardiac arrests
- Utilise data as part of a learning needs analysis
- Inappropriate MET calls should be dealt with sensitively so that staff are not discouraged to call the MET in the future

CLINICAL HANDOVER

The role of accurate, appropriate and succinct clinical handover in the management of the deteriorating patient cannot be overestimated. In recent years the importance of a systematic and structured clinical handover has been recognised. Many systems have been developed that attempt to standardise medical and nursing handover processes. One such system is ISOBAR, which has been

Table 1.1 Medical emergency team (MET) calling criteria, Joondalup Health Campus

Acute changes in	Physiology
Airway	Threatened
Breathing	• **Respiratory arrest** • Respiratory rate <8 breaths/min • Respiratory rate >36 breaths/min
Pulse oximetry; saturation <90% despite oxygen administration	
Circulation	• **Cardiac arrest** • Heart rate <40 beats/min • Heart rate >140 beats/min • Systolic blood pressure <90 mmHg
Neurology	• Sudden fall in level of consciousness • Fall of Glasgow Coma Scale score >2 points
Urine output	• <50 ml total over 4 hours
OR	
Staff member is seriously concerned about the patient	

Reproduced by kind permission of Brendon Burns.

recognised to be applicable for interprofessional handover and transferable between clinical settings (Yee et al. 2009):

I identification of the patient
S situation and status of patient
O observations of the patient
B background and history
A action, agreed plan and accountability
R responsibility and risk management

CLASSIFICATION AND PROVISION OF CRITICAL CARE
'Critical care without walls'
Comprehensive Critical Care (DoH 2000) recommended that critical care should be delivered encapsulating the philosophy 'critical care without walls', i.e. the needs of the critically ill must be met, no matter where such patients are physically located within the hospital. Critical care should be mobile, offering advice, assistance and education outside the traditional confines of the ICU (Baudouin and Evans 2002).

Classification of critical care
Classification of critical care patients should focus on the level of care that individual patients require, regardless of their location (DoH 2000). This approach sees a shift of emphasis away from defining patient needs in terms of hospital geography, e.g. ICU, HDU, etc., and towards a classification system that describes escalating levels of care for individual patients, independent of their location within the hospital (Table 1.2) (Gwinnutt 2008).

The Intensive Care Society (2009) has provided more detailed explanations and definitions of the classification levels. These definitions facilitate the assessment and quantification of the hospital-wide demand for the different levels of care, removing geographical location from being the defining factor for patients accessing critical care (Adam & Osborne 2005).

Provision of critical care
ICU bed provision in the UK currently has one of the lowest numbers of ICU beds in the developed world (3.5 per 100000) compared with Germany (24.6) and the USA (20.0). The demand

Table 1.2 Classification of critical care patients

Level	Description
Level 0	Patients whose needs may be met through normal ward care in an acute hospital
Level 1	Patients at risk of their condition deteriorating, or those recently relocated from higher levels of care, whose needs can be met on an acute ward with additional advice and support from the critical care team
Level 2	Patients requiring more detailed observation or intervention including support for a single failing system or postoperative care and those 'stepping down' from higher levels of care
Level 3	Patients requiring advanced respiratory support alone or basic respiratory support together with support of at least two organ systems. This level includes all complex patients requiring support for multiorgan failure

Department of Health (2000).

for ICU beds will inevitably increase in the future due to advances in medical technology, epidemics such as H1N1 and SARS (severe acute respiratory syndrome), natural disasters, conflict, but also for preventive reasons, such as the recognition of the necessity to transfer high-risk patients to critical care areas early in the course of their illness (Adhikari et al. 2010). Unlimited expansion of critical care beds may not necessarily be economically viable, but the focus on the development of preventive and therapeutic interventions for the sickest patients may hold the key to the future availability of critical care beds (Adhikari et al. 2010).

TRAINING HEALTHCARE STAFF
Several studies have demonstrated that both medical and nursing staff lack the necessary knowledge, skills and confidence to manage acutely ill patients and often do not follow a systematic approach to assessing them (Nolan et al. 2005). In addition, deficiencies in acute care often involve simple interventions, e.g. treating prob-

lems affecting airway, breathing and circulation (McQuillan et al. 1998). The combination of poor early recognition and lack of key skills in responding to acute deterioration probably contributes to poor patient outcome (Adam and Osborne 2005).

There have been several educational initiatives to improve multidisciplinary knowledge, skills and attitudes concerning the management of the critically ill patient (Kause et al. 2004), some of which are described below.

ALERT course

The ALERT (Acute Life-threatening Events – Recognition and Treatment) course was developed at Portsmouth University in 1999 with the aim of improving acute care of both 'at-risk' and critically ill adult patients. It was specifically designed to address the anxieties and areas of perceived weakness in the management of the acutely ill patient, previously identified by ward nurses and pre-registration house officers. It has several aims:

- A reduction in avoidable cardiac arrests
- A reduction in avoidable hospital deaths
- A reduction in avoidable ICU admissions
- Better recognition of the 'at-risk' or acutely ill patient
- Better clinical management of the 'at-risk' or acutely ill patient
- Better partnership and teamwork between health-care professionals
- Better written and verbal communication.

A simple assessment and management system is described which can be used for ill patients with a wide range of underlying clinical conditions, both medical and surgical. The course is mainly designed to train pre-registration house officers and junior nurses. However, other staff groups, e.g. medical students, senior house officers and senior nurses, may also find it helpful.

The 1-day ALERT course has been designed so that medical and nursing staff can train together using a common approach. It is designed on sound principles of adult education – active involvement, personal motivation, experience-centred learning, relevance to practice, regular feedback, clear goals and the use of reflective practice. For further information see www.port.ac.uk.

Advanced Trauma Life Support (ATLS) course
The 2.5-day ATLS course, developed by the American College
of Surgeons in the 1980s, has now been adopted in over 30 countries worldwide. It teaches a simple systematic approach to the
management of trauma patients, treating the most life-threatening
injury. A highly interactive course, it combines lectures, discus-
sions, interactive tutorials, skills teaching and simulated patient
management scenarios (moulage). For further information: Royal
College of Surgeons of England, tel: 020 7869 6309, email: atls@
rcseng.ac.uk.

Advanced Life Support (ALS) course
The Resuscitation Council (UK) ALS course aims to teach the
theory and practical skills to effectively manage cardiorespiratory
arrest, peri-arrest situations and special circumstances. There is
a big emphasis on prevention of cardiopulmonary arrest. The
2-day course comprises lectures, practical skill stations, workshops
and assessments. Candidates are sent a course manual to read 4
weeks before the course. For further information see www.resus.
org.uk.

Immediate Life Support (ILS) course
The ILS course is mainly designed to equip the first responder with
the necessary skills to manage a cardiac arrest while awaiting the
arrival of the cardiac arrest team. In particular, there is a big
emphasis on cardiac arrest prevention and the ABCDE approach
to assess an acutely ill patient. For further information see
www.resus.org.uk.

Care of the Critically Ill Surgical Patient (CCrISP)
This 2.5-day course is designed to advance the practical, theoretical
and personal skills necessary for the care of critically ill surgical
patients. It is aimed at surgeons and those dealing with surgical
patients who are completing basic surgical training. All partici-
pants on the course should have completed at least 1 year of basic
surgical training (not including house jobs), commenced 6 months
general surgery and ideally completed an ATLS course, although
this is not a prerequisite.

START Surgery

The Systematic Training in Acute Illness Recognition and Treatment for Surgery (START Surgery) course is designed for surgical foundation trainees. It is designed to advance the practical, theoretical and personal skills necessary for the care of critically ill surgical patients. For further information see www.rcseng.ac.uk.

CONCLUSION

Critically ill patients have a high morbidity and mortality. Prognosis following an in-hospital cardiopulmonary arrest is poor. Prompt recognition and early appropriate management of critically ill patients are essential to prevent deterioration. Track-and-trigger systems and efficient, easily accessed escalation procedures should be in place to identify at-risk patients and alert expert help. Healthcare staff should be appropriately trained in the recognition and management of the deteriorating patient.

REFERENCES

Australian Commission on Safety and Quality in Health Care (2010) *National Concensus Statement: Eessential elements for recognising and responding to clinical deterioration*. Commonwealth of Australia: ACSQHC.

Adam, S. & Osborne, S. (2005) *Critical Care Nursing Science and Practice*, 2nd edn. Oxford: Oxford University Press.

Adhikari, N. K. J., Fowler, R. A., Bhagwanjee, S. & Rubenfeld, G. D. (2010) Critical care and the global burden of critical illness in adults. *The Lancet*, **376**, 1339–1346.

Baba-Akbari Sari, A., Sheldon, T. A., Cracknell, A., et al. (2006) Extent, nature and consequences of adverse events: results of a retrospective casenote review in a large NHS hospital. *Quality and Safety in Health Care*, **16**, 434–439.

Baudouin, S. & Evans, T. (2002) Improving outcomes for severeley ill medical patients. *Clinical Medicine*, **2**(2), 92–94.

Beaumont, K., Luettel, D. & Thomson, R. (2008) Deterioration in hospital patients: early signs and and appropriate actions. *Nursing Standard*, **23**(1), 43–48.

Calzavacca, P., Licari, E., Tee, A., et al. (2008) A prospective study of factors influencing the outcome of patients after a Medical Emergency Team review. *Intensive Care Medicine*, **34**, 2112–2116.

Cuthbertson, B. H. (2007) The impact of critical care outreach: is there one? *Critical Care*, **11**, 179.

de Vries, E. N., Ramrattan, M. A., Smorenburg, S. M., Gouma, D. J. & Boermeester, M. A. (2007) The incidence and nature of in-hospital adverse events: a systematic review. *Quality and Safety in Health Care*, **17**, 216–223.

Department of Health (2000) *Comprehensive Critical Care: A review of adult critical care services*. London: DH.

Department of Health for Critical Care Stakeholders Forum: National Outreach Forum (2007) Clinical Indicators for Outreach Sevices. Available online at: www.dh.gov.uk/en/Publicationsandstatistics/ Publications/PublicationsPolicyAndGuidance/DH_072769 (accessed 14 September 2011).

Donahue, L. A. & Endacott, R. (2010) Track, trigger and teamwork: Communication of deterioration in acute medical and surgical wards. *Intensive and Critical Care Nursing*, **26**, 10–17.

Fieselmann, J. F., Hendryx, M. S., Helms, C. M. & Wakefield, D. S. (1993) Respiratory rate predicts cardiopulmonary arrest for internal medicine patients. *Journal of General Internal Medicine*, **8**, 354–360.

Franklin, C. & Matthew, J. (1994) Developing strategies to prevent in-hospital cardiac arrest: analysing responses of physicians and nurses in the hours before the event. *Critical Care Medicine*, **22**, 244–247.

Galhotra, S., Devita, M. A., Simmons, R. L. & Dew, M. A. (2007) Mature rapid response system and potentially avoidable cardiopulmonary arrests in hospital. *Quality and Safety in Health Care*, **16**, 260–265.

Gao, H., Harrison, D. A., Parry, G. J., Daly, K., Subbe, C. P. & Rowan, K. (2007) The impact of the introduction of critical care outreach services in England: a multicentre interrupted time-series analysis. *Critical Care*, **11**, R113.

Gao, H., McDonnell, A., Harrison, D. A., et al. (2007) Systematic review and evaluation of physiological track and trigger warning systems for identifying at-risk patients on the ward. *Intensive Care Medicine*, **33**, 667–679.

Goldhill, D. R. (2001) The critically ill: follow your MEWS. *Quarterly Journal of Medicine*, **94**, 507–510.

Goldhill, D., Worthington, L., Mulcahy, A., Tarling, M. & Sumner A. (1999) The patient-at-risk team: identifying and managing seriously ill ward patients. *Anaesthesia*, **54**, 853–860.

Goldhill, D., McNarry, A., Hadjianastassiou, V. & Tekkis, P. (2004) The longer patients are in hospital before Intensive Care admission the higher their mortality. *Intensive Care Medicine*, **30**, 1908–1913.

Gwinnutt, C. L. (2008) *Clinical Anaesthesia*, 3rd edn. Oxford: Wiley Blackwell.

Harrison, D. A., Gao, H., Welch, C. A. & Rowan, K. M. (2010) The effects of critical care outreach services before and after critical care: A matched-cohort analysis. *Journal of Critical Care*, **25**, 196–204.

Herlitz, J., Bang, A., Alsen, B. & Aune, S. (2002) Characteristics and outcome among patients suffering from in hospital cardiac arrest in relation to whether the arrest took place during office hours. *Resuscitation*, **53**, 127–133.

Hodgetts, T. J., Kenward, G., Vlackonikolis, I., et al. (2002) Incidence, location and reasons for avoidable in-hopsital cardiac arrest in a district general hospital. *Resuscitation*, **54**, 115–123.

Holder, P. & Cuthbertson, B. H. (2005) Critical care without the intensive care unit. *Clinical Medicine*, **5**, 449–451.

Intensive Care Society (2009) Levels of Critical Care fro Adult Patients. Aavailble online at: www.ics.ac.uk/intensive_care_professional/ standards_and_guidelines/levels_of_critical_care_for_adult_ patients (accessed 14 September 2011).

Jones, D., Egi, M., Bellomo, R. & Goldsmith, D. (2007) Effect of the medical emergency team on long-term mortality following major surgery. *Critical Care*, **11**, 12.

Kause, J., Smith, G. & Prytherch, D. R. (2004) A comparison to antecedents to cardiac arrests, deaths and emergency intensive care admissions in Australia, New Zealand and the United Kingdom – the ACADEMIA study. *Resuscitation*, **62**, 275–282.

Kause, J., Smith, G., Prythyerch, D., Parr, M., Flabouris, A. & Hillman, K. (2004) A comparison of antecedents to cardiac arrests, dethas and emergency intensive care admissions in Australia and New Zealand, and the United Kingdom – the ACADEMIA study. *Resuscitation*, **62**, 275–282.

McQuillan, P., Pilkington, S., Allan, A., et al. (1998) Confidential enquiry into the quality of care before admission to intensive care. *British Medical Journal*, **316**, 1853–1858.

Meaney, P. A., Nadkarni, V. M., Kern, K. B., Indik, J. H., Halperin, H. R. & Berg, R. A. (2010) Rhythms and outcomes of adult in-hospital cardiac arrest. *Critical Care Medicine*, **38**, 101–108.

National Confidential Enquiry into Patient Outcome and Death (2005) *An Acute Problem?* London: NCEPOD.

National Institute for Health and Clinical Excellence (2007) *Acutely ill patients in hospital*. London: NICE.

National Patient Safety Agency (2007) *Safer Care for the Acutely Ill Patient: Learning from serious incidents*. London: NPSA.

Nolan, J., Deakin, C. & Soar, J. (2005) European Resuscitation Council Guidelines for Resuscitation 2005: Section 4. Adult Advanced Life Support. *Resuscitation*, **675S**, S39–S86.

Odell, M., Victor, C. & Oliver, D. (2009) Nurses' role in detecting deterioration in ward patients: systematic literature review. *Journal of Advanced Nursing*, **65**, 1992–2006.

Peberdy, M., Ornato, J. P., Larkin, G. L., et al. (2008) Survival from in-hospital cardiac arrest during nights and weekends. *Journal of the American Medical Association*, **299**, 785–792.

Resuscitation Council UK (2010) *Adult Advanced Life Support Algorithm*. London: Resuscitation Council UK.

Resuscitation Council (UK) (2011) *Immediate Life Support* 3rd edn. London: Resuscitation Council UK.

Schein, R. M. H., Hazday, N., Pena, M., Ruben, P. H. & Sprung, C. L. (1990) Clinical antecedents to in-hospital cardiac arrest. *Chest*, **98**, 1388–1392).

Schmid-Mazzoccoli, A., Hoffman, L. A., Wolf, G. A., Happ, M. B. & Devita, M. A. (2008) The use of medical emergency teams in medical and surgical patients: impact of patient, nurse and organisational characteristics. *Quality and Safety in Healthcare*, **17**, 377–381.

Sharpley, J. T. & Holden, J. C. (2004) Introducing an early warning scoring system in a district general hospital. *Nursing in Critical Care*, **9**(3), 98–103.

Skrifvars, M. B., Nurmi, J., Ikola, K., Saarinen, K. & Castren, M. (2006) Reduced survival following resuscitation in patients with documented clinically abnormal observations prior to in-hospital cardiac arrest. *Resuscitation*, **70**, 215–222.

Wolfe, B. (2008) Implementing an ICU outreach team model. *Canadian Association of Critical Care Nurses*, **19**(1), 24–29.

Yee, K. C., Wong, M. C. & Turner, P. (2009) 'HAND ME AN ISOBAR': a pilot study of an evidence-based approach to improving shift-to-shift clinical handover. *Medical Journal Australia*, **190**(11), S121–S124.

Assessment of the Critically Ill Patient

2

LEARNING OBJECTIVES

At the end of the chapter the reader will be able to:

☐ outline the ABCDE approach
☐ outline the initial approach to the patient
☐ describe the assessment of the airway
☐ describe the assessment of breathing
☐ outline the assessment of circulation
☐ describe the assessment of disability
☐ outline the importance of exposure

INTRODUCTION

Cardiopulmonary arrests occurring in patients in unmonitored ward areas are usually neither sudden nor unpredictable and are rarely caused by primary cardiac disease (Nolan et al. 2005). These patients have often slowly and progressively deteriorated physiologically, involving hypoxia and hypotension, which has not been recognised by ward staff or, if it has, has been poorly treated (Kause et al. 2004). If adverse physiological signs, e.g. tachycardia, tachypnoea or hypotension, are identified early, and patients are effectively treated, cardiopulmonary arrest may then be prevented (Adam and Osborne 2005). Assessment and the ability to observe and interpret findings, thereby influencing decision-making and management, lie at the core of the nursing profession (Farnsworth and Curtis 2007). Nurses are with patients

Monitoring the Critically Ill Patient, Third Edition.
Philip Jevon, Beverley Ewens.
© 2012 Blackwell Publishing Ltd. Published 2012 by Blackwell Publishing Ltd.

more consistently than other health-care professionals and are therefore more likely to detect deterioration (Gonce Morton and Rempher 2009).

The Resuscitation Council UK (2011) has provided guidance on the assessment of the critically ill patient. Adapted from the ALERT course (Smith 2003), these guidelines follow a logical and systematic ABCDE approach.

The aim of this chapter is to understand the assessment of the critically ill patient.

ABCDE APPROACH

The ABCDE approach can be used when assessing and treating all critically ill patients. The guiding principles are as follows (Resuscitation Council UK 2011):

- Follow a systematic approach, based on airway, breathing, circulation, disability and exposure (ABCDE) to assess and treat the critically ill patient.
- Undertake a complete initial assessment; reassess regularly.
- Always treat life-threatening problems first, before proceeding to the next part of the assessment.
- Always evaluate the effects of treatment and/or other interventions.
- Recognise the circumstances when additional help is required; request it early and utilise all members of the multidisciplinary team. This will enable assessment, instigating monitoring, intravenous (IV) access, etc. to be undertaken simultaneously.
- Ensure effective communication. **Call for help early**.

The ABCDE approach can be used by all health-care practitioners, irrespective of their training, experience and expertise in clinical assessment and treatment: clinical skills and knowledge will determine what aspects of the assessment are undertaken (Resuscitation Council UK 2011):

> The underlying aim of the initial interventions should be seen as a 'holding measure' to keep the patient alive, and produce some clinical improvement, in order that definitive treatment may be initiated.

INITIAL APPROACH TO THE PATIENT

Ensure that it is safe to approach the patient: check the environment and remove any hazards. Measures should also be taken to minimise the risk of cross-infection (see box at end of chapter).

Ask the patient a simple question

Ask the patient a simple question, e.g. 'How are you, sir [or madam]?' The patient's response or lack of response can provide valuable information. A normal verbal response implies that the patient has a patent airway, is breathing and has cerebral perfusion; if the patient can speak only in short sentences, he or she may have extreme respiratory distress and failure to respond is a clear indicator of serious illness (Resuscitation Council UK 2011). If there is an inappropriate response or no response, the patient may be critically ill.

If the patent is unconscious: summon help from colleagues immediately.

General appearance of the patient

Note the general appearance of the patient, e.g. whether he or she appears comfortable or distressed, content or concerned, and also their colour.

Vital sign monitoring

Equipment for vital sign monitoring, e.g. pulse oximetry, electrocardiogram (ECG) monitoring and continuous non-invasive blood pressure monitoring, should be attached as soon as it is safely possible (Resuscitation Council UK 2011).

ASSESSMENT OF AIRWAY

If the patient is talking he or she will have a patent airway. In complete airway obstruction, there are no breath sounds at the mouth or nose. In partial obstruction, air entry is diminished and often noisy. The familiar look, listen and feel approach can detect if the airway is obstructed.

Look

Look for the signs of airway obstruction. Airway obstruction leads to paradoxical chest and abdominal movements ('see-saw' respirations) and the use of the accessory muscles of respiration. Central cyanosis is a late sign of airway obstruction.

Listen

Listen for signs of airway obstruction. Certain noises will assist in localising the level of the obstruction (Smith 2003):

- *Gurgling*: fluid in the mouth or upper airway
- *Snoring*: tongue partially obstructing the pharynx
- *Crowing*: laryngeal spasm
- *Inspiratory stridor*: 'croaking respirations' indicating partial upper airway obstruction, e.g. foreign body, laryngeal oedema
- *Expiratory wheeze*: noisy musical sound caused by turbulent flow of air through narrowed bronchi and bronchioles, more pronounced on expiration; causes include asthma and chronic obstructive pulmonary disease (COPD).

Feel

Feel for signs of airway obstruction. Place your face or hand in front of the patient's mouth to determine whether there is movement of air.

Causes of airway obstruction

Causes of airway obstruction include the following (Smith 2003; Gwinnutt 2006):

- *Tongue* (this is the most common cause of airway obstruction in a semiconscious or unconscious patient; relaxation of the muscles supporting the tongue can result in it falling back and blocking the pharynx)
- Vomit, blood and secretions
- Foreign body
- *Tissue swelling* (causes include anaphylaxis, trauma and infection)
- *Laryngeal oedema* (due to burns, inflammation or allergy occurring at the level of the larynx)

- *Laryngeal spasm* (due to foreign body, airway stimulation or secretions/blood in the airway)
- *Tracheobronchial obstruction* (due to aspiration of gastric contents, secretions, pulmonary oedema fluid or bronchospasm).

Treatment of airway obstruction

> Treat airway obstruction as a medical emergency and obtain expert help immediately; untreated, airway obstruction leads to a lowered PaO_2 and risks hypoxic damage to the brain, kidneys and heart, cardiac arrest, and even death (Resuscitation Council UK 2011).

Once airway obstruction has been identified, treat appropriately. Simple methods, e.g. suction, lateral position, insertion of oropharyngeal airway, are often effective. Administer oxygen as appropriate.

Monitoring the patient's airway is described in more detail in Chapter 3.

ASSESSMENT OF BREATHING

The familiar; look, listen and feel approach can be used to assess breathing, or to detect signs of respiratory distress or inadequate ventilation (Smith 2003).

Look

Look for the general signs of respiratory distress: tachypnoea, sweating, central cyanosis, use of the accessory muscles of respiration, abdominal breathing (Resuscitation Council UK 2011).

Calculate the respiratory rate over 1 minute. A respiratory rate that is high or rapidly increasing is a significant predictor of deterioration or impending adverse events, i.e. cardiac arrest, unplanned admission to intensive care unit (ICU) or death (Farnsworth and Curtis 2007). The normal respiratory rate in adults is approximately 12–20/min (Resuscitation Council UK 2011). Tachypnoea is usually one of the first indicators of respiratory distress and should be compared with the patient's normal rate (Gonce Morton and Rempher 2009). Work of breathing is as important a factor as respiratory rate when assessing respiratory function (Gonce Morton and Rempher 2009).

Bradypnoea is an ominous sign and possible causes include drugs (e.g. opioids), fatigue, hypothermia, head injury and central nervous system (CNS) depression. Sudden bradypnoea in a patient with respiratory distress could quickly be followed by respiratory arrest.

Assess the depth of breathing. Ascertain whether chest movement is equal on both sides. Asynchronous movement of the chest suggests unilateral disease, e.g. atelectasis, flail chest, pneumothorax and the respiratory effort required decreases the quality of respiration at the expense of increased work of breathing and often precedes ventilatory support (Gonce Morton and Rempher 2009). Kussmaul's breathing (air hunger) is characterised by deep rapid respirations due to stimulation of the respiratory centre by metabolic acidosis, e.g. in ketoacidosis and chronic renal failure (Jevon 2008).

Assess the pattern (rhythm) of breathing. Cheyne–Stokes breathing pattern (periods of apnoea alternating with periods of hyperpnoea) can be associated with deep cerebral lesions and metabolic encephalopathy (Venkatesh 2009).

Note the presence of any chest deformity because this could increase the risk of deterioration in the patient's ability to breathe normally (Resuscitation Council UK 2011). If the patient has a chest drain *in situ*, check that it is patent and functioning effectively. The presence of abdominal distension could limit diaphragmatic movement, thereby exacerbating respiratory distress.

Document the inspired oxygen concentration (percentage) being administered to the patient and the peripheral oxygen saturation (SpO_2) reading of the pulse oximeter (normally 97–100%). The pulse oximeter does not detect hypercapnia and if the patient is receiving oxygen therapy, the SpO_2 may be normal in the presence of a very high $PaCO_2$ (Resuscitation Council UK 2011).

Listen

Listen to the patient's breath sounds a short distance from his or her face. Normal breathing is quiet. Rattling airway noises indicate the presence of airway secretions, usually either because the patient is unable to cough sufficiently or is unable to take a deep breath in (Smith 2003). Stridor or wheeze suggests partial, but significant, airway obstruction (see above).

If you are able, auscultate the chest: the depth of breathing and the equality of breath sounds on both sides of the chest should be evaluated. Any additional sounds, e.g. crackles, wheeze and pleural rubs, should be noted. Bronchial breathing indicates consolidation (pneumonia), fibrosis, neoplasm or abscess (Farnsworth and Curtis 2007); absent or reduced sounds suggest a pneumothorax or pleural fluid (Smith 2003).

Feel

Perform chest percussion. Causes of different percussion notes include the following (Gonce Morton and Rempher 2009):

- *Resonant or hollow*: air-filled lung
- *Dull (medium intensity and pitch)*: atelectasis, consolidation, pulmonary oedema, pulmonary haemorrhage
- Hyper-resonant (loud low pitched): pneumothorax, emphysema
- *Tympanitic (high pitched)*: asthma, large pneumothorax.

Check the position of the trachea. Place the tip of the index finger into the suprasternal notch, let it slip either side of the trachea and determine whether it fits more easily into one or other side of the trachea (Ford et al. 2005). Deviation of the trachea to one side indicates mediastinal shift (e.g. pneumothorax, lung fibrosis or pleural fluid).

Palpate the chest wall to detect surgical emphysema or crepitus, caused by pneumothorax, burst pockets of alveoli or positive end respiratory pressure (Gonce Morton and Rempher 2009).

Efficacy of breathing, work of breathing and adequacy of ventilation

- *Efficacy of breathing* can be assessed by air entry, chest movement, pulse oximetry, arterial blood gas analysis and capnography.
- *Work of breathing* can be assessed by respiratory rate and accessory muscle use, e.g. neck and abdominal muscles.
- *Adequacy of ventilation* can be assessed by heart rate, skin colour and mental status.

Causes of compromised breathing

Causes of compromised breathing include the following:

- Respiratory illness, e.g. asthma, COPD, pneumonia
- Lung pathology, e.g. pneumothorax
- Pulmonary embolism
- Pulmonary oedema
- CNS depression
- Drug-induced respiratory depression.

Treatment of compromised breathing

If the patient's breathing is compromised, position him or her appropriately (usually upright), administer oxygen and if possible treat the underlying cause. Expert help should be summoned. Assisted ventilation may be required. During the initial assessment of breathing, it is essential to diagnose and effectively treat immediately life-threatening conditions, e.g. acute severe asthma, pulmonary oedema, tension pneumothorax or massive haemothorax (Resuscitation Council UK 2011).

Assessment and monitoring of the patient's breathing are discussed in more detail in Chapter 3.

ASSESSMENT OF CIRCULATION

In most medical and surgical emergencies, if shock is present, treat for hypovolaemic shock until proven otherwise (Smith 2003). Administer intravenous (IV) fluid to all patients who have tachycardia and cool peripheries, unless the cause of the circulatory shock is obviously cardiac (cardiogenic shock) (Resuscitation Council UK 2011). In surgical patients, haemorrhage should be rapidly excluded. The familiar look, listen and feel approach can be used for the assessment of circulation.

Look

Look at the colour of the hands and fingers. Signs of cardiovascular compromise include cool and pale peripheries.

Measure the capillary refill time (CRT). A prolonged CRT (>2 s) could indicate poor peripheral perfusion, although other factors, e.g. cool ambient temperature, poor lighting and old age, can also do this (Resuscitation Council UK 2011). Look for other signs of a poor cardiac output, e.g. reduced conscious level and, if the patient has a urinary catheter, oliguria (urine volume <0.5 ml/kg per h) (Smith 2003).

Examine the patient for signs of external haemorrhage from wounds or drains or evidence of internal haemorrhage (Ewens 2008). Concealed blood loss can be significant, even if drains are empty (Smith 2003).

Listen

Measure the patient's blood pressure. A low systolic blood pressure suggests shock. However, even in shock, the blood pressure can still be normal, because compensatory mechanisms increase peripheral resistance in response to reduced cardiac output (Verrinder and Kinsman 2007). A low diastolic blood pressure suggests arterial vasodilatation (e.g. anaphylaxis or sepsis). A narrowed pulse pressure, i.e. the difference between systolic and diastolic pressures (normal pulse pressure is 35–45 mmHg), suggests arterial vasoconstriction (e.g. cardiogenic shock or hypovolaemia) (Resuscitation Council UK 2011).

Auscultate the heart. Although abnormalities of the heart valves can be detected, auscultation of the heart is rarely helpful in the initial assessment (Smith 2003).

Feel

Assess the skin temperature of the patient's limbs to determine whether they are warm or cool, the latter suggesting poor peripheral perfusion. Palpate peripheral and central pulses. Assess for presence, rate, quality, regularity and equality (Smith 2003). A thready pulse suggests a poor cardiac output, whereas a bounding pulse may indicate sepsis (Resuscitation Council UK 2011). Assess the state of the veins: if hypovolaemia is present the veins could be under-filled or collapsed (Smith 2003).

Causes of circulatory compromise

Causes of circulatory problems include:

- acute coronary syndromes
- cardiac arrhythmias
- shock, e.g. hypovolaemia, septic and anaphylactic shock

- heart failure
- pulmonary embolism.

Treatment of circulatory compromise

The specific treatment required for circulatory compromise will depend on the cause; fluid replacement, haemorrhage control and restoration of tissue perfusion will usually be necessary (Resuscitation Council UK 2011).

The immediate treatment for a patient presenting with acute coronary syndrome, includes oxygen, aspirin 300 mg, sublingual glyceryl trinitrate and morphine; reperfusion therapy will need to be considered dependent upon risk stratification (Resuscitation Council UK 2011). If shock is present, two large-bore cannulas (12–14 gauge) should be inserted and an IV fluid challenge will usually be required (Ewens 2008).

Assessment and monitoring of the patient's circulation are discussed in more detail in Chapters 4 and 5.

ASSESSMENT OF DISABILITY

Assessment of disability involves evaluating CNS function. Undertake a rapid assessment of the patient's level of consciousness using the AVPU method (Fig. 1.4) (the Glasgow Coma Scale can also be used). Causes of altered conscious level include hypoxia, hypercapnia, cerebral hypoperfusion, the recent administration of sedatives/analgesic medications and hypoglycaemia (Resuscitation Council UK 2011). Therefore:

- Review ABC to exclude hypoxaemia and hypotension
- Check the patient's drug chart for reversible drug-induced causes of altered conscious level
- Undertake bedside glucose measurement to exclude hypoglycaemia
- Examine the pupils (size, equality and reaction to light)

Resuscitation Council UK (2011)

Causes of altered conscious level

Causes of altered conscious level include:

- severe hypoxia
- poor cerebral perfusion

- drugs, e.g. sedatives, opioids
- cerebral pathology
- hypercapnia
- hypoglycaemia
- alcohol

Treatment of altered conscious level

The first priority is to assess ABC: exclude or treat hypoxia and hypotension (Resuscitation Council UK 2011). If drug-induced altered conscious level is suspected and the effects are reversible, administer an antidote, e.g. naloxone for opioid toxicity. Administer glucose if the patient is hypoglycaemic.

Assessment and monitoring of the patient's conscious level are discussed in more detail in Chapter 6.

EXPOSURE

Full exposure of the patient may be necessary in order to undertake a thorough examination and ensure that important details are not overlooked (Smith 2003). In particular, the examination should concentrate on the part of the body that is most likely to be contributing to the patient's ill status, e.g. in suspected anaphylaxis, examine the skin for urticaria. The patient's dignity should be respected and heat loss minimised.

In addition:

- Undertake a full clinical history.
- Review the patient's case notes, observations chart and medications chart.
- Study the recorded vital signs: trends are more significant than one-off recordings.
- Ensure that prescribed medications are being administered.
- Review the results of laboratory, ECG and radiological investigations.
- Consider the level of care the patient requires (e.g. ward, high dependency unit [HDU], ICU).
- Record in the patient's case notes details of assessment, treatment and response to treatment.

Resuscitation Council UK (2011)

Minimising the risk of cross-infection

Measures to minimise the risk of cross-infection should be taken. It is estimated that during 2005 there were at least 300 000 hospital-acquired infections (HAIs) per year, with 9% of patients being affected at any one time, and a cost to the NHS of £1 billion per year (Poole 2011). The principal route of HAIs is via the hands and effective hand hygiene is recognised as the most effective intervention to prevent cross-infection and is the simplest (Cantrell et al. 2009; Petty 2009).

The National Institute for Health and Clinical Excellence (NICE 2003) has issued guidance governing the principles of good practice relating to hand washing (which is currently being updated):

- Hands must be decontaminated immediately before each patient and every episode of direct patient contact or care after any activity or contact that could potentially result in hands becoming decontaminated.
- Hands that are visibly soiled, or potentially grossly contaminated with dirt or organic material, must be washed with liquid soap and water.
- Hands must be decontaminated, preferably with an alcohol-based hand rub unless hands are visibly soiled, between caring for different patients and between different care activities for the same patient.
- Before regular hand decontamination begins, all wrist and ideally hand jewellery should be removed. Cuts and abrasions must be covered with waterproof dressings. Fingernails should be kept short, clean and free from nail polish and no artificial nails should be used.
- An effective handwashing technique involves three stages: preparation, washing and rinsing, and drying. Preparation requires wetting hands under tepid running water before applying liquid soap or an antimicrobial preparation. The handwash solution must come into contact with all surfaces of the hand. The hands must be rubbed together vigorously for a minimum of 10–15 seconds, paying particular attention to the tips of the fingers, the thumbs and the areas between the fingers. Hands should be rinsed thoroughly before drying with good-quality paper towels.
- When decontaminating hands using an alcohol hand rub, hands should be free from dirt and organic material. The hand rub solution must come into contact with all surfaces of the hand. The hands must be rubbed together, paying particular attention to the tips of the fingers, the thumbs and the areas between the fingers, until the solution has evaporated and the hands are dry.
- An emollient hand cream should be applied regularly to protect skin from the drying effects of regular hand decontamination. If a particular

soap, antimicrobial hand wash or alcohol product causes skin irritation an occupational health team should be consulted.

Universal precautions to blood and bodily fluids
Blood is the single most important source of the transmission of human immunodeficiency virus (HIV) and hepatitis B virus (Jevon 2010). Universal precautions should apply to blood, semen, vaginal secretions and cerebrospinal, synovial, pleural, peritoneal, pericardial and amniotic fluids, and any body fluid containing visible blood. Disposable gloves should be worn.

Sharps
Particular care should be taken with sharps because both HIV and the hepatitis B virus have been contracted by health-care workers following needle-stick injuries.

CONCLUSION
Most cardiopulmonary arrests occurring in hospital are predictable. Recognition and the effective treatment of critically ill patients are paramount. The ABCDE approach of assessing the critically ill patient has been described and the importance of calling for help early has been emphasised.

REFERENCES
Adam, S. & Osborne, S. (2005) *Critical Care Nursing Science and Practice*, 2nd edn. Oxford: Oxford University Press.
Cantrell, D., Shamriz, O., Cohen, M., J., Stern, Z., Block, C. & Brezis, M. (2009) Hand hygiene compliance by physicians: Marked heterogeneity due to local culture? *American Journal of Infection Control*, **37**, 301–305.
Ewens, B. (2008) Shock. In: *Jevon, P., Humphreys, M. & Ewens, B. (eds), Nursing Medical Emergency Patients*. Oxford: Wiley-Blackwell.
Farnsworth, L. & Curtis, K. (2007) Patient assessment and essential nursing care. In: Curtis, K., Ramsden, C. & Friendship, J. (eds), *Emergency and Trauma Nursing*. Marickville: NSW: Mosby Elsevier.
Ford, M., Hennessey, I. & Japp, A. (2005) *Introduction to Clinical Examination*. Oxford: Elsevier.
Gonce Morton, P. & Rempher, K. (2009) Patient assessment: Respiratory system. In: Gonce Morton, P. & Fontaine, D. K. (eds), *Critical Care Bursing. A holistic approach*, 9th edn. Philadelphia: PA: Lippincott Williams & Wilkins.

Gwinnutt, C. (2006) *Clinical Anaesthesia*, 2nd edn. Oxford: Blackwell Publishing.

Jevon, P. (2008) Endocrine emergencies. In: Jevon, P., Humphreys, M. & Ewens, B. (eds), *Nursing Medical Emergency Patients*. Oxford: Wiley-Blackwell.

Jevon, P. (2010) *Advanced Cardiac Life Support*. Oxford: Wiley-Blackwell.

Kause, J., Smith, G., Prytherch, D. et al. (2004) A comparison of antecedents to cardiac arrests, deaths and emergency intensive care admissions in Australia and New Zealand, and the United Kingdom – the ACADEMIA study. *Resuscitation*, **62**, 275–282.

National Institute for Health and Clinical Excellence (2003) *Head Injury, Triage, Assessment, Investigation and Early Management of Head Injury in Infants, Children and Adults*. London: NICE.

Nolan, J., Deakin, C. & Soar, J. (2005) European Resuscitation Council Guidelines for Resuscitation 2005: Section 4. Adult Advanced Life Support. *Resuscitation*, **675S**, S39–S86.

Petty, W. C. (2009) PACU why hand washing is vital. *Journal of Peri Anaesthesia Nursing*, **24**, 250–253.

Poole, M. F. (2011) Plan protection from infection. *Occupational Health*, **63**(1), 29–31.

Resuscitation Council UK (2011) *Immediate Life Support*, 3rd edn. London: Resuscitation Council UK.

Smith, G. (2003) *ALERT Acute Life-Threatening Events Recognition and Treatment*, 2nd edn. University of Portsmouth, Portsmouth.

Venkatesh, B. (2009) Disorders of consciousness. In: Bersten, A. D. & Soni, N. (eds), *Oh's Intensive Care Manual*, 6th edn. Philadelphia: PA: Butterworth Heinemann Elsevier.

Verrinder, A. & Kinsman, L. (2007) Physiology for emergency care. In: Curtis, K., Ramsden, C. & Friendship, J. (eds), *Emergency and Trauma Nursing*. Marickville: NSW: Mosby Elsevier.

Monitoring Respiratory Function

3

LEARNING OBJECTIVES

At the end of the chapter the reader will be able to:

☐ describe how to assess the *efficacy of breathing, work of breathing* and *adequacy of ventilation*

☐ discuss the importance of a *comprehensive assessment* of the patient

☐ outline important *associated features of dyspnoea*

☐ describe how to undertake *peak expiratory flow rate measurements*

☐ discuss the principles of *pulse oximetry*

☐ discuss the principles of *arterial blood gas analysis*

☐ discuss the principles of *capnography (end-tidal CO_2)*

☐ discuss the monitoring priorities of a *ventilated patient*

☐ discuss the monitoring priorities of a patient with a *temporary tracheostomy*

☐ outline the monitoring priorities of a patient with a *pleural drain*

INTRODUCTION

Early recognition of respiratory dysfunction and the institution of appropriate measures are vital to support gas exchange and prevent cellular oxygen debt, anaerobic metabolism and varying degrees of tissue and organ damage (Smyth 2005).

Respiratory function requires careful and close monitoring to ensure that the most appropriate treatment is administered and

Monitoring the Critically Ill Patient, Third Edition.
Philip Jevon, Beverley Ewens.
© 2012 Blackwell Publishing Ltd. Published 2012 by Blackwell Publishing Ltd.

Table 3.1 Definitions of respiratory terminology

Term	Definition
Dyspnoea	Difficulty in breathing
Orthopnoea	Dyspnoea necessitating an upright, sitting position for its relief
Tachypnoea	Abnormally rapid rate of breathing (>20 per minute) (Torrance and Elley 1997)
Bradypnoea	Abnormally slow rate of breathing (<12 per minute) (Torrance and Elley 1997)
Hypoxia	Inadequate oxygen at cellular level
Hypoxaemia	Low oxygen levels in the blood
Anoxia	Lack of oxygen, local or systemic

any response to it is accurately evaluated. Table 3.1 shows the basic definitions of respiratory terminology and Table 3.2 some of the most common causes of dyspnoea (breathing difficulty).

In particular it is important to be able to recognise when the patient's respiratory status is compromised. The familiar *look, listen* and *feel* approach should be used to evaluate the efficacy of breathing, work of breathing and adequacy of ventilation (Steen 2010). The patient's general appearance, history and presenting symptoms, together with the characteristics of the dyspnoea, are also important. In addition, peak flow measurements, pulse oximetry and blood gas analysis are helpful in monitoring respiratory function.

The aim of this chapter is to understand the principles of monitoring respiratory function.

ASSESSMENT OF THE EFFICACY OF BREATHING, WORK OF BREATHING AND ADEQUACY OF VENTILATION
Efficacy of breathing
The efficacy of breathing can be assessed as shown in the following:

- *Air entry*: look, listen and feel for signs of breathing. If possible, auscultate the chest to determine the amount of air being

Table 3.2 Causes of dyspnoea (not exhaustive).

Cause	Examples
Respiratory	Asthma, chronic obstructive pulmonary disease (COPD), pneumonia, tuberculosis, pleural effusion, pneumothorax, carcinoma of the lung, pulmonary embolism, mechanical (e.g. fractured ribs – flail segment)
Cardiac	Left ventricular failure and pulmonary oedema, congestivecardiac failure
CNS	Head injury, raised intracranial pressure, drugs (e.g. opiates); aggravating factors, e.g. exercise, cold air, smoking, coughing
Neuromuscular	Guillain–Barré syndrome, myasthenia gravis, muscular dystrophies
Diabetes	Hyperventilation in ketoacidosis
Pregnancy	
Obesity	
Anaemia	

Adapted from Jevon and Ewens (2007).

inspired/expired in the apices and bases. A silent chest is an ominous sign.

- *Chest movement*: is chest movement equal, bilateral and symmetrical? The depth of inspiration should be noted (Simpson 2006).
- *Pulse oximetry*: continuous peripheral oxygen saturation monitoring.
- *Arterial blood gas analysis*: the definitive method to assess the effectiveness of ventilation.

Work of breathing
Healthy spontaneous breathing without a stethoscope is quiet (Moore 2007). Signs of increased work of breathing include a rise in *respiratory rate, noisy respirations* and *use of accessory muscles*.

Respiratory rate
Changes to the rate and depth of respiration can be indicative of many conditions (Trim 2005). A rise in the respiratory rate has

been recognised as one of the first indicators of deterioration and antecedent to adverse events (Schein et al. 1990; Buist et al. 1999; Goldhill et al. 1999; McGloin et al. 1999; Rich 1999; Crispin and Daffurn 2000). The normal respiratory rate in adults is approximately 12 breaths/min; tachypnoea >12 breaths/min (Trim 2005) is usually one of the first indications of respiratory distress (Resuscitation Council UK 2011). Respiratory dysfunction before an adverse event is associated with increased mortality (Considine 2005). Bradypnoea (<10 breaths/min – Simpson 2006) may be an ominous sign and possible causes include drugs, e.g. opiates, fatigue, hypothermia and central nervous system (CNS) depression. The following disturbed breathing patterns are also significant:

- *Kussmaul's breathing (air hunger)*: deep rapid respirations due to stimulation of the respiratory centre by metabolic acidosis, e.g. in ketoacidosis or chronic renal failure.
- *Cheyne–Stokes breathing pattern*: periods of apnoea alternating with periods of hyperpnoea; causes include left ventricular failure, renal failure, increased intracranial pressure (ICP), drug overdose (Simpson 2006) and cerebral injury; usually seen in the end-stages of life.
- *Hyperventilation*: often associated with anxiety states.

Noisy respirations
The following symptoms are also indicative of breathing difficulty and can be heard without the aid of a stethoscope (Jevon and Ewens 2000):

- *Stridor*: 'croaking' respiration that is louder during inspiration; caused by laryngeal or tracheal obstruction, e.g. foreign body, laryngeal oedema or laryngeal tumour.
- *Wheeze*: noisy musical sound caused by turbulent flow of air through narrowed bronchi and bronchioles, more pronounced on expiration; causes include asthma and chronic obstructive pulmonary disease (COPD).
- *'Rattly' chest*: e.g. chest infection, pulmonary oedema and sputum retention.
- *Gurgling*: caused by fluid in the upper airway.

- *Snoring*: snoring sounds may be associated with the tongue blocking the airway in an unconscious patient.

Accessory muscle use

The use of accessory muscles is a further indication of breathing difficulty. When this is present in patients with asthma or COPD this is indicative of a severe exacerbation (Jenkins and Johnson 2010).

Adequacy of ventilation

The assessment of heart rate, skin colour and the patient's mental status can help provide an indication of the adequacy of ventilation. Hypoxaemia can affect the following (Jevon and Ewens 2000):

- *Heart rate*: initially tachycardia (a non-specific sign), but severe hypoxaemia can cause bradycardia.
- *Skin colour*: initially pallor; hypoxia causes catecholamine release and vasoconstriction; central cyanosis is a late and often pre-terminal sign of hypoxaemia (if the patient is anaemic, severe hypoxaemia may not cause cyanosis).*
- *Mental status*: agitation (may be an early sign), drowsiness, confusion and impaired consciousness.

    *If the patient has COPD or congenital heart disease, cyanosis may be 'constant'.

COMPREHENSIVE ASSESSMENT OF THE BREATHLESS PATIENT

Occasional breathlessness is a common human experience and may be a normal reaction to exercise or it can be a symptom of serious pathology. A respiratory rate of >24 breaths/min indicates the potential for respiratory failure and is a medical emergency (Jenkins and Johnson 2010).

It is therefore important that a thorough assessment is undertaken to arrive at a comprehensive assessment of the patient's condition. This includes all other vital sign measurements because the assessment of one system is not to be taken in isolation.

Onset

The onset of the breathlessness provides vital information to the possible aetiology (Jenkins and Johnson 2010). If the onset is rapid (i.e. minutes to hours) it usually indicates speedily evolving pathology, e.g. acute pulmonary oedema (APO), anaphylaxis, acute asthma, pneumothorax, pulmonary embolism or a cardiac arrhythmia (Jenkins and Johnson 2010). A slower onset of breathlessness (i.e. hours to days) may indicate infections or exacerbation of COPD (Jenkins and Johnson 2010).

Severity

It is important to establish what is normal for the patient and the effect of the breathlessness on the patient (Jevon and Ewens 2000). Can the patient talk with ease? How far can the patient walk without having to stop? Can the patient climb the stairs Is the patient orthopnoeic? Is the patient platypnoeic (i.e. sitting up exacerbates the breathlessness, and may be indicative of pulmonary emboli – Jenkins and Johnson 2010)? If orthopnoea is present how many pillows does the patient sleep with? Does breathlessness affect the patient's daily activities or occupation? Does the patient require oxygen at home?

Timing

Severe asthma and left ventricular failure are more common at night. Occupation-related asthma is worse when the patient is at work and improves when the patient is at home (Jevon and Ewens 2000). Bronchitis is more common in the winter months.

Finger clubbing

Finger clubbing can indicate pulmonary or cardiovascular disease such as pulmonary fibrosis, lung cancer, bronchiectasis; clinical features often include loss of nail bed angle, an increased curvature of the nail and swelling of the terminal part of the digit, this is usually as a result of chronic hypoxaemia but its absence does not exclude disease (Simpson 2006; Jenkins and Johnson 2010).

Shape of the chest

The normal chest is bilaterally symmetrical, although it can be distorted by disease of the ribs or spinal vertebrae as well as by

underlying lung disease. In kyphosis (forward bending) or scoliosis (lateral bending) of the vertebral column, lung movement can
be severely restricted. A barrel chest is sometimes associated with
chronic bronchitis and emphysema (Jevon and Ewens 2000).

Chest percussion

Percussion of the chest wall causes the chest wall and underlying
tissues to move (Simpson 2006), which in turn helps to establish
whether the underlying tissues are air filled, fluid filled or solid
(Bickley and Szilagyi 2009). As a result audible sounds and palpa-
ble vibrations are felt. Percussion is performed by placing one
hand on the chest with the fingers separated; the other hand is used
as a hammer to tap the interphalangeal joint, moving down the
chest at 3- to 4-cm intervals (Simpson 2006). Comparison should
be made between the left and right sides of the chest.

Hyper-resonance (loud sound) to percussion is caused by an
increase in air in the chest, e.g. emphysema or pneumothorax.
Dense sound to percussion can be caused by thickening of the chest
wall, lung consolidation or pleural effusion.

Auscultation of the chest

**Normal breath sounds are categorized as: vesicular, bronchove-
sicular and bronchial** (Moore 2007):

- *Vesicular*: low pitched or soft, heard through inspiration and
  expiration without pause, heard over most of the lung fields
  (Moore 2007; Bickley and Szilagyi 2009).
- *Bronchovesicular*: moderate in pitch, heard in anterior region
  near the main bronchi and sometimes separated by a silent
  interval (Moore 2007; Bickley and Szilagyi 2009).
- *Bronchial*: louder and higher in pitch, separated by a pause and
  longer on expiration (Bickley and Szilagyi 2009).
- Adventitious sounds are abnormal breath sounds from the
  above, including crackles and wheezing (Moore 2007).

Diminished breath sounds can be caused by poor ventilation,
e.g. airway obstruction or respiratory depression, or by increased
separation of the stethoscope from the bronchial tree, e.g. obesity,
pleural effusion, pneumothorax or bronchial tumour. Fine late
inspiratory crackles may be heard, e.g. pulmonary oedema; coarse

early inspiratory crackles are heard in bronchitis and bronchiecta-sis (Simpson 2006); a coarse rubbing sound indicates pleural inflammation.

Medications
Medications that the patient is currently taking may be significant, e.g. beta blockers can exacerbate asthma and left ventricular failure. Drugs such as amiodarone and methotrexate can cause pneumo-nitis or pulmonary fibrosis (Jenkins and Johnson 2010).

Halitosis
This may indicate poor oral hygiene or could be a sign of an infec-tion of the upper respiratory tract.

Patient's position and emotional state
Does the patient need to sit in a particular position, e.g. supported by a bed table to facilitate breathing? Is the patient orthopnoeic? A breathless patient will be anxious.

Past medical history and family medical history
All previous illnesses, operations, hospital admissions and inves-tigations, particularly those that are respiratory related, e.g. COPD, should be noted (Booker 2004). Has the patient been prescribed any respiratory-related medication, e.g. inhalers or oxygen? If so the frequency and effectiveness of its use should be noted. Any respiratory disease in the patient's family should be noted.

Occupational and social history
When assessing respiratory disease, both past and present occupa-tions together with any exposure to dust, asbestos, coal or animals could be significant. Smoking history, past and present consump-tion, should be noted, together with any exposure to infection, e.g. tuberculosis. The type of living accommodation may be significant, e.g. stairs, damp environment, lack of a working lift in a block of flats.

Patient's age
Certain respiratory diseases are more likely to occur at particular times of life: <30 years – asthma, pneumothorax, cystic fibrosis,

congenital heart disease; >50 years – chronic bronchitis, COPD, carcinoma of the lung, pneumoconiosis, ischaemic heart disease.

Recent travel
Patients who have recently arrived from the Asian subcontinent may have been exposed to tuberculosis or recently identified viruses such as avian influenza.

Allergies
Any allergies should be recorded both in the patient's medical and nursing notes and on the prescription administration chart. It is also relevant to ascertain in what form the allergy manifests, e.g. tongue swelling or pruritus, and whether the patient carries an adrenaline injection for self-administration (e.g. EpiPen). Dependent on individual hospital policy the patient may be required to wear a red armband in addition to the above precautions.

ASSOCIATED SYMPTOMS OF DYSPNOEA
Chest pain
Respiratory-related chest pain or pleuritic pain is usually sharp in nature and aggravated by deep breathing, coughing or movement of the trunk and can be intermittent or transient (Bickley and Szilagyi 2009; Jenkins and Johnson 2010). It is often localised to one particular area (Jevon and Ewens 2000) and may be present in pneumonia, pleuritis or systemic inflammatory disease (Jenkins and Johnson 2010).

Cough
A cough is a common respiratory symptom. It occurs when deep inspiration is followed by an explosive expiration. A cough that is worse at night is suggestive of asthma or heart failure, while a cough that is worse after eating is suggestive of oesophageal reflux. The timing and duration of the cough is important (Bickley and Szilagyi 2009; Jenkins and Johnson 2010):

- *Dry cough*: laryngitis, left ventricular failure or mitral stenosis
- *Dry cough may become productive:* tracheobronchitis, viral pneumonia, bacterial pneumonia, pulmonary tuberculosis, lung cancer, pulmonary emboli may be due to a chest infection

- *Chronic cough*: asthma, post nasal drip, chronic bronchitis, lung abscess
- *Irritating chronic dry cough*: may be due to oesophageal reflux
- *Chronic cough with production of large volumes of purulent sputum*: may be due to bronchiectasis
- *Change in the character of a chronic cough*: may be due to a serious underlying pathology, e.g. carcinoma of the lung
- *Cough with haemoptysis (streaked with blood or bloody):* bacterial pneumonia, chronic bronchitis, pulmonary tuberculosis, bronchiectasis.

Sputum

Sputum is a key clinical feature of respiratory disease and can provide valuable information for the assessment of a breathless patient, including evaluation of care (Bickley and Szilagyi 2009). If sputum is produced, its colour and consistency should be noted:

- *White mucoid sputum*: seen in asthma and chronic bronchitis
- *Purulent green or yellow sputum*: may indicate respiratory infection
- *Blood present*: may indicate carcinoma of the lung, pulmonary embolism, recent upper airway trauma or coagulation disorder
- *Frothy white or pink sputum*: seen in pulmonary oedema
- *Thick, mucoid sputum*: feature of asthma, usually at the end of an attack (Bickley and Szilagyi 2009)
- *Frothy white, sometimes blood-stained sputum*: associated with acute pulmonary oedema (Moore 2007)
- *Foul-smelling sputum*: indication of respiratory tract infection
- *Black specks*: common causes include smoking, smoke inhalation and coal dust (Moore 2007).

The patient's history is important when determining the significance of sputum production at a particular time of day, e.g. chronic expectoration in the morning over a number of years may be suggestive of smoking-induced bronchitis whereas variable morning or nocturnal expectoration may be suggestive of asthma (Law 2000).

Important coexisting clinical features

A number of important coexisting clinical features may be associated with respiratory problems, including (Jevon and Ewens 2000):

- *Fever*: respiratory infection
- *Poor appetite and weight loss*: carcinoma of the lung, chronic infection
- *Swollen and painful calf*: deep vein thrombosis and pulmonary embolism
- *Ankle swelling*: congestive cardiac failure, deep vein thrombosis
- *Palpitations*: cardiac arrhythmias

MEASUREMENT OF PEAK EXPIRATORY FLOW RATE

Peak expiratory flow rate (PEF) or peak flow is the maximum flow rate, in litres per minute, attained on forced expiration from a position of full inspiration and is a useful baseline measurement of airflow obstruction (Jenkins and Johnson 2010). It is a simple test to ascertain the severity of a patient's asthma and can provide the practitioner with a guide to the level of airflow resistance within the bronchioles. This resistance can be caused by inflammation and/or bronchospasm. PEF measurement is expressed as a percentage of the patient's previous best value or of a predicted best value, if this is not available (British Thoracic Society Scottish Collegiate Guidelines Network 2009). Peak flow is not a measure of fitness or the strength of the patient's chest muscles.

Indications

Recordings should be undertaken four times a day (best of three attempts – Booker 2007), both before and after the administration of bronchodilators (Booker 2004). The results are crucial to the patient's treatment and are an aid to asthma diagnosis (Miller 2005), an indicator of how well the patient's asthma is responding to treatment and an aid to measuring the recovery from an asthma attack (Booker 2007).

Normal range for PEF measurement

The reference range for PEF is dependent on age, gender and height (Booker 2007). PEF measurements are not a stand-alone reading during an exacerbation of asthma, but are taken into account with other observations such as respiratory rate, SpO_2, arterial blood gas analysis, work of breathing and ability to complete sentences. However, during a severe exacerbation of asthma the recording of PEF may not be possible and may even worsen a patient's condition, whereupon other clinical signs and symptoms are sufficient to aid management decisions:

- *PEF >50–75% of best predicted*: moderate exacerbation
- *PEF 33–50% of best predicted*: acute severe attack
- *PEF <33% of best predicted*: life-threatening attack.

Procedure

1. Explain the procedure to the patient.
2. Assemble the necessary equipment – mini-Wright flowmeter is one of the most commonly available (Booker 2007), clean mouthpiece and ensure that the flowmeter is set at zero.
3. If possible stand the patient up.
4. Ask the patient to take a deep breath in and place the peak flowmeter in the mouth, holding it horizontally and closing the lips.
5. Ask the patient to breathe out in a short sharp 'huff'.
6. Note the recording on the flow meter and then return it to zero.
7. Ask the patient to repeat the procedure twice.
8. Record the best of the three recordings.
9. Clean the equipment as per manufacturer's instructions between patients.

(Adapted from Booker 2007)

PULSE OXIMETRY

Pulse oximetry is widely regarded as one of the greatest advances in clinical monitoring (Giuliano and Higgins 2005) since the invention of the ECG (Fox 2002) and is an essential monitoring and diagnostic tool in both critical care and ward areas (Mathews 2005). It is a simple, non-invasive bedside method of measuring arterial oxygen saturation in peripheral blood vessels (Booker 2008), expressed as SpO_2 (Welch 2005). Pulse oximetry was developed in the 1980s; before this time oxygenation assessment relied on subjective and unreliable physical assessment of the skin for cyanosis (Giuliano and Higgins 2005), which when present is an indicator of advanced hypoxaemia (Giuliano 2006).

Pulse oximetry measures only the extent to which haemoglobin is saturated with oxygen and does not provide information on oxygen delivery to the tissues or ventilatory function (Higgins 2005). Nevertheless, it is an invaluable monitoring tool in a variety of clinical settings, as long as its uses and limitations are fully understood (Jevon and Ewens 2000; Giuliano 2006).

Role of pulse oximetry

Hypoxaemia is common in all aspects of medical practice and without appropriate treatment will lead to cellular death and organ dysfunction.

Cyanosis is a late sign of hypoxaemia and the oxygen saturation must decrease to 80–85% before any changes in skin colour become apparent (Giuliano and Higgins 2005). In addition, manifestations of hypoxaemia, including restlessness, confusion, agitation, cyanosis, combative behaviour and tachycardia (McEnroe Ayres and Stucky Lappin 2004), may be missed or wrongly interpreted.

Pulse oximetry will immediately alert the practitioner to a fall in arterial oxygen saturations and the development of hypoxaemia, before visual recognition of cyanosis, which is not always present (Jenkins and Johnson 2010). In clinical practice an oxygen saturation of less than 90% is of grave concern.

> The absence of cyanosis does not exclude severe hypoxaemia; it will not be present if there is abnormal haemoglobin, very low SpO_2 levels or there is poor peripheral perfusion (Pullen 2010).

The mechanics of pulse oximetry

Pulse oximetry (Fig. 3.1) is a differential measurement based on the spectrophotometric absorption method using the Beer–Lambert law for optical absorption (Welch 2005).

The pulse oximeter probe consists of two light-emitting diodes (one red and one infrared) on one side of the probe. These emit red and infrared light via a relatively translucent area of the body and

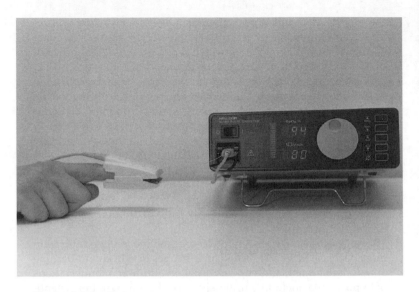

Fig. 3.1 Pulse oximeter.

detect the amount of light passing through the capillary bed (Booker 2008). The ratio of infrared light absorbed by oxyhaemoglobin and the red light absorbed by haemoglobin provides the data used to calculate the SpO_2 (Booker 2008). The more oxygenated the blood, the more red light and the less infrared light pass through (Giuliano 2006). By calculating the ratios of red to infrared light over time, oxygen saturation is calculated (Giuliano 2006).

Uses of pulse oximetry
Pulse oximetry is known as the fifth vital sign (British Thoracic Society 2008) and has become an integral component of standard vital sign recording, along with respiratory rate, blood pressure, pulse rate and temperature in all acute settings.

Advantages of pulse oximetry
Pulse oximetry is an inexpensive, non-invasive and portable method of continuous measurement of arterial oxygen saturation

which facilitates the early detection of hypoxaemia and reduces the need for arterial blood gas sampling (Booker 2008).

Normal values for oxygen saturation

All critically ill patients require immediate administration of high concentration oxygen. When stable, oxygen should be titrated against arterial blood gases (British Thoracic Society 2008). Oxygen saturation targets in the acutely ill patient should be 94–98% or 88–92% in those patients at risk of hypercapnia, e.g. COPD or morbid obesity (British Thoracic Society 2008). However, low oxygen saturation levels, i.e. <94%, may be normal in some patients and do not need oxygen therapy if their condition is stable (British Thoracic Society 2008).

Procedure for pulse oximetry

The following preliminary points should be observed:

- Wash and dry hands
- Ensure that the probe is clean
- Remove nail varnish or artificial nails
- Select a probe appropriate for the sensor site, duration of monitoring and patient activity levels (Pullen 2010)
- Explain the procedure to the patient.

Select an appropriate site with an adequate pulsating vascular bed. Sites include finger (most popular), ear lobe, toe, nose and forehead, and avoid areas of oedema or on an extremity where non-invasive blood pressure monitoring is being taken (Pullen 2010). The probe should be secured, but without the use of restrictive tape, to ensure blood flow and reduce the risk of pressure sores (Booker 2008). The following precautions must be taken during the procedure:

- Ensure that the trace is reliable and corresponds to pulse rate, i.e. oxygen saturation measurements are accurate (Fig. 3.2).
- Ensure careful positioning to ensure that the sensor is opposite the probe (Booker 2008).
- Ensure that the alarms on the pulse oximeter are set within locally agreed limits and according to the patient's condition.

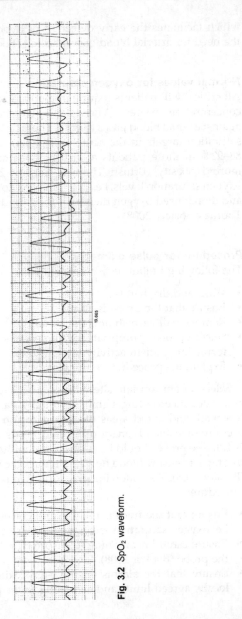

Fig. 3.2 SpO₂ waveform.

- Regularly monitor the probe site for complications, e.g. burns and joint stiffness, and regularly vary the site.
- Ensure that the patient's pulse rate correlates with the pulse oximetry display (Pullen 2010).
- Regularly monitor the patient's vital signs as per monitoring plan.
- Document the readings on a track-and-trigger system (British Thoracic Society 2008) and escalate as appropriate.

Interpreting plethysmographic waveforms
The quality of the pulse and circulation at the point where SpO_2 is being measured is reflected in the plethysmographic waveform (Fig. 3.2); the strength of the pulse is proportional to the amplitude of the waveform (Booker 2008).

Causes of inaccuracy
Inaccurate readings can be caused by any of the factors listed below:

- *Carbon monoxide poisoning*: false high readings (British Thoracic Society 2008).
- *Methaemoglobinaemia* (changes in the structure of iron in haemoglobin) and carboxyhaemoglobin (in carbon monoxide exposure) present in high doses can give false high or low readings (Pullen 2010).
- *Poor vascular perfusion*: pulse oximeter requires pulsatile blood flow to evaluate oxygen saturation.
- *Venous pulsation*: e.g. tricuspid valve failure, securing the probe too tightly (Booker 2008) heart failure, inflating blood pressure cuff distal to the probe, resulting in a false low reading.
- *Poor vascular perfusion*: e.g. in hypovolaemia, hypotension, septicaemia, hypothermia, cardiogenic shock or peripheral vascular disease, resulting in a false low reading.
- *Cardiac arrhythmias* such as atrial fibrillation can cause inadequate and irregular perfusion, resulting in a false low reading (Pullen 2010).
- *Factors that affect light absorption*: skin pigmentation, dried blood, high levels of bilirubin , nail polish with a blue pigment in and intravenous dyes, e.g. indocyanine green (Booker 2008).

- *Bright external light,* particularly fluorescent lighting can give a false high reading (Booker 2008).
- Low *oxygen saturations* (Booker 2008).
- *Patient movement,* e.g. shivering; although modern pulse oximeters can minimise the interference from patient movement (Gwinnutt 2006).

Limitations

Although pulse oximetry measures oxygen saturation and can detect hypoxaemia, it does not provide an indication of the adequacy of ventilation and carbon dioxide retention.

Davidson and Hosie (1993) reported a case of a postoperative patient who had a normal oxygen saturation (95%), but had abnormally high carbon dioxide levels causing a life-threatening respiratory acidosis. Failure to detect hypoventilation in such a patient is an example of a false sense of security generated by a single physiological variable being within safe limits (Hutton and Clutton-Brock 1993). If hypercapnia is suspected arterial blood gas analysis should always be performed.

Troubleshooting

It is important to ensure a reliable trace at all times. If it is difficult to secure an acceptable trace:

- Warm and rub the skin to improve circulation
- Try a different probe site, e.g. ear lobe
- Try a different probe/different pulse oximeter.

Complications

Pulse oximetry is very safe; complications are uncommon and are rarely serious if they do occur. Nevertheless complications have been reported:

- *Ischaemic pressure necrosis* (Fox 2002): in the reported case the patient was septic, hypotensive and had pre-existing arterial disease. In addition an arterial line was *in situ* in the radial artery, which may have further compromised the distal circulation.
- *Blister injuries at the probe site*: caused by a faulty probe cable; intermittent shortening resulted in excess electrical current supply to the light-emitting diode causing overheating.

- *Mechanical injury*: if the patient is unable to flex his or her finger; in unconscious or semiconscious patients the probe may inhibit voluntary use of the finger, resulting in stiffness. Changing the probe site regularly is therefore advocated (Booker 2008). This is potentially a problem for patients on intensive care units (ICUs) where prolonged monitoring occurs.

Best practice – pulse oximetry

- Remove anything that could impair the translucence of the sensor site.
- Position the probe without excessive force, i.e. avoid the use of adhesive tape.
- Ensure that an accurate trace is obtained.
- Be aware of any past or presenting history which may give aberrant results.
- Note any activity associated with a lower and higher SpO_2 reading.
- Note the use of supplementary oxygen.
- Compare results with previous readings and assess for any trends.
- Always rely on clinical judgement rather than an SpO_2 reading in isolation.
- Regularly monitor and alternate probe site.
- Ensure that the digit used is regularly flexed to avoid mechanical injury.

ARTERIAL BLOOD GAS ANALYSIS

Arterial blood gas (ABG) analysis is one of the most common tests performed in the critically ill patient and has become an essential skill for all health-care practitioners (Simpson 2004). It provides clinicians with valuable information about a patient's respiratory function and metabolic state (Simpson 2004; Allen 2005) and as such forms an integral component of monitoring the critically ill patient. It is important to remember that, as with all assessment methods, ABG interpretation should not be taken in isolation (Simpson 2004).

Procedure for arterial blood sampling

There are two methods of arterial blood sampling, from either a one-off arterial puncture or 'stab' or an arterial cannula. An arterial 'stab' is usually taken from the radial artery (Woodrow 2004), because it is most accessible. The femoral artery is also sometimes used.

The following procedure for arterial blood sampling is based on recommendations by Driscoll et al. (1997):

1. Ensure that the three-way tap is closed to air. This is to prevent back-flow of blood and blood spillage.
2. Remove cap from three-way tap, clean the open port with an alcohol swab and connect a sterile 5-ml syringe.
3. Turn the tap to connect the artery to the syringe and aspirate 5 ml of blood. This will ensure that the sample of blood used for analysis is fresh and does not contain 'flush solution'. The tap is now 'off' to the flush solution.
4. Turn the tap off to the syringe; remove and discard the syringe.
5. Replace with a heparinised syringe and turn the tap to connect it to the artery.
6. Slowly aspirate the required amount of blood (Fig. 3.3) and then turn the tap off to the syringe. It is important to aspirate the blood slowly because this will help to prevent spasm in the vessel (Dougherty and Lister 2011).
7. Remove the syringe and reapply a new sterile cap, ensuring that it is securely attached.
8. Flush the tubing and watch for return of reliable arterial trace on the monitor. Ensure that the infuser cuff is inflated to 300 mmHg (Dougherty and Lister 2011).
9. Insert blood into the blood gas analyser according to manufacturer's recommendations, being sure to include the patient's identification, temperature and any supplementary oxygen being administered (Fig. 3.4).
10. Document the results and inform medical staff if appropriate.

Indications for ABG analysis
Indications for ABG analysis include:

- respiratory compromise
- post cardiopulmonary arrest
- metabolic conditions, e.g. diabetic ketoacidosis (DKA)
- sudden or unexplained deterioration

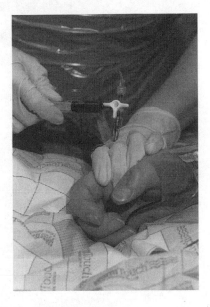

Fig. 3.3 Arterial blood sampling.

- evaluation of interventions, e.g. changes in invasive ventilation settings
- titration of non-invasive ventilation
- before major surgery as a baseline to facilitate postoperative comparison
- major trauma.

Principles of ABG analysis

Oxygen supply to the tissues is dependent on how oxygen disassociates itself from the haemoglobin (Hb) molecule to be made available for the tissues. This, in turn, is dependent on blood pH, body temperature and partial pressure of carbon dioxide ($PaCO_2$) of the blood (Foxall 2008). As the blood becomes more acidotic, warmer and with a higher $PaCO_2$, the oxygen dissociation curve shifts to the right and reduces the oxygen-carrying capacity of Hb (Elliott et al. 2007). Although less oxygen can be picked up by the

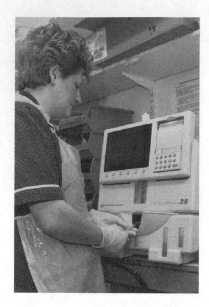

Fig. 3.4 Blood gas machine.

lungs, more can be released to the tissues (Elliott et al. 2007). Conversely, a shift to the left results in the Hb molecule having a greater affinity to oxygen but less can be released to the tissues. Therefore this may result in poor oxygenation despite an adequate PaO_2.

When a sample of arterial blood is processed by a blood gas analyser it provides not only an invaluable and accurate insight into the patient's respiratory function but also a window into their metabolic status.

The levels of blood gases are dependent on three variables: blood supply, ventilation and diffusion. Therefore if there is a poor blood supply to the alveoli but adequate ventilation, insufficient diffusion will lead to retention of PCO_2, e.g. pulmonary embolus. Conversely if there is a good blood supply to the alveoli but poor ventilation, gaseous exchange will also be compromised, e.g. COPD, pneumonia and asthma. Both of these imbalances will lead to a perfusion–ventilation (V/Q) mismatch or a 'shunt' (Smyth 2005). Blood gas units of measurement are kilopascals (kPa) or millimetres of mercury (mmHg). Both units are currently in use (to convert kPa to mmHg: kPa × 7.5 = mmHg and to convert mmHg to kPa: mmHg ÷ 7.5 = kPa).

Parameters measured by a blood gas analyser

- The pH: 7.35–7.45. Measures overall acid–base balance of the blood sample and is affected by both respiratory and metabolic function (Foxall 2008). Acid–base balance is the maintenance of hydrogen ion (H^+) balance that enables normal cell function (Foxall 2008). H^+ and pH levels have an inverse ratio, i.e. one increases as the other decreases (Simpson 2004). Small changes in pH are life threatening (Allen 2005) so the body relies on compensatory mechanisms to counteract dramatic changes in pH. Buffers in the body act as chemical sponges, which absorb excess alkali or acid (Allen 2005).

- PaO_2: 10–12.0 kPa (75–90 mmHg). This is the measurement of partial pressure of oxygen dissolved in the blood sample, not how much oxygen is in the blood (Foxall 2008). Arterial PO_2 (PaO_2) is dependent on the alveolar PO_2 (PaO_2) (Resuscitation Council UK 2011). PaO_2 is always less than PaO_2 and the extent of this difference is dependent on the incidence of lung disease. Increases in the difference indicate V/Q mismatch (Simpson 2004). A person with normal lungs breathing air (FiO_2 0.21) at sea level should have a PaO_2 >11 kPa (80 mmHg) and breathing an oxygen concentration of 50% (FiO_2 0.5) at sea level will result in a PaO_2 of approximately 40 kPa (300 mmHg) (Resuscitation Council UK 2011). When a patient is receiving supplementary oxygen, a normal PaO_2 will not necessarily indicate adequate ventilation as small increases in FiO_2 will overcome any hypoxaemia caused by under-ventilation (Resuscitation Council UK 2011). A PaO_2 level <8 kPa (60 mmHg) is considered a diagnosis of hypoxaemia (British Thoracic Society 2008). Critically ill patients have increased oxygen demands because of the pathological demands of the body. It is critical that these increased oxygen demands are met to maintain adequate tissue oxygenation and prevent cell death.

- $PaCO_2$: 4.5–6.0 kPa (34–45 mmHg). This is the measurement of partial pressure of dissolved carbon dioxide in the blood (more soluble than oxygen). To be carried to the lungs to be exhaled carbon dioxide is transported in a plasma solution as carbonic acid (H_2CO_3). If the patient has too little or too much carbon dioxide this will have an effect on the acidity or alkalinity of the blood (Foxall 2008). Carbon dioxide concentration provides information about the adequacy of ventilation (Foxall 2008). Carbon dioxide is a waste product of tissue metabolism and the respiratory centres in the brain stem are stimulated in a response to high levels of carbon dioxide (Foxall 2008). The respiratory centres in the brain stem are sensitive to H^+ concentration (Resuscitation Council UK 2011). Therefore, as the carbon dioxide rises the respiratory centres are stimulated to increase respiratory rate and depth and reduce carbon dioxide levels, and conversely, when there is hyperventilation and carbon dioxide reduces, the respiratory centres are stimulated to reduce respiratory rate and depth:

$$CO_2 + H_2O = H_2CO_3 = HCO_3^- + H^+$$

Carbon dioxide + Water → Carbonic acid → Bicarbonate + hydrogen ions

- Bicarbonate (HCO_3^-) (22–26 mmol/l): the major buffering systems in the body involve bicarbonate, protein and phosphate; however, bicarbonate is the most important. Buffers have two qualities: they bind free hydrogen ions when they are in excess (acidosis) and donate hydrogen ions when they are too low (alkalosis) (Foxall 2008).
- Base excess (BE) (−2 mmol to +2 mmol): base excess is the quantity of acid or base required to restore the blood to a pH of 7.4 (Woodrow 2004; Resuscitation Council UK 2011). A negative value indicates a deficit of base (or excess of acid) and a positive value indicates an excess of base (or deficit of acid) (Resuscitation Council UK 2011).
- SaO_2 (92–99%): arterial oxygen saturation is the percentage of oxygen that has combined with the Hb molecule. Oxygen com-

Table 3.3 Normal ranges for arterial blood gas results

Parameter	Normal range
pH	7.35–7.45
PO_2	10.0–12.0 kPa (75–90 mmHg)
PCO_2	4.5–6.0 kPa (34–45 mmHg)
Bicarbonate (HCO_3^-)	22–26 mmol/l
SaO_2	>95%
Base excess	−2 to +2

(Foxall, 2008)

bines with Hb in sufficient amounts to meet the needs of the body, while at the same time releasing oxygen to meet tissue demands (Foxall 2008).

- Other values: most analysers measure electrolytes, e.g. sodium (Na^+), potassium (K^+), calcium (Ca^{2+}) and chloride (Cl^-), Hb and lactate, which can be useful for a 'quick check'. In most ICUs these values are accepted as accurate and treatment is titrated according to them. However, if aberrant values are obtained it will be necessary to obtain laboratory analysis for comparison.

Normal ranges for ABG analysis are shown in Table 3.3.

Systematic analysis of ABG results

Foxall (2008) recommends three principles in analysing ABG results:

- Consider the patient's clinical history and physical examination.
- Systematically analyse the results.
- Integrate the clinical findings with interpretation of the data.

A systematic approach for the analysis of ABGs is a prerequisite for objective assessment and the Resuscitation Council UK suggest a five-step approach, as follows

Step I: assess oxygenation

- Is the patient hypoxic?
- What supplementary oxygen are they receiving?

Step 2: determine pH level
Is there an acidosis (pH < 7.35) or alkalosis (pH > 7.45) present?

Step 3: determine the respiratory component
Is the $PaCO_2$ low (<4.7 kPa, <35 mmHg) or high (>6.0 kPa, >45 mmHg)? If the carbon dioxide is low this may indicate either a primary respiratory alkalosis or a secondary respiratory compensation for a metabolic acidosis. If the carbon dioxide is high this may indicate either a primary respiratory acidosis or a secondary compensation for a metabolic alkalosis.

Step 4: determine metabolic component
Is the bicarbonate low (<22 mmol/l) or high (>26 mmol/l)? If the bicarbonate is low this may indicate a primary metabolic acidosis or a secondary renal compensation for a respiratory alkalosis. If the bicarbonate is high this may indicate a primary metabolic alkalosis or a secondary metabolic compensation for a respiratory acidosis. It is not necessary to evaluate BE because the level of BE and bicarbonate mirror each other.

Step 5
Combine the findings from steps 2, 3 and 4 and determine what the primary disturbance is and whether there are any compensatory mechanisms evident.

Best practice – arterial blood gas analysis

Consider the patient's clinical history and physical examination
Systematically analyse the results
Integrate the clinical findings with interpretation of the data
Never remove supplementary oxygen when taking an arterial blood sample for analysis. It is important to assess the patient's response to supplementary oxygen and the withholding of oxygen in the compromised patient is dangerous practice
The changes in acid–base disorders are summarised in Table 3.4

Classification of imbalance
Acid–base balance disturbance occurs when there are either too many H^+ (acidosis) or too few (alkalosis) (Foxall 2008). If this

Table 3.4 Summary of changes in acid–base disorders (Resuscitation Council UK, 2011)

Acid–base disorder	pH	$PaCO_2$	HCO_3^-
Respiratory acidosis	↓		N
Metabolic acidosis	↓	N	↓
Respiratory alkalosis		↓	N
Metabolic alkalosis		N	
Respiratory acidosis with metabolic compensation	↓[a]		
Metabolic acidosis with respiratory compensation	↓[a]	↓	↓
Respiratory alkalosis with metabolic compensation	[a]	↓	↓
Metabolic alkalosis with respiratory compensation	[a]		
Mixed metabolic and respiratory alkalosis	↓		↓
Mixed metabolic and respiratory alkalosis		↓	

[a]If the compensation is virtually complete the pH may be normal (N).

imbalance has a respiratory cause the metabolic system will aim to compensate as will the respiratory system if there is a metabolic imbalance.

There are four classifications of imbalance with or without compensation:

- *Respiratory* acidosis
- *Metabolic* acidosis
- *Respiratory* alkalosis
- *Metabolic* alkalosis.

Respiratory acidosis

Respiratory acidosis occurs when the pH of blood falls below 7.35 (Foxall 2008) and is caused by inadequate ventilation, leading to the retention of carbon dioxide and an increase in free hydrogen ions. Predisposing factors include:

- Exacerbation of COPD
- Pulmonary oedema
- Pneumonia
- Mechanical disruption to ventilation, e.g. diaphragmatic rupture, fractured sternum
- Neurological disorder, e.g. intracranial events and neuromuscular disorders

- Over-sedation, i.e. opioids or sedatives
- Self-poisoning.

An example of respiratory acidosis without metabolic compensation:

pH 7.24
$PaCO_2$ 8.0 kPa (60 mmHg)
PaO_2 7.5 kPa (56 mmHg)
HCO_3^- 24 mmol/l
BE 0
SaO_2 94%

It is vital that there is a fine balance between acids and bases to provide the optimum neutral environment for cell function. In the above example, the buffer system provided by the kidneys should counterbalance the free H^+ as a result of excessive carbon dioxide production. Compensation for acidosis or alkalosis is achieved by the other system (i.e. the renal system will compensate for respiratory derangement and the respiratory system for metabolic derangement). The lungs, however, provide a much quicker compensatory mechanism than the kidneys, which can take hours or even days to compensate adequately.

An example of respiratory acidosis with metabolic compensation:

pH 7.37
$PaCO_2$ 7.3 kPa (55 mmHg)
PaO_2 9.6 kPa (72 mmHg)
HCO_3^- 32 mmol/l
BE +6
SaO_2 95%

In this example there is an increase in the amount of HCO_3^- reabsorbed by the kidneys which act as a buffer for the excessive free H^+. The compensation is said to be adequate only if the pH has returned to within normal limits, as in this example.

Metabolic acidosis
This involves excess fixed acid production, i.e. lactate or loss of HCO_3^-. Causes include:

- diarrhoea
- cardiac arrest
- diabetic ketoacidosis
- renal failure
- distributive shock
- salicylate poisoning.

Example of metabolic acidosis without respiratory compensation:

pH 7.20
$PaCO_2$ 4.7 kPa (35 mmHg)
PaO_2 10.0 kPa (75 mmHg)
HCO_3^- 16 mmol/l
BE −12
SaO_2 96%

The lack of circulating HCO_3^- has resulted in a metabolic acidosis reflected in a base deficit of −12.

Example of metabolic acidosis with respiratory compensation:

pH 7.35
$PaCO_2$ 2.7 kPa (20 mmHg)
PaO_2 11.8 kPa (88 mmHg)
HCO_3^- 12 mmol/l
BE −14
SaO_2 97%

The respiratory system has compensated by reducing the level of carbon dioxide by hyperventilation, thereby reducing the level of circulating free H^+.

Respiratory alkalosis
Respiratory alkalosis is caused by the over-excretion of carbon dioxide, leading to a reduction in free H^+ and an alkalotic state. Predisposing factors include:

- hyperventilation in hysteria
- excessive mechanical ventilation.

Example of respiratory alkalosis without metabolic compensation:

pH 7.50
$PaCO_2$ 2.5 kPa (19 mmHg)
PaO_2 8.6 kPa (65 mmHg)
HCO_3^- 22 mmol/l
BE +1
SaO_2 92%

Example of respiratory alkalosis with metabolic compensation:

pH 7.44
$PaCO_2$ 2.6 kPa (19 mmHg)
PaO_2 8.9 kPa (67 mmHg)
HCO_3^- 15 mmol/l
BE −9
SaO_2 93%

The patient excretes bicarbonate ions via the renal system in order to reduce the presence of alkaline buffers in the blood further.

Metabolic alkalosis

Metabolic alkalosis is caused by a loss of acids or an increase in alkaline buffers, i.e. bicarbonate. Causes include:

- gastrointestinal disorders, e.g. severe vomiting
- overdose of antacids
- diuretics.

An example of metabolic alkalosis without respiratory compensation:

pH 7.67
$PaCO_2$ 4.2 kPa (31 mmHg)
PaO_2 13.1 kPa (97 mmHg)
HCO_3^- 38 mmol/l
BE +15
SaO_2 98%

There is an increase in circulating bicarbonate, i.e. an excess of alkaline leading to an alkalosis.

An example of metabolic alkalosis with respiratory compensation:

pH 7.45
$PaCO_2$ 7.6 kPa (57 mmHg)
PaO_2 12.4 kPa (93 mmHg)
HCO_3^- 32 mmol/l
BE +4
SaO_2 96%

The respiratory system retains carbon dioxide in order to create more available free H^+ to balance the excess alkaline production, thereby maintaining the equilibrium.

PRINCIPLES OF CAPNOGRAPHY

Measuring end-tidal carbon dioxide ($ETCO_2$) is helpful when monitoring the critically ill patient. There is virtually no carbon dioxide in inspired air; but as $ETCO_2$ concentration is very similar to $PaCO_2$, measuring $ETCO_2$ does provide an indication as to the adequacy of ventilation (Urden et al. 2006).

Capnometry is the measurement of expired carbon dioxide (Myers 2006). It can simply be undertaken by attaching a colorimetric detector (Fig. 3.5) to the tracheal tube: a pH-sensitive indicator strip turns yellow in the presence of exhaled carbon dioxide, thus confirming correct tracheal tube placement (Andrews and Nolan 2006). This colorimetric detector device is frequently used during cardiopulmonary resuscitation to help ascertain that the tracheal tube has been inserted into the trachea. New capnography devices are now available for patients who are awake and spontaneously breathing.

Electronic capnometry, using infrared light technology, is more accurate and reliable than colorimetric capnometry, particularly in patients with circulatory shock (Salem 2001). It works on the principle that carbon dioxide absorbs infrared light in proportion to its concentration (Gwinnutt 2006). It produces a capnogram, a waveform that shows the proportion of carbon dioxide in exhaled air (Mosby 2006). This method of monitoring is referred to as capnography.

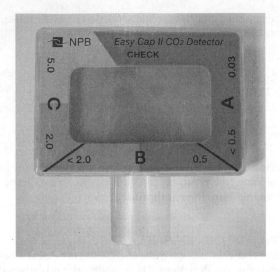

Fig. 3.5 A colorimetric carbon dioxide detector.

The use of capnography has expanded over recent years and it is currently used in a variety of acute care settings. It provides comprehensive information on ETCO$_2$, with a continuous characteristic waveform (Fig. 3.6) being displayed (Andrews and Nolan 2006). It provides clinicians with information about ventilation and assists in clinical diagnosis, e.g. pulmonary embolism (Ahrens and Sona 2003). It is particularly helpful in the critically ill patient because it can alert the nurse to hypoventilation even when the patient's pulse oximetry readings are normal (Woomer and Berkheimer 2003). Capnography is also a helpful monitoring tool if pulse oximetry is malfunctioning (Kober et al. 2004).

Indications for capnography include (Gonce Morton and Rempher 2009):

- monitoring when weaning from ventilation
- during the transport of critically ill patients
- during anaesthesia
- during cardiopulmonary resuscitation
- after tracheal tube insertion to confirm correct placement.

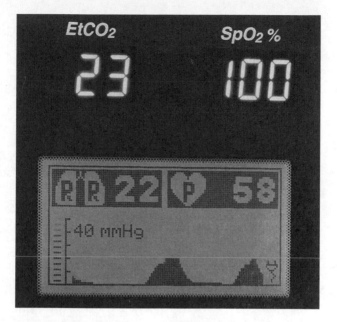

Fig. 3.6 A characteristic end-tidal CO_2 waveform (Proact Medical Ltd).

Changes in the waveform produced enable correlation with clinical conditions, e.g. airflow obstruction.

In patients with a low cardiac output or chest disease, the gap between the arterial carbon dioxide and $ETCO_2$ levels increases; care must therefore be taken when interpreting $ETCO_2$ concentrations in these circumstances (Gwinnutt 2006). Arterial blood gas analysis enables the $ETCO_2$ to be calibrated against the $PaCO_2$: the capnography can then be used as an indirect, continuous monitor of $PaCO_2$, and therefore ventilation (Andrews and Nolan 2006).

MONITORING PRIORITIES OF A VENTILATED PATIENT

Mechanical ventilation is a major supportive treatment for critically ill patients and as such is a frequent occurrence in the ICU

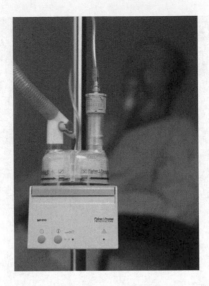

Fig. 3.7 Humidifier (Fisher and Paykell).

(Newmarch 2006) (Fig. 3.8). The use of an endotracheal or tracheostomy tube, via a closed circuit, ensures the delivery of guaran-
teed fraction of inspired oxygen (FiO_2) and delivery of gas under
a pre-set constant pressure or at a pre-set tidal volume (Newmarch
2006).

There are many physical, as well as psychological, parameters
to be monitored, all of which must be fully understood by the
nurse caring for these patients. The primary physiological changes
taking place concern the cardiovascular system. As mechanical
ventilation (MV) is totally converse to normal physiological breathing, cardiovascular effects can be ongoing and therefore continuous, consistent monitoring is essential. During spontaneous
breathing air is 'sucked in' under a negative pressure, whereas
with MV air is delivered under a positive pressure (Manno 2005).
As air is delivered under a positive pressure, venous return to the
right side of the heart is impeded, reducing preload and, consequently, cardiac output (Manno 2005). In addition, the fall in

cardiac output leads to a reduction in renal blood flow which stimulates the release of antidiuretic hormone (ADH) causing fluid retention and oedema.

The classification of ventilators depends on the methods used to cycle from the inspiratory phase to the expiratory phase (Newmarch 2006). If the ventilator mode is pressure cycled, inspiratory pressure is set, rate is set and volume is dependent on the patient's lung compliance. If the mode is volume cycled, the tidal volume is pre-set, rate is set and peak inspiratory pressure varies dependent on the patient's degree of lung compliance. The most frequently used ventilator modes are:

- *SIMV (volume or pressure cycled)*: synchronised intermittent mandatory ventilation delivers a pre-set volume or pressure, at a pre-set rate and is synchronised with the patient's own respiratory effort (Schumacher and Chernecky 2005). A comparison between the patient's breath and mandatory breaths will be demonstrated and should be recorded. This is the most commonly used ventilator mode and can be used as a weaning mode.
- *CMV – controlled mandatory ventilation*: delivers gas at a pre-set volume and rate and does not synchronise with spontaneous breaths (Manno 2005).
- *Pressure support ventilation (PSV)*: spontaneous mode where a pre-set inspiratory pressure augments the patient's breath. The patient controls the rate and volume of ventilation (Schumacher and Chernecky 2005).
- *Pressure control ventilation (PC)*: gas is delivered at a pre-set rate and inspiratory pressure and the volume is determined by the patient's lung compliance.
- *Bilevel positive airway pressure (BIPAP)*: a pressure-controlled ventilation allows the patient to breathe spontaneously anywhere in the cycle and provides high and low positive end expiratory pressure (Manno 2005).
- *Continuous positive airway pressure (CPAP)*: provides a constant positive airway pressure in spontaneous mode (frequently seen with PSV) and promotes gaseous exchange by opening alveoli and increasing functional residual capacity (Schumacher and Chernecky 2005).

- *Positive end-expiratory pressure (PEEP)*: same principle as CPAP but in non-spontaneous mode.

Parameters to be monitored during mechanical ventilation
During mechanical ventilation careful note should be taken of the following measurements, which should be recorded hourly and after any alterations in settings:

- *Respiratory rate*: the number of breaths delivered by the ventilator per minute (Manno 2005) and any spontaneous breaths.
- *Tidal volume* (VT): volume of air per expired breath. This should be the same or slightly more than the preset VT. Aim for 6–8 ml/kg, i.e. maximum for a 70 kg person should be 560 ml/breath. A decrease in mortality has been demonstrated with patients with acute lung injury using these lower tidal volumes (Brower et al. 2000). If the inspired VT does not correlate with the expired VT in volume-cycled ventilation, check for leaks in the circuit, check that the cuff on the endotracheal tube is inflated sufficiently and check the ventilator (inner valves, etc.). If VT is high, the patient is probably breathing spontaneously. Increases in tidal volumes could also be due to added gas into the circuit, i.e. when nebulising drugs.
- *Minute volume (MV)*: amount exhaled each minute. It should always be the same as pre-set tidal volume multiplied by the pre-set rate (VT × rate = MV).
- *Peak inspiratory pressure*: peak pressure at which the tidal volume is delivered or is pre-set in pressure-cycled ventilation. Measured in centimetres of water, it must always be at the lowest possible to ensure adequate ventilation. This will lessen the cardiovascular side effects of MV and reduce the risks of barotrauma.
- *PEEP*: this should range between 5 and 20 cmH$_2$O. PEEP is over and above inspiratory pressure, i.e. if pressure is set at 20 cmH$_2$O and PEEP at 5 cmH$_2$O, the peak inspiratory pressure will be 25 cmH$_2$O.
- *FiO$_2$*: fraction of inspired oxygen expressed as a fraction of a whole, i.e. 40% = FiO$_2$ 0.4.
- *Inspiratory to expiratory ratio (I:E ratio)*: each breath has three components: inspiration, pause and expiration. Alteration of

the I:E ratio manipulates alveolar gas exchange, normal I:E ratio is 1:2 (Newmarch 2006).

- *ETCO₂ levels* (if used).
- *Humidifier temperature*: should be 37°C at the patient end (Fig. 3.7).
- Ensure that all high and low alarm limits are set appropriately and monitored regularly.

NEVER SILENCE A VENTILATOR ALARM UNLESS YOU ARE SURE OF THE CAUSE.

Monitoring the endotracheal tube

The following are key principles of the management of a patient with an endotracheal tube:

- Maintain patency: ventilation should be closely monitored and suction should be immediately available.

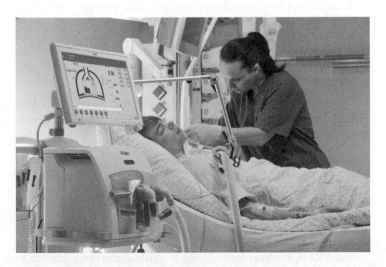

Fig 3.8 Ventilated patient (Drager Medical).

- Secure the endotracheal tube to the patient's face and head with either adhesive or cotton tape.
- Alter the position of the tube daily at the lips to prevent pressure ulceration.
- Document the length at which the tube is cut and tied at the lips and check regularly for migration from these markers.
- Ensure continuous ECG with respiratory waveform.
- Ensure continuous pulse oximetry to detect hypoxaemia.
- Apply regular endotracheal suction, either with or without hyperinflation, to prevent sputum retention and maintain patency of the tube.
- Regularly auscultate for breath sounds to ensure equal inflation. The possibility of the tip of the tracheal tube slipping into the right main bronchus causing unilateral ventilation can therefore be excluded.
- Regular oral toilet, preferably with a soft toothbrush and toothpaste, will help to maintain oral hygiene and prevent proliferation of bacteria.
- Secure/support ventilator tubing to prevent excess weight on the endotracheal tube.
- Check emergency equipment, i.e. intubation equipment, suction and manual re-breathe circuits at least once a shift in case of accidental extubation.
- Use endotracheal tubes with high-volume, low-pressure cuffs to minimise the risk of tracheal stenosis/ischaemia and regularly check cuff pressures with cuff manometers.

The nurse should be alert to the possible complications of endotracheal intubation. The acronym DOPE is helpful in detecting problems:

Displacement of tube
Obstruction of tube
Pneumothorax
Equipment

Other complications of tracheal intubation include oesophageal or right main bronchus intubation, herniation of the cuff, damage to vocal folds, tracheal stenosis, tracheal ulceration and damage to soft palate and lips.

MONITORING THE PATIENT RECEIVING
NON-INVASIVE VENTILATION

The use of non-invasive ventilation (NIV) to avoid endotracheal intubation was first described in 1989 (Keenan et al. 2005). It has now become a frequent occurrence in ICUs, HDUs and wards, primarily to avoid the use of invasive ventilation. There are many different terminologies that describe NIV depending on machines used (Woodrow 2003): CPAP, non-invasive positive pressure ventilation (NIPPV), nasal ventilation (NV), and the most frequently used BiPAP. The British Thoracic Society recommends the term NIV, which incorporates all of the above (BTS 2010).

NIV is delivered via a face or nasal mask and is considered first line treatment in cardiogenic pulmonary oedema and persistent hypercapnic respiratory failure. NIV gives the patient breathing assistance by delivering a pressured gas through a tight-fitting mask (Preston 2001). By supporting patients with NIV, work of breathing is reduced, tidal volume is increased, and oxygenation and hypercapnia improve (Preston 2001). Bilevel NIV consists of the following parameters:

- Inspiratory positive airway pressure (IPAP)
- Expiratory positive airway pressure (EPAP).

BTS guidelines (2010) recommend the use of bilevel NIV for:

- COPD with respiratory acidosis (pH 7.25–7.35)
- hypercapnic respiratory failure secondary to chest wall deformity, e.g. scoliosis, thoracoplasty, neuromuscular disease
- cardiogenic pulmonary oedema that is unresponsive to CPAP alone
- weaning patients from mechanical ventilation.

Bilevel NIV alternates between IPAP and EPAP. The higher level of inspiratory pressure occurs during inspiration (IPAP) and increases tidal volume, helping to reduce carbon dioxide levels and the work of breathing (Woodrow 2003). The lower level of pressure occurs at the end of expiration (EPAP) maintaining a positive pressure, thereby recruiting alveoli and preventing atelectasis to improve oxygenation (Woodrow 2003). Typical pressures to commence bilevel NIV would be IPAP of $10\,cmH_2O$ and EPAP of $5\,cmH_2O$, titrated according to the patient's response.

When monitoring a patient receiving bilevel NIV the following precautions should be observed:

- Take arterial blood gases (ABG); after 1 hour, some improvement should be recognised. If carbon dioxide levels and respiratory acidosis have not significantly improved in 4–6 hours invasive ventilation should be commenced (BTS 2010).
- Monitor vital signs regularly; continuous SpO_2 is vital (NICE 2010).
- Monitor and record levels of IPAP, EPAP, respiratory rate, FiO_2, tidal volume and minute volume.
- Administer regular eye and mouth care as high-pressure gas can be very drying.
- A full facemask should be used in the first 24 hours (Royal College of Physicians 2008).
- The patient should have minimal breaks from NIV during the first 24 hours of treatment (Royal College of Physicians 2008).
- If a nasogastric tube is inserted, use a fine bore to minimise leak from the mask (NICE 2010).
- Be aware that the masks can be claustrophobic for some patients. When condition has stabilised, regular breaks from the mask for oral toilet, diet and fluids can be given, but supplementary oxygen must be administered.
- Monitor chest wall movement (BTS 2010).

PRINCIPLES OF MONITORING A PATIENT WITH A CHEST DRAIN

A chest drain can be used to manage a variety of thoracic conditions. They are used to remove air (pneumothorax), blood (haemothorax) , pus (empyema) or other fluid (hydropneumothorax) from the pleural cavity in patients with collapsed lungs, malignancies, chest trauma or after surgery (National Patient Safety Agency 2008).

The drain insertion should ideally be performed under ultrasound guidance, the insertion site should be within the midaxillary safe triangle (fourth to sixth intercostal spaces) (NPSA 2008), a small-bore chest tube (<14 Fr) is recommended (BTS 2010). Suction should not be routinely used because of the high risk of pulmonary oedema (BTS 2010).

When monitoring a patient with a chest drain the following precautions should be observed:

- Monitor the patient's vital signs, in particular in relation to the patient's respiratory status.
- Request a chest radiograph after insertion of chest drain to check its position and ensure that the lung has reinflated (BTS 2010).
- Administer prescribed analgesia for pain (Hilton 2004).
- Secure the drain to prevent movement; however, large amounts of tape and dressing are unnecessary and a transparent dressing and one anchor tape are recommended (BTS 2010).
- Regularly examine the insertion site for signs of infection and culture as necessary (Sullivan 2008)
- Regularly check the fluid level, because an underwater sealed drain operates as a one-way valve allowing air to bubble out through the water during expiration and coughing but not permitting air to be drawn back in (Sullivan 2008).
- Observe and record the amount, consistency and colour of any drainage regularly.
- Observe the level of water in the tubing. It should fluctuate with respirations; a gradual decrease in fluctuation could indicate re-expansion of the lung whereas a sudden decrease suggests that the tube is blocked (Elliott et al. 2007). Bubbling is another sign that air is being evacuated from the pleural space; it should decrease as the lung reinflates. The continuation of bubbling suggests a continued leak in the visceral pleura (BTS 2010). Also check that there are no loose connections in the system. If a blocked tube is suspected, check that the cause is not a kinked tube. The tubing may need to be replaced. 'Milking' the tube is not recommended because this causes unnecessary fluctuations in intrapleural pressures.
- Monitor any suction used ensuring that the prescribed suction level is maintained; high-volume low-grade suction is recommended (10–20 cm H_2O) and can be used to help remove air or

fluid from the chest cavity (Sullivan 2008; BTS 2010). Note that if a chest drain is connected to a suction unit that has been switched off it is equivalent to it being clamped off and could therefore result in a tension pneumothorax.

- Clamp the drain close to the chest wall only when changing the bottle/container or after accidental disconnection. A bubbling chest drain should never be clamped (BTS 2010).
- Ensure that the drainage bottle is kept below the level of the patient's chest to prevent fluid re-entering the pleural space (Sullivan 2008).
- Assess patient for pain during insertion, when in situ and during the removal process (Hunter 2008; Sullivan 2008).

PRINCIPLES OF MONITORING THE PATIENT WITH A TEMPORARY TRACHEOSTOMY

A tracheostomy is an opening in the anterior wall of the trachea inferior to the cricoid cartilage (Neville Regan and Dallachiesa 2009). Patients who require a temporary tracheostomy are a frequent occurrence in the critically ill population both within critical care units and during their recovery phase in ward areas. Insertion of a tracheostomy tube is a surgical procedure that is performed either in the operating theatre (surgical tracheostomy) or in the ICU (percutaneous dilational tracheostomy).

Indications for a temporary tracheostomy include:

- upper airway obstruction (Barnett 2008)
- elective head and neck surgery (Russell and Matta 2004)
- prolonged oral intubation (>14 days)
- inability to wean from mechanical ventilation (Neville Regan and Dallachiesa 2009)
- inability to maintain own airway (Neville Regan and Dallachiesa 2009)
- neurological trauma or disease (Parker et al. 2010).

Monitoring priorities of the patient with a temporary tracheostomy

A patient who has been in intensive care and subsequently required a temporary tracheostomy will often have suffered a severe and protracted illness resulting in severe debilitation. These patients will have significantly impaired muscle strength and physical energy reserve and remain susceptible to infection. Therefore, these vulnerable patients require continuous monitoring in the post intensive care period. Monitoring should focus on maintaining the patency of the tracheostomy tube and the early detection of complications that may occur. A tracheostomy tube that has a removable inner tube for cleaning purposes can significantly reduce the serious complication of a blocked tube and compromised airway (Barnett 2008).

Monitoring principles are:

- Continual observation: ensure that the patient is located in a highly visible area of the ward.
- Monitor the position and patency of the tube: continually observe the patient for signs of respiratory distress, ensuring that they have access to call buttons and communication aids.
- Regular physiological monitoring: respiratory rate, heart rate, blood pressure, SpO_2, temperature, level of consciousness.
- Monitor the temperature and water level of the humidifier, ensuring that any water traps are empty and positioned lower than the head height of the patient.
- Observe and record the amount, colour and consistency of secretions on tracheal suction (suction as required, for the shortest duration possible – Neville Regan and Dallachiesa 2009).
- Observe the amount and consistency of sputum in the inner tube when cleaned with sterile 0.9% NaCl and clean according to requirements (at *least* three times a day) (Neville Regan and Dallachiesa 2009).
- Monitor microbiological results from sputum samples.
- Monitor nutritional status; keep a food diary if not receiving enteral nutrition.
- Regularly observe the tracheal stoma for signs of infection, irritation or granulation (Barnett 2008). Contact a wound specialist if there is risk of stoma breakdown (Neville Regan and Dallachiesa 2009).

Name..Unit number..............................

Date of tracheostomy...................................Tube size/type...........................

Criteria for use of purple cap (all must be Yes)

Relevant multidisciplinary team members aware	Yes/No
Oxygen saturations maintained ie 92--95%	Yes/No
Strong spontaneous cough	Yes/No
Cuff is deflated	Yes/No
Patient aware of procedure	Yes/No
Fenestrated tube with inner tube	Yes/No
Tube has been downsized	Yes/No

<u>Weaning process</u>

Day 1	Discuss -- Apply cap at 08:00 for up to 12 hours, give humidified oxygen by mouth if required. Remove cap overnight. Monitor respiratory rate and saturations 10 minutes after occlusion and hourly for first 4 hours -- then 4 hourly. Re-apply cap following suction via tracheostomy.
Day 2	Cap from 08:00 as above plan to occlude during daylight hours if tolerated. Discuss with physiotherapists or OR team. Monitor respiratory rate and saturations 4 hourly.
Day 3	If cap is tolerated for daylight hours discuss with multidisciplinary team ie. medical team, physiotherapists and OR team re: decannulation. <u>Tracheostomy to be removed by a practitioner who has achieved the tracheostomy competencies,</u> a dry dressing and non-porous tape, i.e. sleek, applied over the stoma until healed. Inform Speech Therapist re: swallowing assessment.

Date/ Time	Speaking valve ON	Speaking valve OFF	Cap ON	Cap OFF	Comments	Signed

<u>REMOVE CAP IMMEDIATELY IF:</u>

- Patient becomes breathless and/or distressed
- Patient becomes sweaty or clammy
- Saturations drop to a level lower than before capping
- Patient requires frequent suction to clear secretions
- Patient becomes confused and/or agitated

Fig. 3.9 Tracheostomy weaning chart.

Best practice – temporary tracheostomies

Have available at the bedside a tracheostomy tube of the same size and type that the patient has *in situ* and a size below (Neville Regan and Dallachiesa 2009)

Have available at the bedside tracheal dilating forceps

Ensure that the tracheostomy tube is securely fixed with tape or foam tracheostomy holder and regularly changed, particularly if soiled

Clean the tracheostomy site with saline as required using a clean technique and with two nurses

Use aseptic technique for suctioning the tracheostomy tube and wear personal protective equipment (PPE) (Barnett 2008)

Be aware of emergency procedures if the tube becomes dislodged, including appropriate details of personnel to contact

Be aware of who has overall responsibility for the management of the tracheostomy (e.g. ear, nose and throat [ENT] team)

Ensure that the tracheostomy tube is changed according to hospital policy by trained practitioners

Utilise a tracheostomy chart (Fig. 3.9) which monitors the patient's progress towards de-cannulation

Ensure that emergency equipment is at the bedside, i.e. a re-breathe circuit with both a catheter mount and a facemask for emergencies (Edgtton-Winn and Wright 2005)

SCENARIOS

Scenario 1

Barbara, a 65-year-old woman weighing 95 kg had undergone an open cholecystectomy 3 days ago. Her postoperative recovery was protracted and she was still requiring assistance to mobilise. Barbara was a known hypertensive and had type 2 diabetes controlled by diet.

She had returned from the shower and was resting on her bed when she experienced an acute episode of breathlessness. She was attended by her nurse who immediately called for help, applied oxygen at 4 litres via a facemask and performed an assessment;

Continued

A – airway was patent but Barbara was talking in short sentences

B – respiratory rate was 32/min with increased work of breathing. $SpO2$ was 90% on supplementary oxygen. Upon auscultation reduced air entry was identified in both lung bases

C – heart rate 140/min and irregular, BP 110/65 mmHg, capillary refill time >3 s, core temperature 38.6°C

D – Barbara's AVPU score was A for alert

E – nil of note

Barbara was attached to the cardiac monitor; the rhythm was identified as atrial fibrillation (AF). The nurse inserted a cannula into Barbara's right antecubital fossa vein and primed an IV giving set with a 500 ml bag of 0.9%.NaCl

On arrival of the medical emergency team (MET) Barbara's nurse gave a concise history of events to the team, including reason for admission and past medical history. Barbara was transferred to a non re-breather mask at 15 l oxygen, as her SpO_2 remained at 90%. Blood was taken for a full haematological and biochemical screen, including cardiac biomarkers and arterial blood gas analysis. A chest radiograph was undertaken and also a 12-lead ECG which confirmed AF and excluded any recent ischaemic changes. A comprehensive physical assessment and review of documentation was then undertaken by the MET. A diagnosis of bilateral chest infection and bilateral lower lobe consolidation with some atelectasis was confirmed on radiograph. Blood gases demonstrated:

pH 7.37
$PaCO_2$ 4.0 kPa (30 mmHg)
PaO_2 7.0 kPa (mm 52.5Hg)
HCO_3^- 24 mmol/l
BE −1
SaO_2 89%

What do these results demonstrate?
Blood gas analysis demonstrates a type 1 respiratory failure, resulting in hypoxaemia in the absence of carbon dioxide retention.

Barbara was commenced on an amiodarone infusion of 300 mg over 1 hour for her recent-onset AF and commenced on the antibiotic co-amoxiclav 1.2 g i.v. three times daily. As her hypoxaemia was not improving on the ward she was transferred to the high dependency unit where non-invasive ventilation was commenced. Her family was informed and events documented.

Arterial blood gases were repeated after one hour of CPAP and demonstrated:

pH 7.38
PaCO$_2$ 3.8 kPa (28.5 mmHg)
PaO$_2$ 8.7 kPa (65 mmHg)
HCO$_3^-$ 24 mmol/l
BE −2
SaO$_2$ 93%

Barbara required CPAP +10 cmH$_2$O for 24 hours which was then slowly weaned off. Her AF reverted to sinus rhythm during the following 10 hours and she was stepped back down to the ward 3 days after her admission to HDU. She was followed up by the outreach team until her discharge on day 9 after her surgery.

Scenario 2

Clive, a 62-year-old man with a history of chronic asthma, presented to his GP with an acute exacerbation that had not responded to his usual inhaled bronchodilators and steroid medications. He was so acutely ill at his GP's that an ambulance was called and Clive was transferred to his nearest emergency department (ED). On admission to the ED he was immediately transferred to a resuscitation bay and commenced on cardiac monitoring. An assessment demonstrated:

A – airway was patent with an audible wheeze
B – Clive's respiratory rate was 38/min, SpO$_2$ 88% with increased work of breathing and very limited chest expansion
C – BP 160/100, heart rate 150, sinus tachycardia, core temperature 36.8°C
D – Clive responded to voice on the AVPU scale
E – nil of note

Clive had a peripheral cannula inserted by his GP and already had an infusion of salbutamol in progress. The decision was made on clinical presentation to intubate and ventilate Clive without further delay. A rapid sequence induction was performed using suxamethonium, (muscle relaxant), propofol (sedative) and fentanyl (opiate). A nasogastric tube was inserted at the time for stomach decompression. His intubation was uneventful and he was attached to the portable ventilator and
Continued

commenced on an infusion of propofol and fentanyl. A chest radiograph was taken as well as a full haematological and biochemical screen, including arterial blood gas analysis:

pH 7.11
$PaCO_2$ 10.8 kPa (81 mmHg)
PaO_2 6.8 kPa (51 mmHg)
HCO_3^- 32 mmol/l
BE +5
SaO_2 84%

What do these results tell you?
Blood gas analysis demonstrates a severe type 2 respiratory failure resulting in hypoxaemia, carbon dioxide retention and severe respiratory acidosis without metabolic compensation. Carbon dioxide retention is rare in exacerbation of asthma but is an indication for ventilation because it demonstrates hypoventilation usually related to extreme fatigue.

A chest radiograph demonstrated a typical chronic airway disease appearance with no areas of collapse. Regular nebulised salbutamol, Pulmicort (budesonide) and ipratropium were commenced as well as hydrocortisone 200 mg four times daily. A urinary catheter was inserted and intravenous fluid commenced. The ventilator settings were:

Mode: pressure controlled ventilation
Peak pressure: 25 cmH$_2$O
$FiO2$ .7
PEEP 5 cmH$_2$O

However, due to high airway pressures, Clive's tidal volumes were only 250 ml, inadequate for effective ventilation (6–8 ml/kg). The pressure control was increased to 40 cmH$_2$O and an urgent request for an ICU bed was made. He was transferred on to ICU shortly after this and connected to an ICU ventilator. Clive was very difficult to ventilate due to his severe bronchospasm and resultant high airway pressures. Any adjustments to Clive's position resulted in desaturation and destabling of his condition. Clive continued with this instability over the next 2 days. He was started on enteral nutrition and received full nursing care with minimal handling and repositioning. Gradually the bronchospasm improved and by day 5 his ventilation had reduced and he was ready for weaning. He weaned quickly from the ventilator and was extubated on day 6. He was discharged to the HDU the following day and to the ward the next day. He was followed up by the outreach team on the ward and was discharged home at day 12.

CONCLUSION
Monitoring respiratory function requires accurate assessment of the efficacy of breathing, work of breathing and adequacy of ventilation together with a comprehensive patient assessment. Peak expiratory flow rate measurements, pulse oximetry and arterial blood gas analysis also contribute to the monitoring process.

REFERENCES
Ahrens, T. & Sona, C. (2003) Capnography application in acute and critical care. *AACN Clinical Issues*, **14**, 123–132.

Allen, K. (2005) Four step method of interpreting arterial blood gas analysis. *Nursing Times*, **101**(1), 42.

Andrews, F. & Nolan, J. (2006) Critical care in the emergency department: monitoring the critically ill patient. *Emergency Medicine Journal*, **23**, 561–564.

Barnett, M. (2008) A practical guide to the management of a tracheostomy. *Journal of Community Nursing*, **22**(12), 24–26.

Bickley, L. (2009) *Bates' Guide to Physical Examination and History Taking*, 10th edn. Philadelphia, PA: Lippincott Williams & Wilkins.

Booker, R. (2004) The effective assessment of acute breathlessness in a patient. *Nursing Times*, **100**(24), 61.

Booker, R. (2007) Peak expiratory flow measurement. *Nursing Standard*, **21**(39), 42–43.

Booker, R. (2008) Pulse oximetry. *Nursing Standard*, **22**(30), 39–41.

British Thoracic Society (2008) *Guideline for Emergency Oxygen Ooxygen Use in Adult Patients: Executive summary*. London: BTS.

British Thoracic Society (2010) *BTS Pleural Disease Guideline*. London: BTS.

British Thoracic Society Scottish Collegiate Guidelines Network (2009) *British Guideline on the Management of Asthma*. London: BTS.

Brower, R., Matthay, M., Morris, A., et al. (2000) Ventilation with lower tidal volumes as compared with traditional tidal volumes for acute lung injury and the acute respiratory distress syndrome. *New England Journal of Medicine*, **342**, 1301–1308.

Buist, M.D., Jarmolowski, E., Burton, P., et al. (1999) Recognising clinical instability in hospital patients before cardiac arrest or unplanned admission to intensive care. *Medical Journal of Australia*, **324**, 22–25.

Considine, J. (2005) The role of nurses in preventing adverse events related to respiratory dysfunction: literature review. *Journal of Advanced Nursing*, **49**, 624–633.

Crispin, C. & Daffurn, K. (2000) Nurses' response to acute severe illness. *Australian Critical Care*, **11**, 131–133.

Davidson, J.A. & Hosie, H.E. (1993) Limitations of pulse oximetry: respiratory insufficiency – a failure of detection. *British Medical Journal*, **307**, 372–373.

Dougherty, L., Lister, S. (2011) The Royal Marsden Hospital Manual of Clinical Procedures. Chichester: Wiley-Blackwell.

Driscoll, P., Brown, T., Gwinnutt, C., et al. (1997) *A Simple Guide to Blood Gas Analysis*. London: BMJ Publishing Group.

Edgtton-Winn, M. & Wright, K. (2005) Tracheostomy: a guide to nursing care. *Australian Nursing Journal*, **13**(5), 17–20.

Elliott, D., Aitken, L., & Chaboyer, W., eds (2007) *Critical Care Nursing*. Marickville: NSW: Mosby Elsevier.

Fox, N. (2002) Pulse oximetry. *Nursing Times*, **98**(40), 65–67.

Foxall, F. (2008) Blood Gas Analysis. An easy learning guide. Cumbria: M&K Publishing.

Giuliano, K.K. (2006) Knowledge of pulse oximetry among critical care nurses. *Dimensions of Critical Care Nursing*, **25** 1), 44–49.

Giuliano, K.K. & Higgins, T.L. (2005) New generation pulse oximetry in the care of critically ill patients. *American Journal of Critical Care*, **14**(1), 26–37.

Goldhill, D.R., White, S.A. & Sumner, A. (1999) Physiological values and procedures in the 24 hours before ICU admission from the ward. *Anaesthesia*, **54**, 529–534.

Gwinnutt, C. (2006) *Clinical Anaesthesia*, 2nd edn. Oxford: Blackwell Publishing.

Higgins, D. (2005) Pulse oximetry. *Nursing Times*, **101**(6), 34.

Hilton, P. (2004) Evaluating the treatment options for spontaneous pneumothorax. *Nursing Times*, **100**(28), 32.

Hunter, J. (2008) Chest drain removal. *Nursing Standard*, **22**(45), 35–38.

Hutton, P. & Clutton-Brock, T. (1993) The benefits and pitfalls of pulse oximetry. *British Medical Journal*, **307**, 457–458.

Jenkins, P. F. & Johnson, P. H. (2010) *Making sense of acute medicine*. London: Hodder Arnold.

Jevon, P. & Ewens, B. (2000) Pulse oximetry. *Nursing Times*, **96**(26), 43–44.

Jevon, P. & Ewens, B. (2007) *Monitoring the Critically Ill Patient*. Oxford: Wiley-Blackwell.

Keenan, S.P., Powers, C.E. & McCormack, D.G. (2005) Noninvasive positive-pressure ventilation in patients with milder chronic obstructive pulmonary disease exacerbations: a randomised controlled trial. *Respiratory Care*, **50**, 610–616.

Kober, A., Schubert, B., Bertalanffy, P. et al. (2004) Capnography in non-tracheally intubated emergency patients as an additional tool in pulse oximetry for prehospital monitoring of respiration. *Anesthesia & Analgesia*, **98**, 206–210.

Law, C. (2000) A guide to assessing sputum. *Nursing Times* **96**(24), *Respiratory Care Supplement* 7–10.

McEnroe Ayers, D.M. & Stucky Lappin, J. (2004) Act fast when your patient has dyspnoea. *Nursing*, **34**(7), 36–41.

McGloin, H., Adam, S.K. et al. (1999) Unexpected deaths and referrals to intensive care of patients on general wards. Are some cases potentially preventable? *Journal of the Royal College of Physicians*, **33**(3), 255–259.

Manno, M.S. (2005) Managing mechanical ventilation. *Nursing*, **35**(12), 36–41.

Mathews, P.J. (2005) The latest in respiratory care. *Nursing Management, Supplement: Critical Care Choices*, **18**, 20–21.

Miller, M. (2005) Changes in measuring peak expiratory flow. *Practice Nursing*, **16**, 449–503.

Moore, T. (2007) Respiratory assessment in adults. *Nursing Standard*, **21**(49), 48–58.

Myers, T., ed. (2006) *Mosby's Medical Dictionary*, 7th edn. St Louis, MI: Mosby.

National Patient Safety Agency. (2008) *Risks of chest drain insertion*. London: NPSA.

Neville Regan, E. & Dallachiesa, L. (2009) How to care for a patient with a tracheostomy. *Nursing*, **39**(8), 34–39.

Newmarch, C. (2006) Caring for the mechanically ventilated patient: part 2. *Nursing Standard*, **20**(18), 55–64.

National Institute for Health and Clinical Excellence (2010) *Chronic Obstructive Pulmonary Disease*. London: NICE.

Parker, V., Giles, M., Shylan, G., et al. (2010) Tracheostomy management in acute care facilities – a matter of teamwork. *Journal of Clinical Nursing*, **19**, 1275–1283.

Preston, R. (2001) Introducing non-invasive positive pressure ventilation. *Nursing Standard*, **15**(26), 42–45.

Pullen, R. L. (2010) Using pulse oximetry acurately. *Nursing*, **40**(4), 63.

Resuscitation Council UK (2011) *Advanced Life Support*, 5th edn. London: Resuscitation Council UK.

Rich, K. (1999) Inhospital cardiac arrest: pre-event variables and nursing response. *Clinical Nurse Specialist*, **13**, 147–155.

Royal College of Physicians (2008) *The Use of Non-invasive Ventilation in the Management of Patients with Chronic Obstructive Pulmonary Disease admitted to Hospital with Acute Type II Respiratory Failure*. London: RCP.

Russell, C. & Matta, B. (2004) *Tracheostomy. A multi professional handbook*. London: Greenwich Medical Ltd.

Salem, M. (2001) Verification of endotracheal tube position. *Anesthesiology Clinics of North America*, **19**, 813–839.

Schein, R. M. H., Hazday, N., Pena, M. et al. (1990) Clinical antecedents to in-hospital cardiac arrest. *Chest*, **98**, 1388–1392.

Schumacher, L. & Chernecky, C. C. (2005) *Real World Nursing Survival Guide: Critical care and emergency nursing*. Philadelphia, PA: Saunders.

Simpson, H. (2004) Interpretation of arterial blood gases: a clinical guide for nurses. *British Journal of Nursing*, **13**, 522–528.

Simpson, H. (2006) Respiratory assessment. *British Journal of Nursing*, **15**, 484–488.

Smyth, M. (2005) Acute respiratory failure: Part 2. Failure of ventilation: Exploring the other cause of acute respiratory failure. *American Journal of Nursing*, **105**, 72AA–72DD.

Steen, C. (2010) Prevention of deterioration in acutely ill patients in hospital. *Nursing Standard*, **24**(49), 49–57.

Sullivan, B. (2008) Nursing management of patients with a chest drain. *British Journal of Nursing*, **17**, 388–393.

Torrance, C. & Elley, K. (1997) Respiration, technique and observation 1. *Nursing Times*, **43**(suppl).

Trim, J. (2005) Respirations. *Nursing Times*, **101**(22), 30–31.

Urden, T., Stacy, K. M., & Lough, M. E., eds (2006) *Thelan's Critical Care Nursing. Diagnosis and management*, 5th edn. St Louis, MI: Mosby Elsevier.

Welch, J. (2005) Pulse oximeters. *Biomedical Instrumentation and Technology*, March/April, 125–130.

Woodrow, P. (2003) Using non-invasive ventilation in acute ward settings: part 1. *Nursing Standard*, **17**(18), 39–44.

Woodrow, P. (2004) Arterial blood gas analysis. *Nursing Standard*, **18**(21), 45–52, 54–55.

Woomer, J. & Berkheimer, D. (2003) Using capnography to monitor ventilation. *Nursing*, **33**(4), 42–43.

Monitoring Cardiovascular Function 1: ECG Monitoring

4

LEARNING OBJECTIVES

At the end of the chapter the reader will be able to:

☐ describe the common features of a *cardiac monitor*
☐ describe how to set up *ECG monitoring*
☐ discuss the potential *problems* that may be encountered with ECG monitoring
☐ describe the *ECG* and its *relationship to cardiac contraction*
☐ describe a systematic approach to *ECG interpretation*
☐ define and classify *cardiac arrhythmias*
☐ *recognise* important cardiac arrhythmias

INTRODUCTION

Electrocardiograph (ECG) monitoring is one of the most valuable diagnostic tools in modern medicine. It is essential if disorders of the cardiac rhythm are to be recognised, and can help with diagnosis and alert health-care staff to changes in a patient's condition. However, ECG monitoring must be meticulously undertaken. Consequences of poor technique include misinterpretation of arrhythmias, mistaken diagnosis, wasted investigations and mismanagement of the patient. Nurses must understand the principles of ECG monitoring, including troubleshooting and recognition of important arrhythmias.

The aim of this chapter is to understand the principles of ECG monitoring.

Monitoring the Critically Ill Patient, Third Edition.
Philip Jevon, Beverley Ewens.
© 2012 Blackwell Publishing Ltd. Published 2012 by Blackwell Publishing Ltd.

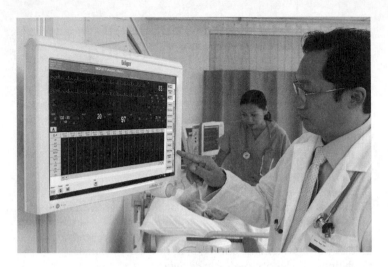

Fig. 4.1 Bedside cardiac monitor (Drager Medical).

COMMON FEATURES OF A CARDIAC MONITOR

The bedside cardiac monitor (Fig. 4.1) or oscilloscope provides a continuous display of the patient's ECG and has the following common features (Resuscitation Council UK 2010):

- *Screen for displaying the ECG trace*: a dull/bright switch can be adjusted if the ECG recording and background is too light or too dark.
- *ECG printout facility*: this is particularly useful for recording cardiac arrhythmias and is invaluable for both diagnostic and treatment purposes. The ECG printouts can also complement the patient's records.
- *Heart rate counter*: most calculate the heart rate by counting the number of QRS complexes in a minute.
- *Monitor alarms*: can alert the nurse to changes in the heart rate that are outside pre-set limits. If the monitor alarms are to be relied on, they should be on and set within safe parameters (agreed locally), based on the patient's clinical condition. More advanced monitors can identify important cardiac arrhythmias and set off the alarm accordingly.

- *Lead select switch*: lead II is usually the most popular lead for ECG monitoring.
- *ECG gain*: this can alter the gain or size of the ECG complex; if it is set too low or too high the ECG trace may be unclear and misinterpreted.
- *Digital processing of the ECG*: potential for electronic analysis.

SETTING UP ECG MONITORING

The following measures should be observed when setting up ECG monitoring (Jevon 2009):

1. Explain the procedure to the patient.
2. Prepare the skin: ensure that the skin is dry, not greasy; if necessary use an alcohol swab and/or abrasive pad to clean (Resuscitation Council UK 2010). If necessary, shave off any excess hair. This will also make it less uncomfortable for the patient when the electrodes are removed.
3. Attach the electrodes following locally agreed guidelines. Switch the cardiac monitor on and select the required monitoring lead.
4. Ensure that the ECG trace is clear. Rectify any difficulties encountered (see below).
5. Ensure that alarms are set within safe parameters following locally agreed guidelines and according to the patient's clinical condition.
6. Ensure that the cardiac monitor can clearly be seen.
7. Document in the patient's notes that ECG monitoring has commenced.

Correct chest and limb electrode placement (Fig. 4.2) is crucial for obtaining accurate information from any monitoring lead (Thompson 2010). The electrode placement and monitoring lead selected for ECG monitoring will depend on the following factors:

- *Monitoring system* (e.g. three- or five-wire monitoring system). If a five-wire system is being used a suggested ECG electrode placement is red (right shoulder), yellow (left shoulder), green (left lower thorax/hip region), black (right lower thorax/ hip region) and white on the chest in the desired V position, usually V1 (Jevon 2009). If a three-wire system is being used a

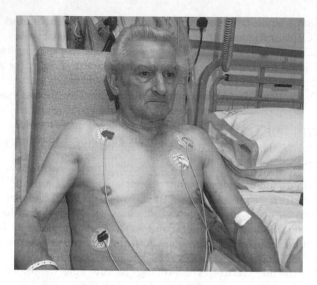

Fig. 4.2 Suggested ECG electrode placement using a five-wire monitoring system.

suggested ECG electrode placement is red (right shoulder), yellow (left shoulder) and green (left lower thorax/hip region), although this system is much less commonly used in clinical practice.

- *Goals of monitoring*, e.g. if arrhythmia diagnosis is the goal.
- *Patient's clinical situation*, e.g. in cardiopulmonary resuscitation, the precordium should be left unobstructed in case defibrillation is required (Resuscitation Council UK 2010).

EASI 12-lead ECG monitoring

The conventional 12-lead ECG using 10 electrodes attached to the limbs and chest is recognised as the current medical standard for the identification, analysis and confirmation of many cardiac abnormalities including cardiac arrhythmias and cardiac ischaemia/infarction.

If 12-lead ECG monitoring is undertaken on a continual basis, the benefits include:

- Facilitating the accurate recognition of cardiac arrhythmias
- Enabling the monitoring of the mid-precordial leads which is particularly important for the detection and management of ischaemia
- Enabling the recording of *transient* ECG events of particular diagnostic or therapeutic importance
- Enabling the differentiation between post-PTCA (percutaneous transluminal coronary angioplasty) ischaemia and occlusion.

Unfortunately the use of a conventional 12-lead ECG system using 10 electrodes for continuous cardiac monitoring is cumbersome and generally not practical in the clinical area. However, the EASI system, a new concept in 12-lead ECG monitoring, requires the use of only 5 electrodes (Fig. 4.3):

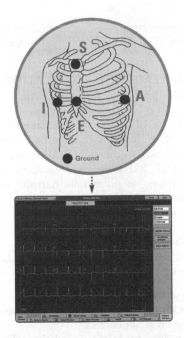

Fig. 4.3 EASI 12-lead ECG monitoring system. (Reproduced by permission of Philips.)

- **E** electrode on the lower sternum at the level of the fifth intercostal space
- **A** on the left midaxillary line on the same level as the E electrode
- **S** electrode on the upper sternum
- **I** on the right midaxillary line on the same level as the E electrode..

A fifth ground electrode can be placed anywhere.

The EASI system for 12-lead ECG monitoring using only 5 electrodes is less cumbersome and more practical than the standard 10-electrode system. It is therefore more comfortable for the patient. In addition it will not interfere with such procedures as cardiac auscultation, cardiopulmonary resuscitation (CPR), defibrillation and echocardiography.

> ECG monitoring should *complement not replace* basic nursing observations of the patient. Treat the patient not the monitor.

POTENTIAL PROBLEMS WITH ECG MONITORING

There are potential problems that can occur when undertaking ECG monitoring and it is important to realise that standardisation is possible only if the ECG is performed in a standard way each time (Thompson 2010). It has been identified in the literature that there is a wide variation in the identification of correct lead placement (McCann et al. 2007) leading to inaccurate diagnosis and patients being exposed to potentially harmful therapeutic interventions (Rajaganeshan et al. 2008). Potential problems that may be encountered include the following.

The 'flat-line' trace

Check the patient immediately. However, the most likely cause is mechanical. Check:

- the condition of the patient
- that the correct monitoring lead is selected (usually lead II)
- that the ECG gain is set correctly
- that the electrodes are 'in date' and the gel sponge is moist, not dry

- that the electrodes are properly connected
- that the leads are plugged into the monitor.

Poor-quality ECG trace
If the ECG trace quality is poor, check:

- all the connections
- the brightness display
- that the electrodes are 'in date' and the gel sponge is moist, not dry (Jevon 2009)
- that the electrodes are properly attached.

If there are still difficulties obtaining a clear ECG trace, wiping the skin with an alcohol wipe may help. As electrodes tend to dry out after about 3 days, they should be changed at least that often although every 24 hours may be optimum to maintain skin integrity (Perez 1996).

Interference and artefacts
Poor electrode contact, patient movement and electrical interference, e.g. from bedside infusion pumps, can cause a 'fuzzy' appearance on the ECG trace. Interference can be minimised by applying the electrodes over bone rather than muscle (Resuscitation Council UK 2006). The patient should also be reassured and kept warm.

Wandering baseline
A wandering baseline (ECG trace going up and down) is almost always caused by poor electrode contact to the skin (Thompson 2010). If respiration is the cause and the problem is not transient, serial ECG recordings should be taken in both inspiratory and expiratory phases (Thompson 2010).

Small ECG complexes
Sometimes the ECG complexes may be too small and unrecognisable. Possible causes include pericardial effusion, obesity and hypothyroidism. However, sometimes it can be caused by a technical problem. Check that the ECG gain is correctly set and that lead II is being monitored. Repositioning the electrodes or selecting another monitoring lead sometimes helps (Jevon 2009).

Incorrect heart rate display

If the ECG complexes are too small, a false low heart rate may be displayed. Large T waves, muscle movement and interference can be mistaken for QRS complexes, resulting in a false high heart rate being displayed. The nurse must be alert to the possibility of inaccurate heart rate readings, which can in particular be caused by poor electrode contact and interference (Jevon 2009). To minimise the potential for inaccuracies, a reliable good-quality ECG trace should be obtained.

Skin irritation

ECG electrodes can cause skin irritation and contact dermatitis has been well reported in the literature (Rühlemann et al. 2010). The electrode sites should be regularly examined and if the patient's skin appears irritated select another electrode placement.

False alarms

Frequent false alarms will undermine the rationale for setting alarms and can also cause undue anxiety for the patient. It is important to ensure that the alarms are correctly and sensibly set and that the ECG is accurate, reliable and of a high standard.

Best practice – ECG monitoring

Ensure adequate skin preparation
Use ECG electrodes that are in date, with moist gel sponge
Position ECG electrodes and select monitoring lead following locally agreed protocols
Set cardiac monitor alarms according to the patient's clinical condition
Ensure that the ECG trace is accurate
Ensure that the cardiac monitor is visible

THE ECG AND ITS RELATIONSHIP TO CARDIAC CONTRACTION

The ECG functions in four stages as follows (Fig. 4.4):

1. The sinus node fires and the electrical impulse spreads across the atria. This results in atrial contraction (P wave).

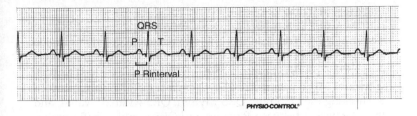

Fig. 4.4 The ECG and its relation to cardiac contraction (PQRST complex).

2. On arriving at the atrioventricular (AV) junction the impulse is delayed, allowing the atria time to contract fully and eject blood into the ventricles. This brief period of absent electrical activity is represented on the ECG by a straight (isoelectric) line between the end of the P wave and the beginning of the QRS complex. The P–R interval represents atrial depolarisation and the impulse delay in the AV junction before ventricular depolarisation.
3. The impulse is then conducted down to the ventricles through the bundle of His, right and left bundle branches and Purkinje fibres, causing ventricular depolarisation and contraction (QRS complex).
4. The ventricles then repolarise (T wave).

SYSTEMATIC APPROACH TO ECG INTERPRETATION

It is important to develop a systematic approach to ECG interpretation and to apply it consistently: this will minimise the risk of missing something important (Aehlert 2011).

The following systematic approach to ECG interpretation enables the practitioner to interpret most ECG traces and arrive at a reliable diagnosis on which to base effective treatment. The six-stage approach is as follows (Resuscitation Council UK 2006):

1. Electrical activity: present?
2. QRS rate: normal, slow or fast?
3. QRS rhythm: regular or irregular?
4. QRS width: normal or wide?
5. P waves: present?
6. P waves and QRS: associated or disassociated?

Electrical activity

If there is no electrical activity present, assuming that the patient has a pulse, check that the leads and electrodes are correctly attached, that the ECG gain is not too low and that the correct monitoring lead has been selected, e.g. lead II. If electrical activity is present and recognisable QRS complexes can be seen, proceed to checking the QRS rate, QRS rhythm, QRS width, P waves, and the relationship between P waves and QRS complexes (Resuscitation Council UK 2006).

QRS rate

Estimate the QRS rate by counting the number of large (1 cm) squares between adjacent QRS complexes and dividing it into 300, e.g. the QRS rate in Fig. 4.4 is approximately 80/min (300/3.8) (Jevon 2009).

- Normal ventricular rate is 60–100 beats/min.
- Bradycardia – rate <60 beats/min.
- Tachycardia – rate >100 beats/min.

Leach (2004)

If the QRS rhythm is irregular it is preferable to estimate the rate by counting the number of QRS complexes in a 15-second ECG strip and then multiplying it by four.

QRS rhythm

Determine whether the QRS rhythm is regular or irregular. It is important to assess the regularity of the QRS rhythm using an adequate length of ECG rhythm strip (Resuscitation Council UK 2006). Compare R–R intervals by either using a calliper or by marking two consecutive R waves on a piece of paper, and then comparing the marks with other R–R intervals on the ECG rhythm strip.

If it is irregular, establish if there is a common pattern or whether it is very erratic. Causes of an irregular QRS rhythm include sinus arrhythmia, premature complexes and some AV blocks. If the QRS rhythm is very erratic, it is most likely to be atrial fibrillation, particularly if the QRS width is normal (Resuscitation Council UK 2006).

QRS width

Calculate the QRS width. The upper limit of normal is 0.12 seconds or 3 small squares (Resuscitation Council UK 2006). Causes of a wide QRS complex include bundle branch block, ventricular premature contractions and ventricular tachycardia.

P waves

Determine whether P waves are present. They should be upright in lead II and be all of the same morphology. P waves of different morphology indicate a changing atrial pacemaker. P waves may be absent in some conduction disturbances and sometimes they may be difficult to distinguish or indeed be 'hidden' in the QRS in some tachyarrhythmias.

Relationship between the P waves and the QRS complexes

If P waves are present, establish whether a P wave precedes each QRS complex and that each QRS complex is followed by a P wave. Calculate the P–R interval: it should remain constant and the normal range is three to five small squares. A shortened or prolonged P–R interval is indicative of a conduction abnormality. A prolonged P–R interval can be seen in AV block. Complete dissociation between the P waves and QRS complexes is most commonly seen in third-degree or complete AV heart block.

Sinus rhythm

This is illustrated in Fig. 1.3.

QRS rate: 80/min
QRS rhythm: regular
P waves: present and normal
Relationship between P waves and QRS: the P waves precede each
    QRS and the P–R interval is normal
QRS width: normal (<2.5 squares).

The impulse originates in the sinus node at a rate of between 60 and 100 beats/min, is regular and is conducted down the normal pathways with no abnormal delays, i.e. sinus rhythm.

Best practice – ECG interpretation

Assess the patient for adverse signs
Calculate the QRS rate
Ascertain the QRS rhythm
Identify if P waves are present
Assess the relationship between P waves and QRS complexes
Calculate the QRS width
Obtain 12-lead ECG if necessary

DEFINITION AND CLASSIFICATION OF CARDIAC ARRHYTHMIAS

A 'cardiac arrhythmia' can be defined as any ECG rhythm that deviates from normal sinus rhythm. Cardiac arrhythmias can be classified into one of two groups (Meltzer et al. 1977):

1. Arrhythmias resulting from a disturbance in impulse *formation*
2. Arrhythmias resulting from a disturbance in impulse *conduction*.

Some cardiac arrhythmias may have a disturbance in both impulse formation and impulse conduction.

Arrhythmias resulting from a disturbance in impulse formation

These arrhythmias can be classified in respect of their site of origin and the mechanism of the disturbance as shown below (adapted from Jevon 2009).

Site of origin

The following features are significant:

- *SA (sinoatrial) node*: sinus rhythms, e.g. sinus bradycardia, sinus tachycardia
- *Atria*: atrial rhythms, e.g. atrial premature, atrial fibrillation
- *AV junction*: junctional rhythms, e.g. junction rhythm
- *Ventricles*: ventricular rhythms, e.g. ventricular premature beats, ventricular tachycardia.

Mechanism

Features arising from the mechanism of the disturbance are:

- tachycardia >100 beats/min
- bradycardia <60 beats/min
- premature contractions
- flutter
- fibrillation.

Arrhythmias resulting from a disturbance in impulse conduction

A disturbance in conduction relates to an abnormal delay or block of the impulse at any point along the conduction system. They are traditionally categorised according to the site of the defect:

- *SA blocks*, e.g. sinus arrest
- *AV blocks*, e.g. first-, second- and third-degree block
- *Intraventricular blocks*, e.g. right and left bundle-branch blocks.

RECOGNITION OF IMPORTANT ARRHYTHMIAS

When interpreting arrhythmias it is important to assess:

- The haemodynamic effect: clinical signs of a low cardiac output include hypotension, impaired consciousness, chest pain, dyspnoea and heart failure
- Whether there is a risk of cardiac arrest.

Sinus tachycardia

This is illustrated in Fig. 4.5:

Electrical activity and recognisable QRS complexes: present
QRS rate: >100/min (Thompson 2010)
QRS rhythm: regular
QRS width: normal
P waves: present and normal morphology
Relationship between P waves and QRS complexes: P waves precede every QRS complex; P–R interval normal.

The ECG shows the same characteristics as sinus rhythm except that the ventricular (QRS) rate is >100 beats/min. Causes include anxiety, acute blood loss, exercise, shock, pyrexia and drugs, e.g.

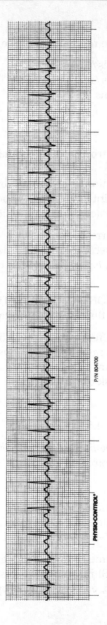

PHYSIO-CONTROL®

P/N 804700

Fig. 4.5 Sinus tachycardia.

hydralazine, nebulised salbutamol, or can be a primary cardiac abnormality (Thompson 2010). It is particularly worrying in the presence of myocardial ischaemia because it increases myocardial oxygen consumption (Thompson 2010). The treatment is to identify and treat the cause which may be hyperthyroidism, blood loss, anxiety, alcohol withdrawal, hypoxaemia or worsening cardiac function (Thompson 2010). Sometimes beta blockers are beneficial, e.g. in acute myocardial infarction.

Sinus bradycardia
Sinus brachycardia is illustrated in Fig. 4.6.

Electrical activity and recognisable QRS complexes: present
QRS rate: 40/min
QRS rhythm: regular
QRS width: normal
P waves: present and normal
Relationship between P waves and QRS complexes: P waves precede each QRS complex and the P–R interval is normal.

ECG shows the same characteristics as sinus rhythm except that the ventricular rate is <60 beats/min. Causes include vagal stimulation, e.g. during tracheal suction, increased intracranial pressure, hypoxia, severe pain, hypothermia and drugs, e.g. beta blockers. Sometimes it is normal for the patient, e.g. an athlete. Treatment often requires oxygen and atropine. Sometimes pacing may be indicated. The treatment required will depend on the risk of developing asystole, rather than the precise classification of the bradycardia (Resuscitation Council UK 2006).

Atrial fibrillation
This is illustrated in Fig. 4.7.

Electrical activity and recognisable QRS complexes: present
QRS rate: 140/min
QRS rhythm: irregular and very erratic
QRS width: normal
P waves: not present, irregular baseline – small, irregular and rapid oscillations
Relationship between P waves and QRS complexes: no P waves present.

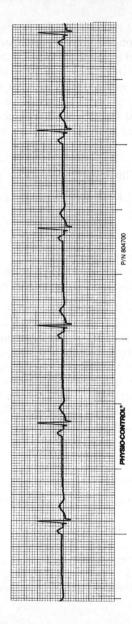

Fig. 4.6 Sinus bradycardia.

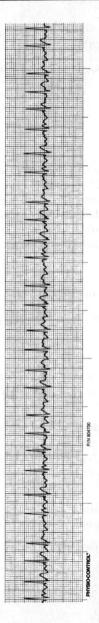

Fig. 4.7 Atrial fibrillation.

PHYSIO-CONTROL®

P/N 804700

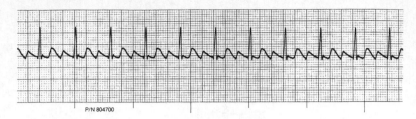
P/N 804700

Fig. 4.8 Atrial flutter.

Atrial fibrillation is characterised by absent P waves, irregular baseline and irregular QRS complexes. The loss of atrial contraction or 'atrial kick' results in a 25% reduction in cardiac output. It is the most common cardiac arrhythmia encountered in clinical practice (Resuscitation Council UK 2006). The ventricular rate can vary and treatment often includes digoxin. Cardioversion is sometimes required.

Atrial flutter
Atrial flutter is illustrated in Fig. 4.8.

Electrical activity and recognisable QRS complexes: present
QRS rate: 100/min
QRS rhythm: regular
QRS width: normal
P waves: flutter 'sawtooth' waves at a rate of 300/min
Relationship between P waves and QRS complexes: has no meaning and is not measured.

Atrial flutter is characterised by the 'sawtooth' flutter waves that usually have a rate of approximately 300/min. The ventricular response depends on the degree of AV block; in the example it is 3:1. Treatment could include digoxin or amiodarone. Cardioversion may be required.

Narrow complex tachycardia
The features of this are shown in Fig. 4.9.

Electrical activity and recognisable QRS complexes: present
QRS rate: 180/min
QRS rhythm: regular
QRS width: normal

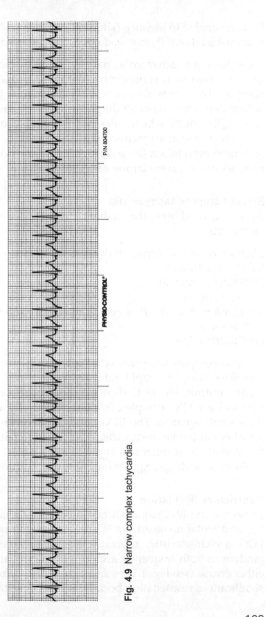

Fig. 4.9 Narrow complex tachycardia.

P waves: unable to identify (situated on T waves?)
Relationship between P waves and QRS complexes: unable to determine.

Unlike sinus tachycardia, narrow complex tachycardia (sometimes referred to as supraventricular tachycardia) starts and ends abruptly. The rate is always >140 beats/min. A 12-lead ECG will help to determine the exact diagnosis. The key issue with this ECG is the QRS width, which rules out the often more serious broad complex (ventricular) tachycardia. Treatment, which will depend on how compromised the patient is, could include vagal manoeuvres, adenosine, amiodarone and cardioversion.

Broad complex tachycardia
Figure 4.10 shows the salient features of broad complex tachycardia.

Electrical activity and recognisable QRS complexes: present
QRS rate: 180/min
QRS rhythm: regular
P waves: not seen
Relationship between P waves and QRS complexes: unable to determine
QRS width: wide.

Broad complex tachycardia usually results from a focus in the ventricles firing at a rapid rate. The patient may or may not lose cardiac output. The ECG shows a rapid heart rate usually >150/min and the QRS complex is characteristically wide (more than three small squares). The ECG configuration can vary depending on where in the ventricles the focus is. If the patient has arrested the definitive treatment is rapid defibrillation. Other treatment could include drugs, e.g. amiodarone and cardioversion.

Ventricular fibrillation
In ventricular fibrillation all coordination of electrical activity in the ventricular myocardium is lost, resulting in cardiac arrest. The ECG is characteristic, a bizarre irregular waveform apparently random in both frequency and amplitude. It can be classified as either coarse (see Fig. 1.1) or fine (Fig. 4.11). Certainly the latter is significant in resuscitation because it can be mistaken for asystole,

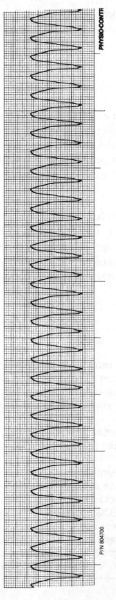

Fig. 4.10 Broad complex tachycardia.

P/N 804700

PHYSIO-CONTR

particularly if there is some interference. The definitive treatment is rapid defibrillation (Resuscitation Council UK 2010).

Asystole

Asystole (see Fig. 1.2) is characteristically an undulating line and rarely a straight line.

In all cases of apparent asystole, the ECG trace should be viewed with suspicion before arrival at a final diagnosis. Check the patient. Other causes of a straight-line ECG trace should be excluded, e.g. incorrect lead setting, disconnected leads and ECG gain incorrectly set. It is important not to miss ventricular fibrillation.

Pulseless electrical activity

Pulseless electrical activity (see Fig. 1.3) is a condition in which the patient is pulseless, but has a normal ECG trace. The diagnosis is made from a combination of the clinical absence of a cardiac output together with an ECG trace that would normally be associated with a good pulse.

Scenario

A 40-year-old man is admitted to the coronary care unit with an acute inferior myocardial infarction. On admission his BP is 120/90, pulse 70/min, sinus rhythm, respirations 15/min and temperature 36.7°C. The cardiac monitor starts to alarm as it has recognised 'asystole'. What would you do?

First of all check the patient. He is conscious, sitting up in bed and smiling. The cardiac monitor is still alarming 'asystole'. What would you do?

The ECG display is a straight line, which the monitor has mistaken for asystole. There must be a mechanical problem. The lead select on the cardiac monitor is checked to ensure that the desired lead has been selected. In addition the ECG gain (size) on the monitor is checked and found to be fine. The leads are checked to ensure that they are still connected. One of the leads has become disconnected from the electrode resulting in a straight line on the ECG. Following reconnection, sinus rhythm 70 beats/min is displayed on the cardiac monitor.

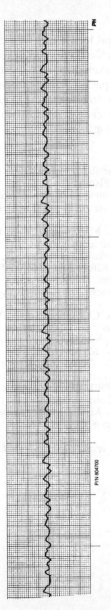

P/N 804700

Fig. 4.11 Ventricular fibrillation (fine).

CONCLUSION

ECG monitoring is central to the care of a critically ill patient. It must be meticulously undertaken in order to avoid misinterpretation of arrhythmias, mistaken diagnosis, wasted investigations and mismanagement of the patient. Nurses need to understand the principles of ECG monitoring, including troubleshooting, and recognise important cardiac arrhythmias. Always remember to treat the patient not the monitor.

REFERENCES

Aehlert, B. L. (2011) *Pocket Reference for ECGs made Easy*, 4th edn. St Louis, MI: Mosby Jems Elsevier.

Jevon, P. (2009) *ECGs for Nurses*, 2nd edn. Oxford: Wiley Blackwell.

Leach, R. (2004) *Critical Care Medicine at a Glance*. Oxford: Blackwell Publishing.

McCann, K., Holdgate, A., Mahammad, R. & Waddington, A. (2007) Accuracy of ECG electrode placement by emergency department clinicians. *Emergency Medicine Australasia*, **19**, 442–448.

Meltzer, L., Pinneo, R. & Kitchell, J. (1977) *Intensive Coronary Care, a Manual for Nurses* 3rd edn. London: Prentice-Hall.

Perez, A. (1996) Cardiac monitoring: mastering the essentials. *Registered Nurse*, **59**(8), 32–9.

Rajaganeshan, R., Ludlam, C. L., Francis, D. P., Parasramka, S. V. & Sutton, R. (2008) Accuracy in ECG lead placement among technicians, nurses, general physicians and cardiologists. *International Journal of Clinical Practice*, **62**, 65–70.

Resuscitation Council UK (2006) *Advanced Life Support*, 5th edn. London: Resuscitation Council UK.

Resuscitation Council UK (2010) *Adult Advanced Life Support Algorithm*. London: Resuscitation Council UK.

Rühlemann, D., Kügler, K., Mydlach, B. & Frosch, P. J. (2010). Contact dermatitis to self-adhesive ECG electrodes. *Contact Dermatitis*, **62**, 314–315.

Thompson, P., ed. (2010) *Coronary Care Manual*, 2nd edn. Chatswood, NSW: Elsevier.

Monitoring Cardiovascular Function 2: Haemodynamic Monitoring

5

LEARNING OBJECTIVES

At the end of the chapter the reader will be able to:

☐ discuss the factors affecting *tissue perfusion*
☐ define and classify *circulatory shock*
☐ describe non-invasive methods of *haemodynamic monitoring*
☐ outline the general principles of monitoring with *transducers*
☐ discuss the principles of *central venous pressure monitoring*
☐ outline and discuss the principles of *pulmonary artery pressure monitoring*
☐ discuss the principles of *cardiac output studies*

INTRODUCTION

Haemodynamics can be defined as the study of blood circulation through the cardiovascular system and haemodynamic monitoring detects cardiovascular insufficiency and guides therapy (Kent and Dowd 2007; Sturgess and Morgan 2009). Haemodynamic monitoring and interpretation of the data are central to the care of a critically ill patient and can be classified as *non-invasive*, *invasive* and *derived* (i.e. data calculated from other measurements).

Interpretation of haemodynamic data must be combined with regular clinical assessment together with effective clinical therapy (Sturgess and Morgan 2009). Knowledge of the evidence underpinning the technology of haemodynamic monitoring and the processes of interpretation is vital to optimize the use and help

Monitoring the Critically Ill Patient, Third Edition.
Philip Jevon, Beverley Ewens.
© 2012 Blackwell Publishing Ltd. Published 2012 by Blackwell Publishing Ltd.

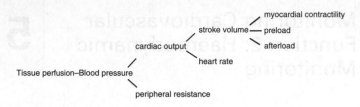

Fig. 5.1 Overview of factors affecting tissue perfusion.

evidence-based decision making (Kent and Dowd 2007). The aim of this chapter is to understand the principles of haemodynamic monitoring.

FACTORS AFFECTING TISSUE PERFUSION

Tissue perfusion is dependent on an adequate blood pressure in the aorta. This pressure is determined by the product of two factors: *cardiac output* and *peripheral resistance* (Kent and Dowd 2007) (Fig. 5.1).

Cardiac output

Cardiac output is the amount of blood ejected from the left ventricle in 1 minute. At rest this is approximately 5000 ml. It is determined by heart rate and stroke volume.

Heart rate

Factors influencing heart rate include baroreceptor activity, the Bainbridge effect, pyrexia, higher centres, intracranial pressure and oxygen and carbon dioxide levels in the blood.

Stroke volume

Stroke volume is the amount of blood ejected from the left ventricle in one contraction. At rest this is approximately 70 ml. It is affected by heart rate, myocardial contractility, preload and afterload (Fig. 5.1).

- *Heart rate*: tachycardia reduces diastolic filling time resulting in a decreased stroke volume.
- *Myocardial contractility* refers to the ability of the heart to function independently of the changes in preload and afterload

Table 5.1 Factors affecting myocardial contractility

Change	Factors
Increased contractility	Drugs with inotropic properties, e.g. dobutamine, dopamine (dose related), digoxin, adrenaline, noradrenaline; circulating catecholamines; calcium; increased preload; hyperthyroidism
Decreased contractility	Drugs with negative inotropic properties, e.g. lignocaine, amiodarone; hypoxia; hypocalcaemia and calcium channel blockers; β-adrenergic blockers, e.g. atenolol; decreased preload; functional deficit, e.g. after myocardial infarction

(Cooke and Thompson 2011). It is commonly referred to as the 'force of contraction'. Inotropic drugs, e.g. dobutamine and adrenaline, can increase myocardial contractility. Table 5.1 lists factors affecting myocardial contractility.

- *Preload* (or end-diastolic volume/pressure) is the load that passively stretches cardiac tissue before the onset of ventricular contraction (Cooke and Thompson 2011). Starling's law of the heart states that 'the force of myocardial contraction is directly proportional to the initial fibre length', i.e. stretched fibres contract more forcefully (not overstretched). Venous return is the main factor determining preload and, as the filling pressure rises, stroke volume increases. However, in an overstretched ventricle, excessive dilatation may result in a fall in stroke volume. In the clinical setting manipulation of the preload is the most efficient method of improving cardiac output because it is associated with only a minimal rise in oxygen consumption. Table 5.2 lists factors affecting preload.
- *Afterload* is the resistance to the outflow of blood provided by the vasculature which must be overcome by the ventricles during contraction. In the clinical setting a rise in afterload, particularly in the failing heart, results in a decrease in cardiac output (Cooke and Thompson 2011). Table 5.3 lists factors affecting afterload.

Peripheral resistance
Peripheral resistance is the resistance that the vessels offer to the flow of blood, i.e. dependent on the extent of dilatation or constriction (Scanlon and Sanders 2007).

Table 5.2 Factors affecting preload

Change	Factors
Increased preload	Volume gain, e.g. fluid overload; renal failure; vasoconstriction (may be caused by drugs, e.g. noradrenaline, adrenaline and dopamine (dose related)); heart failure; hypothermia and anxiety; bradycardia
Decreased preload	Volume loss, e.g. haemorrhage, severe vomiting and polyuria; vasodilatation, e.g. anaphylaxis, septicaemia, pyrexia, neurogenic shock and drugs such as nitrates; impeded venous return, e.g. pulmonary embolism, pericardial tamponade; tachycardia (fall in diastolic filling time)

Table 5.3 Factors affecting afterload

Change	Factors
Increased afterload	Drugs with vasoconstriction properties, e.g. noradrenaline; cardiogenic shock; atherosclerosis
Decreased afterload	Drugs with vasodilator properties, e.g. nitrates, nitroprusside; anaphylaxis; septicaemia; hyperthermia

The smooth muscle in the arterioles is controlled by the vasomotor centre in the medulla. It is in a state of partial contraction caused by continuous sympathetic nerve activity, often referred to as 'sympathetic tone'. An increase in vasomotor activity causes vasoconstriction of the arterioles, resulting in a rise in peripheral resistance. If the cardiac output remains constant the blood pressure will rise. In contrast, a decrease in vasomotor activity causes vasodilatation and a fall in peripheral resistance. If the cardiac output remains constant the blood pressure will fall. The most significant factors affecting vasomotor activity are:

- *Baroreceptor activity* helps to maintain the blood pressure at a constant level. Baroreceptors are located in the aortic arch, carotid arteries and carotid sinus. Baroreceptor activity inhibits the action of the vasomotor centre: a rise in blood pressure increases, and a fall decreases, baroreceptor activity. When moving from a lying to a standing position, the cardiac output will fall. However, baroreceptor activity ensures that the blood pressure remains constant. After prolonged bed rest this mechanism may be lost and the patient may faint.

- *Carbon dioxide* (CO_2): a rise in blood carbon dioxide levels increases vasomotor activity, whereas a fall suppresses it. In ventilated patients care needs to be taken to avoid over-ventilation because this may lead to a fall in carbon dioxide levels with a corresponding fall in blood pressure.
- *Sensory nerves* can influence vasomotor activity, particularly those that are associated with pain. Mild pain can increase vasomotor activity resulting in a rise in blood pressure, whereas severe pain may decrease vasomotor activity and cause a fall in blood pressure.
- *Respiratory centre*: this lies next to the vasomotor centre; an increase in its activity, particularly on inspiration, will result in an increase in vasomotor activity, causing a rise in blood pressure.
- *Oxygen* (O_2): a moderate fall in blood oxygen levels increases vasomotor activity directly and also indirectly via chemoreceptors.
- *Higher centres*: emotional excitement or stress results in a rise in vasomotor activity and a corresponding rise in blood pressure. In some situations inhibition of the vasomotor centre will occur resulting in vasodilatation and a fall in blood pressure, e.g. some people faint at the sight of blood.

There are other factors that affect peripheral resistance including:

- *Angiotensin*: inadequate renal blood flow leads to the release of the enzyme renin which causes the formation of angiotensin, a powerful vasoconstrictor.
- *Blood viscosity*: if the blood viscosity increases, e.g. in polycythaemia, peripheral resistance will also rise.
- *Stimulation of α- and β_2-receptors* (found in the smooth muscle of the arterioles): stimulation of α-receptors, e.g. by noradrenaline, will cause vasoconstriction; stimulation of β_2-receptors, e.g. by salbutamol, will cause vasodilatation.

SHOCK

Shock is a clinical state with characteristic signs and symptoms but can be defined as occurring when there is an imbalance between oxygen demand and supply (McLuckie 2009), resulting in inadequate tissue perfusion (Jenkins and Johnson 2010). A complex physiological phenomenon, shock is a life-threatening condition with a variety of causes. Without treatment it leads to cell starvation, cell death, organ dysfunction, organ failure and mortality rates of >50% (Jenkins and Johnson 2010).

Haemodynamic monitoring will assist nurses in recognising the early signs of shock, facilitate timely management, evaluate treatment response and potentially reverse the early stages of this deadly sequela.

The prognosis of shock will depend on the underlying cause, severity and duration of the shocked state. The patient's age and pre-existing illness (co-morbidity) are also contributing factors. There are four major classifications of shock: cardiogenic, hypovolaemic, distributive and obstructive (Bridges and Dukes 2005).

Hypovolaemic shock

Hypovolaemic shock is characterised by inadequate intravascular volume (Garretson and Malberti 2007). Causes of hypovolaemia are from either internal fluid shifts or external fluid losses (Diehl-Oplinger and Kaminski 2004). Fluid shifts from intravascular compartments to 'third spaces' (intracellular or extracellular compartments), which do not support the circulation, can be the result of intestinal obstruction, vomiting and diarrhoea, pancreatitis, peritonitis, burns and excessive diuretic therapy (Garretson and Malberti 2007) External fluid loss can be caused by haemorrhage, severe vomiting, osmotic diuresis, trauma and surgery (Kent and Dowd 2007).

Cardiogenic shock

Cardiogenic shock is caused by severe heart failure (Leach 2004) usually secondary to ST-elevation acute myocardial infarction (STEMI) but can also follow acute mitral regurgitation, ventricular septal rupture, cardiomyopathies, congestive cardiac failure and trauma (Garretson and Malberti 2007; Kent and Dowd 2007). As a result of a reduced cardiac output, catecholamines (adrenaline and noradrenaline), renin and aldosterone are released, which cause a tachycardia and vasoconstriction, increasing afterload, myocardial workload and oxygen consumption. Haemodynamic readings will demonstrate tachycardia, systolic BP <90 mmHg cardiac index <2.1 l/min per m², pulmonary artery wedge pressure >18 mmHg and increased systemic vascular resistance (SVR) (Kent and Dowd 2007).

Distributive shock

Distributive shock arises from abnormality of the peripheral circulation and can be divided into three different types: neurogenic, anaphylactic and septic (McLuckie 2009). Despite an adequate circulating volume, the vasculature expands and hypovolaemia occurs due to plasma leakage from capillaries (McLuckie 2009).

Although cardiac output could rise, the uptake of oxygen is impaired; there is still a relatively low volume because the intravascular space has increased due to dilatation of the systemic vasculature. In sepsis and anaphylaxis capillaries become permeable because of circulating inflammatory mediators. This permeability causes fluid leakage from the vasculature to the interstitial space, further reducing intravascular volume. Neurogenic shock can be caused by damage to the spinal cord or brain stem, emotional trauma or drugs that cause a reduction of sympathetic impulses causing massive vasodilatation, hypotension, bradycardia and hypothermia (Kent and Dowd 2007).

Haemodynamic readings initially appear normal or show an increase in cardiac output, fall in SVR and low to normal pulmonary artery wedge pressure (PAWP) as a hyperdynamic state develops to compensate for reducing cardiac output.

Obstructive shock

Obstructive shock is caused by circulatory obstruction (Leach 2004). Causes include pulmonary embolism, tension pneumothorax and cardiac tamponade.

Haemodynamic readings show a fall in cardiac output, fall in PAWP and rise in SVR. Pressures in the right side of the heart, pulmonary artery and left chambers equilibrate in diastole, whereas cardiac output falls, SVR rises and PAWP is variable depending on the cause of the obstruction.

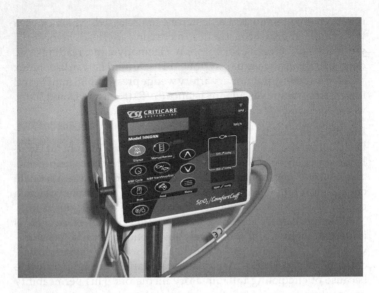

Fig. 5.2 Non-invasive blood pressure monitoring device.

NON-INVASIVE METHODS OF HAEMODYNAMIC MONITORING

This section discusses the various non-invasive methods of haemodynamic monitoring. A non-invasive monitoring device is illustrated in Fig. 5.2.

Assessment of respiratory rate

Respiratory rate is an early significant indicator of cellular dysfunction. This is a sensitive physiological indicator and should be monitored and recorded regularly. Rate and depth of respirations will initially increase in response to cellular hypoxia.

Assessment of pulse and ECG

A rapid, weak, thready pulse is a characteristic sign of hypovolaemia (Bickley and Szilagyi 2009). A full bounding or throbbing pulse may be indicative of anaemia, heart block, heart failure or the early stages of septic shock – the hyperdynamic or compensatory stage

(Jenkins and Johnson 2010). A discrepancy in the volume between central and distal pulses may be caused by a fall in cardiac output (and also cold ambient temperature).

ECG monitoring is an invaluable non-invasive method of continuous monitoring of the heart rate. It can provide the practitioner with an early sign of a fall in cardiac output. The principles of ECG monitoring were discussed in Chapter 4.

Assessment of cerebral perfusion

Altered mental state (Cooke and Thompson 2011), such as a deterioration in conscious level, confusion, agitation and lethargy, is an important determinant of cerebral perfusion and the presence of shock.

Assessment of skin perfusion

Decreased skin perfusion is often characterised by cool peripheries, skin mottling, pallor, cyanosis and delayed capillary refill time (CRT). The following procedure is suggested for the assessment of CRT:

- Explain the procedure to the patient.
- Elevate the digit to the level of the heart (or slightly higher). This will ensure the assessment of arteriolar capillary and not venous stasis refill.
- Apply sufficient pressure to cause blanching to the digit for 5 seconds and then release (Resuscitation Council UK 2006).
- Time how long it takes for the colour of the skin to return to the same colour of the surrounding tissues, i.e. CRT. The normal CRT is <2 s (Gwinnutt 2008).

A sluggish (delayed) CRT (>2 s) suggests poor peripheral perfusion. Other factors that can prolong CRT include a cold ambient temperature, poor lighting and old age (Resuscitation Council UK 2006). CRT as an assessment tool must be used with caution because it is not a specific monitoring aid and used only as a guide.

Assessment of urine output

Urine output can indirectly provide an indication of cardiac output. In health, 25% of the cardiac output perfuses the kidneys. When renal perfusion is adequate, urine output should exceed 0.5 ml/kg per hour (Snyder 2009). Decreased urine output may be an early sign of hypovolaemia because, when cardiac output falls, so does renal perfusion (Gonce Morton 2009). Once urine output is less than approximately 500 ml/day, the kidneys are unable to excrete the waste products of metabolism; uraemia, metabolic acidosis and hyperkalaemia will then develop (Gwinnutt 2008).

In the critically ill patient, acute renal failure is usually caused by inadequate renal perfusion pressure (prerenal failure) caused by, for example, hypovolaemia (Gwinnutt 2008). If diuretics have been administered, e.g. frusemide urine output is not helpful in assessing cardiac output. If the patient is catheterised, ensure that the tube is not blocked or kinked.

Arterial blood pressure measurements

Arterial blood pressure (ABP) is the force exerted by the circulating volume of blood on the walls of the arteries (Wallymahmed 2008). Changes in cardiac output or peripheral resistance can affect the blood pressure. A patient with a low cardiac output can maintain a normal blood pressure by vasoconstriction, whereas a patient who is vasodilated may be hypotensive despite a high cardiac output, e.g. in sepsis. Mean arterial pressure (MAP) is an average pressure reading within the arterial system (Garretson 2005) and is a useful indicator because it can approximate perfusion to essential organs such as the kidneys. MAP is recognised as the main therapeutic endpoint for a patient with sepsis (Giuliano 2006). MAP is also thought to be more relevant because it is least dependent upon measurement site or technique and least altered by dampening, and determines tissue flow by autoregulation (Sturgess and Morgan 2009).

'The adequacy of blood pressure in an individual patient must always be assessed in relation to their premorbid value' (Hinds and Watson 2008). Table 5.4 provides an indication of 'expected' systolic and diastolic blood pressure measurements. Hypotension can lead to inadequate perfusion of vital organs. Hypertension increases myocardial workload and can precipitate cerebral vascular accidents.

Cardiac output is related to pulse pressure, which is the difference between the systolic and diastolic pressures, usually 40–60 mmHg (Gonce Morton 2009). Following a fall in cardiac output the pulse pressure will narrow, resulting in a thready pulse. In the

Table 5.4 Normal intracardiac pressures

Parameter	Normal range
Central venous	0 to +8 mmHg (right atrial level)
Right ventricle	0 to +8 mmHg diastolic +15 to +30 mmHg systolic
Pulmonary capillary wedge pressure	+5 to +15 mmHg
Left atrium	+4 to +12 mmHg
Left ventricle	+4 to +12 mmHg diastolic +90 to +140 mmHg systolic
Aorta	+90 to +140 mmHg systolic +60 to +90 mmHg diastolic +70 to +105 mmHg mean

Reproduced with kind permission of Routledge from Woodrow (2000, p. 212).

early stages of septic shock, the cardiac output can rise, resulting in a wide pulse pressure and bounding pulses.

Factors influencing blood pressure measurements

There are numerous factors that can influence blood pressure, e.g. nicotine, anxiety, pain, position of patient, medications, illicit drugs, alcohol and exercise. It is important to ensure that a standardised approach is used to minimise the impact of extraneous variables on blood pressure (Wallymahmed 2008).

There are no recommendations of which arm to use but initially the BP should be taken in both arms (Heart Foundation 2008). Wide discrepancies between right and left arm blood pressure measurements may be indicative of an aortic aneurysm.

Factors affecting accuracy of blood pressure measurements

The accuracy of blood pressure measurement may be affected by the following factors:

- *Cuff width*: if this is too narrow the blood pressure reading will be falsely high whereas if it is too wide it will be falsely low (British Hypertension Society 2006). The European Standard recommends that the width of the bladder should be 40%, and the length 80–100%, of the limb circumference (British Hypertension Society 2006).

- *Position of the arm*: the arm should be supported in a horizontal position at the level of the heart. Incorrect positioning during the procedure can lead to errors of as much as 10% (Heart Foundation 2008).
- *Deflating the cuff too quickly:* cuff should be deflated at 2–3 mm/ beat (Heart Foundation 2008).

Complications

Complications associated with non-invasive blood pressure devices include limb oedema, friction blisters and ulnar nerve palsy if the cuff is placed too low on the upper arm (British Hypertension Society 2006). If the patient is being heparinised or has a systemic coagulopathy, over-inflation or frequent inflations could cause excessive bruising.

GENERAL PRINCIPLES OF MONITORING WITH TRANSDUCERS

Transducers enable the pressure readings from invasive monitoring of the patient to be displayed on a monitor, i.e. arterial lines or central venous pressure (CVP) lines. To maintain patency of the cannula and tubing and prevent back-flow of blood, a bag of (0.9%) saline should be connected to the transducer tubing and kept under continuous pressure of 300 mmHg (i.e. greater than arterial pressure), thus facilitating a continuous flush at 3 ml/h.

Best practice – monitoring with transducers

Check flush bag each shift – if it runs too low the line will clot off
Ensure that the pressure bag remains inflated at 300 mmHg – to ensure continuous flushing
If flat trace check for breaks in the circuit and air – rectify safely and flush line
If trace remains flat withdraw blood while manipulating limb
Always check the patient – asystole causes a flat trace

Ensuring accuracy

The following precautions will help to ensure accuracy of measurements:

- Keep the transducer level with the zero reference point, usually the midaxilla. Always use the same reference point in order to ensure meaningful comparison.
- Limit the use of three-way taps.
- Remove any air bubbles from the system.
- Calibrate the transducer to atmospheric pressure prior to and regularly during use. This should be undertaken following the manufacturer's recommendations and is typically as follows:
  1. Switch the three-way tap in the tubing open to air (atmospheric pressure) and off to the patient.
  2. Press the zero button on the monitor and observe for 0 to be displayed.
  3. Switch the three-way tap off to air and open to the patient.
  4. Ensure that the transducer is at the zero reference point and observe for the pressure trace on the monitor.

Principles of arterial pressure monitoring

Indications for insertion of an arterial line include the requirement for continuous monitoring of arterial blood pressure in critically ill patients (Garretson 2005), when using potent vasoactive drugs such as adrenaline and noradrenaline, and frequent blood sampling, e.g. blood gas and acid–base analysis.

Best practice – monitoring an arterial line

Ensure arterial line is clearly labelled 'arterial'

The transducer should be level with the phlebostatic axis (bisection of the fourth intercostal space at midpoint between anterior and posterior chest wall)

Limb should be exposed and constantly observed for signs of a decrease in perfusion and disconnection of the cannula (Garretson 2005)

Use transparent dressing so site can be monitored for signs of infection

Ensure that monitor alarms are set following local protocols

If flat trace observed, once asystole excluded, identify and rectify cause of problem

---

Common insertion sites

The radial artery (alternative sites include the brachial, dorsalis pedis and femoral arteries) is usually the site of choice; advantages include:

- superficial position
- readily accessible
- easy to monitor and observe
- easy to apply pressure in the event of bleeding
- minimal restriction to patient movement
- adequate collateral circulation is normally present provided by the ulnar artery (Kent and Dowd 2007).

The arterial waveform

The arterial waveform reflects the pressure generated in the arteries following ventricular contraction and should correlate with the QRS of the ECG (Garretson 2005). Figure 5.3 depicts a typical arterial waveform and its configuration can be described as follows:

- *Anacrotic notch*: presystolic rise during first phase of ventricular systole, before opening of aortic valve (McGee et al. 2009).
- *Peak systolic pressure*: this reflects maximum left ventricular systolic pressure.
- *Dicrotic notch*: reflects aortic valve closure, marking the end of systole and the start of diastole (McGee et al. 2009). It is notably elevated in patients with increased peripheral resistance and decreased cardiac output.
- *Diastolic pressure*: reflects the degree of vasoconstriction or dilatation in the arterial system.

Complications of arterial line insertion

Nurses need to be constantly alert to the possible complications of arterial line insertion. These include exsanguination, ischaemia distal to the cannula and tissue necrosis, inadvertent

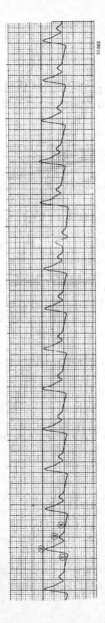

Fig. 5.3 Arterial waveform: (1) anacrotic notch; (2) peak systolic pressure; (3) dicrotic notch; (4) diastolic pressure.

administration of drugs into the artery, air embolus and thrombosis (Table 5.5).

Monitoring priorities of a patient with an arterial line

The following measures should always be observed when a patient with an arterial line is being monitored:

- Ensure that the tubing and cannula are secured.
- Clearly label the tubing 'arterial' with red connections and/or red tubing to help prevent accidental arterial injection of drugs (Kent and Dowd 2007).
- Use a transparent dressing so that any dislodgement or disconnection will be immediately recognised.
- Ensure that the limb is visible at all times to monitor perfusion and maintain a closed circuit.
- Regularly assess tissue perfusion distal to the cannula site. Thrombosis or the development of an adjacent haematoma could jeopardise arterial blood flow. If signs of poor tissue perfusion are present, e.g. if the limb becomes white, cold or painful, inform medical staff immediately – the line will need to be removed.
- Regularly assess the site for signs of infection. Replace dressing if soiled.
- Maintain a bag of 0.9% saline at a pressure of 300 mmHg to help maintain patency and change it following locally agreed protocols.
- Ensure that all connections are secure. Exsanguination from arterial catheters is possible and extra vigilance is required if the femoral artery has been used because the site may not be visible. The arterial line should always be transduced; alarms should be appropriately set to alert the nurse to any disruption in the pressures indicating disconnection.
- Only competent practitioners should undertake arterial blood sampling.
- Use minimum amount of 'taps' to reduce the risk of infection, leakage and inadvertent drug administration.

Table 5.5 Summary of potential problems associated with an arterial cannula

Problem	Cause	Action
'Dampened' trace (see Fig. 5.3) leading to underestimated BP (blunt pressure peak, loss of dicrotic notch)	Loss of pressure or no fluid in the infusion pressure bag	Inflate pressure bag to 300 mmHg Check there is sufficient flushing fluid
	Thrombus/fibrin formation at tip of catheter	Withdraw blood and then flush catheter
	Air in tubing or transducer	Disconnect tubing from catheter and flush through to expel air before reconnecting. If necessary, change transducer
	Too many three-way taps in the circuit	Remove excess taps
	Long length of tubing between catheter and transducer	Shorten tubing
	Poor position of limb, tip of catheter against vessel wall, kinked tubing	Manipulate catheter and/or limb to achieve a better trace
No arterial waveform (straight line)	Taps turned off to patient or transducer	Check taps are on to patient and transducer
	Disconnection of catheter	Check catheter site – reconnect immediately
	Disconnection of transducer cable to monitor	Check connections – reconnect
	Poor catheter position (tip against vessel wall)	Manipulate position, flush catheter
	Asystole	Institute cardiopulmonary resuscitation
Backflow of blood from catheter towards transducer	Loose tap connection within the circuit	Check all connections are secure
	Flush bag pressure too low (below patient's BP)	Inflate bag to 300 mmHg pressure

© Sheila K. Adam and Sue Osborne 1997. Reproduced by permission of Oxford University Press from Adam and Osborne (1997).

Troubleshooting – flat arterial trace

If a flat arterial trace is observed on the monitor check:
- patient is not in asystole
- circuit connections
- circuit for air bubbles and safely remove if present
- tubing in the circuit not kinked
- flush bag has adequate fluid and sufficient pressure is being maintained
- proximal joint as the cannula may be kinked or compressed against the vessel wall – repositioning the joint may be necessary
- patency of the arterial cannula by withdrawing blood
- patient's blood pressure manually

Once the problem has been rectified flush and re-zero line.

Pulse contour analysis

Devices are now available that analyse the shape of the arterial waveform (pulse contour analysis): they can derive stroke volume and determine cardiac output (Gwinnutt 2008). The stroke volume is derived from analysis of the systolic area of the arterial waveform, with corrections for the patient's age and heart rate (British Hypertension Society 2006). Calibration against a simultaneous method, e.g. thermodilution, enables pulse contour analysis to be used on peripheral arterial waveforms (British Hypertension Society 2006).

PRINCIPLES OF CENTRAL VENOUS PRESSURE MONITORING

Central venous pressure reflects right atrial filling pressure and aids assessment of intraventricular volume and right-sided heart function (McGee et al. 2009). Readings are dependent on cardiac function, intravascular volume, vascular tone, intrinsic venous tone, increased intra-abdominal or intrathoracic pressures, and vasopressor therapy (McGee et al. 2009). The normal CVP is 0–8 mmHg (Kent and Dowd 2007). A low CVP reading usually indicates hypovolaemia whereas a high CVP reading has a number of causes, including hypervolaemia, cardiac failure and pulmonary embolism.

Indications for central venous catheters

Indications for central venous catheters include:

- Rapid fluid resuscitation
- Drug and fluid administration, e.g. parenteral nutrition
- Chronically ill patients, who will usually have a peripherally inserted central line (PICC)
- Measurement of central venous pressure
- Poor venous access
- Cardiac pacing
- Post insertion of a pulmonary artery catheter (same site) (McGee et al. 2009).

Central venous catheters are frequently used in the management of critically ill patients for both monitoring and administration of drugs and fluids. The usual sites for insertion of central venous catheters are internal jugular (right and left) and subclavian veins (right or left). The latter is often the preferred site. Although the subclavian has more recognisable landmarks to help the clinician and associated with lower risks of infection compared to other sites, there are fewer risks associated with the insertion at the internal jugular. The femoral vein is sometimes used but generally only as a last resort because of the increased risk of infection (Kent and Dowd 2007).

Central venous catheters can consist of one, three, four or five lumina and choice is dependent upon the severity of the patient's condition and their prime use. Strict asepsis must be adhered to on insertion and during on-going management because migration of skin organisms at the insertion site or direct contamination of the catheter hub by hand contact, contaminated fluids or devices is the source of most catheter-related bloodstream infections (Walz et al. 2010).

There is recent evidence to suggest that antimicrobial-impregnated central venous catheters may reduce the risk of catheter-related bloodstream infections. The most potent of these antimicrobials is silver but other agents have been reported such as antibiotics, e.g. rifampicin and minocycline, and antiseptic agents, e.g. chlorhexidine and silver sulfadiazine (McGee et al. 2009).

Central venous pressure monitoring can be helpful in the assessment of cardiac function, circulating blood volume, vascular tone and the patient's response to treatment. However, CVP can be influenced by a number of factors and should therefore be interpreted together with other systemic measurements. An isolated CVP measurement can be misleading; a trend in readings will demonstrate response to treatment and/or disease progression (Woodrow 2002) and is therefore of more value.

To help ensure validity of the measurements and accuracy of their interpretation, the patient's position should be constant (supine if possible) and the same point of reference (phlebostatic axis) should be used for each reading.

Methods of CVP monitoring
There are two methods of CVP monitoring:

1. *Manometer system*: enables intermittent readings, but is less accurate than the transducer system and infrequently used.
2. *Transducer system*: enables continuous readings that are displayed on a monitor (Gwinnutt 2008).

CVP measurement using a manometer
CVP manometers are no longer used in clinical practice. If a patient's condition necessitates CVP monitoring they should be managed in a higher level of care, i.e. HDU or ICU, where electronic monitoring of invasive pressures is routinely undertaken.

Procedure for CVP measurement using a transducer

1. Explain the procedure to the patient.
2. Ensure patency of the central venous catheter before the procedure.
3. Position the patient, supine if possible. The same position should be used for each measurement.
4. Calibrate (zero) the monitor following the manufacturer's recommendations – this usually involves opening the system to the atmosphere (off to the patient, open to air) and pressing a 'zero' button on the monitor; once zero is displayed the monitor has been calibrated). Zeroing a CVP ensures that the atmospheric pressure at the point of measurement is zero (Woodrow 2002).
5. Observe the CVP trace on the monitor. The waveform on the monitor should be slightly undulating in nature (Fig. 5.4),

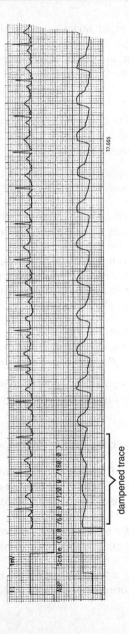

Fig. 5.4 Dampened arterial trace.

reflecting changes in right atrial pressure during the cardiac cycle.

6. Document the reading and report any changes and abnormalities (also calculate mean pressure reading).

The CVP waveform

The CVP waveform reflects changes in right atrial pressure during the cardiac cycle. Figure 5.5 depicts a typical CVP waveform and its configuration can be described as follows:

- *A wave:* right atrial contraction (P wave on the ECG). If the A wave is elevated the patient may have right ventricular failure or tricuspid stenosis.
- *C wave:* tricuspid valve closure (follows QRS complex on the ECG). The distance from A to C should correlate with the P–R interval on the ECG.
- *V wave:* pressure generated to the right atrium during ventricular contraction, despite the tricuspid valve being closed (latter part of the T wave on the ECG). If the V wave is elevated the patient may have tricuspid valve disease.

Normal CVP measurements

Central venous pressure monitoring should normally show measurements as follows (Sturgess and Morgan 2009):

- 0–5 mmHg in spontaneously breathing patients
- 10 mmHg generally the highest acceptable in ventilated patients.

Troubleshooting

The following needs to be considered when monitoring CVP:

- *Occluded catheter*: this will result in a persistently high reading with a dampened trace. Ensure that the catheter is patent.
- *Incorrect calibration*: transducers should be calibrated regularly as per unit guidelines
- *Inconsistent procedure for measurements*: ensure consistent procedure (identical patient position and point of reference) for serial CVP measurements.
- *Infusion(s) in progress*: a falsely high CVP measurement will result if infusion(s) continue to be administered through the

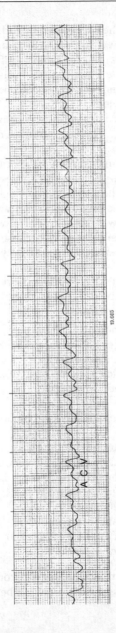

Fig. 5.5 Central venous pressure (CVP) trace: A, C and V waves.

CVP catheter during the procedure. In addition if the infusion fluid contains vasoactive drugs, the resultant 'flush' can cause a sudden period of cardiac instability. Infusion(s) should be temporarily switched off while CVP measurement is undertaken and any vasopressor drugs should be infused through a separate dedicated lumen.

- *Catheter tip in the right ventricle*: this will result in an unexpected high pressure reading. The presenting ventricular waveform will confirm suspicions.
- *Respiratory oscillations*: measurements should be taken at end-expiration, especially if the patient is in respiratory distress or is being ventilated, as the CVP will be artificially higher because of positive intrathoracic pressure (Kent amd Dowd 2007).
- *Erroneous results:* a low CVP may not always mean that the patient is under volume – it may be because of other pathology, e.g. vasodilatation in sepsis (Kent and Dowd 2007)

Complications following CVP line insertion
Nurses should be alert to the possibility of complications following central venous catheter insertion:

- Malposition of the catheter (Fig. 5.6)
- Carotid artery puncture (McGee et al. 2009)
- Pneumothorax, hydrothorax (McGee et al. 2009)
- Damage to sympathetic chain, because of anatomical location of large veins (Kent and Dowd 2007)
- Haemorrhage
- Infection (central line-associated bloodstream infections – CLABSI)
- Intravascular loss of guide wire (Sturgess and Morgan 2009)
- Air embolus: 10–20 ml air entering the venous system is needed before the patient becomes symptomatic, i.e. confusion, light-headedness, anxiety and unresponsiveness; cardiac arrest may occur (Gonce Morton 2009)
- Thrombosis (Sturgess and Morgan 2009)
- Ventricular perforation (McGee et al. 2009)
- Cardiac arrhythmias on insertion.

Management of a patient with a central venous catheter
The precautions listed below should always be observed.

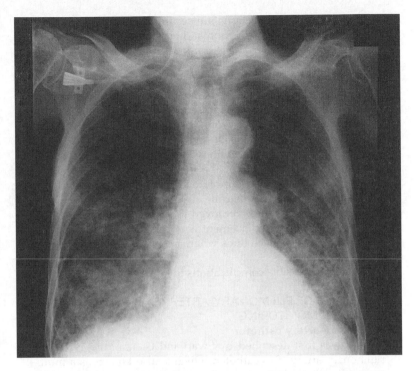

Fig. 5.6 Malposition of the central venous pressure (CVP) catheter – patient with known chronic obstructive pulmonary disease and basal pulmonary fibrosis. The right subclavian line tip is pointing cranially with the tip in the internal jugular vein. (We are grateful to Louise Holland, Consultant Radiologist at the Manor Hospital Walsall for her assistance.)

- Monitor the patient for signs of complications.
- Label central venous catheter with drugs/fluids, etc. being infused in order to minimise the risk of accidental bolus injection.
- If not in use, flush the cannula regularly to help prevent thrombosis. When transducing a CVP line a 500 ml bag of 0.9% saline should be maintained at a pressure of 300 mmHg and changed in accordance with locally agreed protocols.

- Ensure that all connections are secure to prevent exsanguination, introduction of infection and air emboli.
- Change lines and dressing as per local guidelines (usually every 72 hours).
- Observe the insertion site frequently for signs of infection. Transparent dressings should be used to permit continuous monitoring of the site. The incidence of central venous catheter-related infection ranges from 4% to 18%. If infection of the central venous catheter is suspected blood cultures should be taken after removal of the line. The catheter tip should be sent for culture. The length of the indwelling catheter should be recorded and regularly monitored. The dressing should be changed as required, ensuring strict aseptic technique.
- Central lines should be removed as soon as they are no longer required. Routine replacement is not recommended but some clinicians will replace lines when an infective focus cannot be identified.
- Be alert to possible complications identified above.

PRINCIPLES OF PULMONARY ARTERY PRESSURE MONITORING
Pulmonary artery catheter

Since it was first described by Swan and Ganz in the 1970s, the pulmonary artery (PA) catheter, which is also known as a multi-lumen directional flow catheter (Fig. 5.7), has been widely used for the diagnosis and treatment of critically ill patients (Swan and Ganz 1974).

It can be used to evaluate cardiac function and detect problems in the pulmonary vasculature, and enables the clinician to optimise cardiac output and delivery of oxygen while minimising the risk of pulmonary oedema; it also allows the rational use of vasoactive and inotropic drugs (Gonce Morton 2009). The use of the PA catheter is not without risk. Although it has been common in the ICU environment in the last 30 years there have been doubts about its safety. However, a large multi-centre randomised controlled trial (Harvey et al. 2005) concluded that there was no clear evidence of benefit or harm to the critically ill patient managed with a PA catheter. The use of PA catheters should be limited to experienced, well-trained clinicians familiar with the interpretation of data

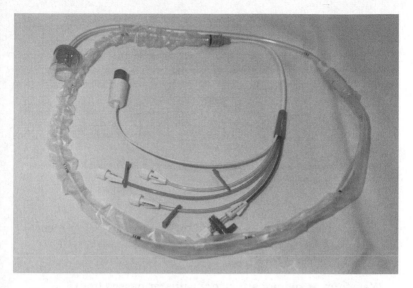

Fig. 5.7 Pulmonary artery catheter.

derived from the catheter, who are able to adjust treatment based on the results obtained.

As a result of doubts surrounding the efficacy of PA catheters, less invasive methods of measuring cardiac output have been developed and these are discussed later.

Indications

Use of PA pressure measurement is indicated for:

- Differentiation of shock states of similar clinical presentation, e.g. cardiogenic shock due to myocardial infarction or MI (pulmonary artery occlusion pressure [PAOP] ↑, CVP normal or ↑, pulmonary artery pressure [PAP] normal) from pulmonary embolus (PAOP normal, CVP ↑, PAP ↑) (Sturgess and Morgan 2009; Jenkins and Johnson 2010)
- Optimising fluid, inotrope and vasopressor therapy (Sturgess and Morgan 2009). Measurement of right atrial pressure, PAP and cardiac output using thermodilution technique and

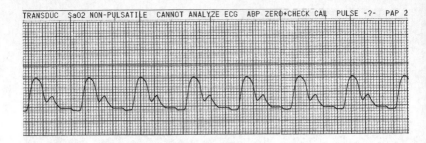

TRANSDUC SaO2 NON-PULSATILE CANNOT ANALYZE ECG ABP ZERO+CHECK CAL PULSE -?- PAP 2

Fig. 5.8 Pressure traces seen as the pulmonary artery catheter passes from the vena cava to the pulmonary artery.

derived values such as SVR and pulmonary vascular resistance (PVR).
- Post cardiac surgery.

Waveform as pulmonary artery catheter passes from the vena cava to the pulmonary artery

Figure 5.8 depicts the pressure traces seen as a pulmonary artery catheter passes from the vena cava to the pulmonary artery. Pulmonary vasculature is more compliant than the systemic vessels, so pulmonary pressures are lower (see Table 5.5) (Woodrow 2008). Pulmonary hypertension is common in ICU patients, e.g. those with acute respiratory distress syndrome (ARDS). If the PAP is low despite a high CVP this is indicative of right-sided heart failure (Woodrow 2008).

Pressures

Using a pulmonary catheter it is possible to measure the pressures in the right atrium (RA), right ventricle (RV) and PA (see Table 5.5):

- *RA pressure*: during ventricular filling is 0–8 mmHg
- *RV pressure*: end-diastolic pressure is 0–8 mmHg, systolic pressure 15–30 mmHg
- *PA pressure*: diastolic 5–15 mmHg, systolic 15–30 mmHg.

A high diastolic pressure indicates right heart failure, pulmonary hypertension or tamponade. High PA pressure indicates left ventricular failure (LVF) or pulmonary hypertension; low PA pressure is suggestive of hypovolaemia.

Cardiac index (CI) is the cardiac output indexed to individual body surface area (Sturgess and Morgan 2009). A normal value is between 2.8 and 4.2l/min per m² (Sturgess and Morgan 2009). These readings may never be completely precise because it is very difficult to weigh and measure a very sick patient accurately. The relevance, however, is in the trend of results that the PA catheter facilitates and the response to treatment administered.

Pulmonary artery occlusion or wedge pressure

If the balloon is inflated in the branch of the PA (<1.5 ml air), the pressure at the tip of the balloon closely approximates the left atrial pressure, which approximates the left ventricular end diastolic pressure (LVEDP) (Sturgess and Morgan 2009).

Procedure

1. Explain the procedure to the patient.
2. Watching the monitor at the same time, slowly inflate the balloon until the characteristic flattened waveform is identified (see Fig. 5.8). The balloon is now 'wedged', i.e. it occludes the blood flow in a branch of the PA.
3. Stop inflating the balloon and allow the trace to run for three respiratory cycles (very important).
4. Freeze the monitor screen and deflate the balloon rapidly.
5. Ascertain the wedge pressure by aligning the cursor control on the monitor to the correct position on the waveform (end-expiration).
6. Unfreeze the monitor screen and ensure that the pulmonary artery waveform is present.

Precautions

Care should be taken to observe the following precautions:

- Do not leave the balloon inflated for longer than three respiratory cycles (15s).
- Do not inflate more than 1.5 ml of air into the balloon.
- Do not flush the catheter if the balloon is inflated.

- If the trace rises sharply during balloon inflation, then the catheter is over-wedged.

Limitations

PAOP/PAWP does not accurately reflect left atrial and ventricular pressure in:

- pulmonary venous obstruction
- mitral stenosis
- left atrial myxoma (very rare).

Normal pulmonary occlusion/wedge range is 6–15 mmHg (Sturgess and Morgan 2009) and should correlate with the pulmonary artery diastolic pressure; a high reading may signify LVF, mitral insufficiency or fluid overload, whereas a low reading may signify hypovolaemia.

Systemic vascular resistance is the measurement of afterload and a critical measurement in the diagnosis and treatment of sepsis. A normal SVR is 900–1400 dynes s/cm^5. Systemic vascular resistance index (SVRI) is indexed to body surface area calculated from weight and height.

Complications

Complications resulting during insertion and use of PA catheter include the following:

- Cardiac arrhythmias
- Valve damage
- Thrombosis
- Pulmonary infarction
- PA rupture – often associated with over-inflation of the balloon during measuring the PAOP/PAWP, pulmonary hypertension, age, abnormal coagulation profile and is usually fatal (Cooke and Thompson 2011)
- Air embolism (Sturgess and Morgan 2009)
- Knotting or kinking of the catheter (Sturgess and Morgan 2009).

CARDIAC OUTPUT STUDIES
Thermodilution
Thermodilution is a method for measuring cardiac output. To assess progress towards desired treatment goals it is important that

readings are taken after interventions, e.g. titration of vasoactive or inotropic drugs or fluid bolus. This process involves a rapid injection of a measured amount of cold fluid (usually 5–10 ml of 5% dextrose) into the right atrium through the proximal lumen of the PA catheter. Its dilution by the blood is calculated by serial changes in PA temperature as the fluid bolus travels through the heart. The cardiac output is calculated on the basis of the temperature change: the rise in solution temperature is inversely related to the functioning of the heart.

Indications

Thermodilution is indicated in clinical situations where the assessment of volaemic status and cardiac output along with haemodynamic variables will help in the diagnosis and management, e.g.:

- Management and diagnosis of all forms of shock
- Impaired right or left ventricular function as seen in cardiac failure
- Measurement of cardiac output
- Measurement of mixed venous saturation
- Diagnosis of ventricular septal defect.

Procedure

1. Explain the procedure to the patient.
2. Draw up the injection fluid.
3. Ensure that the temperature of injection fluid is lower than the body temperature.
4. Flush the proximal port with the injection fluid; the injection fluid displayed on the monitor should be within the accepted range for the monitoring system.
5. Ensure that the monitor is ready.
6. Press the start button on the monitor and inject 5–10 ml smoothly within 4 s (do not hold the syringe barrel, because this could warm the injection fluid). Approximately 15 s later, the cardiac output measurement will be displayed on the monitor. After about 45 s, the monitor will display 'ready' again.
7. Press the start button again and repeat the above procedure. At least three measurements should be made and an average of the three readings calculated.

Troubleshooting

The following problems are associated with thermodilution cardiac output measurements (Adam and Osborne 2005):

- *Difficulty injecting the solution*: the tube may be kinked or occluded or the catheter tip may be positioned against the vessel wall. Unkink, reposition or replace catheter as necessary.
- *Blood temperature not displayed*: the thermistor may be faulty or have a fibrin growth attached. Replace the catheter if necessary.
- *Injection fluid temperature not displayed*: replace the faulty temperature probe.
- *Major discrepancies in serial measurements*: possible causes include poor injection technique, cardiac arrhythmias (causing varying stroke volumes), and vascular disease causing turbulent blood and patient movement. Adhere to procedure described above, do not inject during arrhythmic episodes and limit patient movement during injection.
- *Inappropriately high cardiac output measurements*: possible causes include incorrect injection fluid volume (usually too little or leaking connection), injection fluid temperature too low, poor injection technique and computer error. Adhere to the procedure described above and if indicated check the computer.
- *Inappropriately low cardiac output measurements*: possible causes include incorrect injection fluid volume (usually too much), injection fluid temperature too high, start button on the monitor pressed after starting the injection, computer error, prolonged injection time and concomitant fluid infusion through the distal lumen. Adhere to the procedure described above and if indicated check the computer.

Mixed venous oxygen saturation

Mixed venous oxygen saturation (SvO_2) represents the amount of oxygen that remains after perfusion of the capillary beds and is an indicator of the balance between oxygen delivery ($DO2$) and oxygen consumption ($\dot{V}O2$) (McGee et al. 2009). SvO_2 measurements can be used as a direct guide to tissue hypoxia (Morgan and Venkatesh 2009).

- SvO_2 75%: normal reflecting a desirable balance between global oxygen supply and demand (Morgan and Venkatesh 2009).
- SvO_2 ≤75%: low. If the oxygen delivery drops or if tissue oxygen demand rises this can lead to a low measurement. If SvO_2 <30% then oxygen delivery is insufficient to meet the oxygen needs of the tissues.
- SvO_2 ≥75%: high, can be difficult to interpret. Causes include sepsis, hyperthyroidism and severe liver disease (Morgan and Venkatesh 2009).

Methods for SvO_2 measurements

SvO_2 measurement may be performed in two ways:

1. *Intermittent* blood sampling from the distal PA catheter or *continuously* through a fibreoptic PA catheter
2. A co-oximeter is also required because blood gas machines are unable to calculate lower SvO_2.

Non-invasive methods of measuring cardiac output

As a result of the invasive nature of PA catheters and their associated complications, it may be preferable to use non-invasive methods if available, to measure cardiac function.

NICO

NICO is a non-invasive device (Fig. 5.9) that calculates cardiac output by a modified Fick equation, based on partial carbon dioxide re-breathing. Cardiac output data are derived from sensors that measure flow, airway pressure and carbon dioxide concentration. As a result of this, use of the NICO is limited to the patient who is mechanically ventilated.

PiCCO

PiCCO is continuous pulse contour cardiac analysis and provides derived haemodynamic data via a femoral or axillary artery catheter and a central venous catheter.

Transthoracic echocardiography

Echocardiography is a non- or minimally invasive method of measuring cardiac function and structure, primarily after an MI.

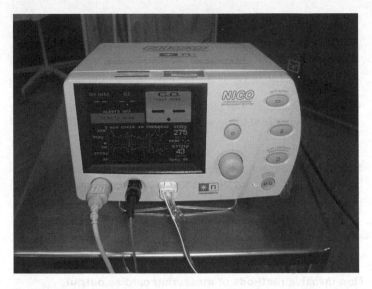

Fig. 5.9 Non-invasive cardiac output monitor.

Echocardiography also forms part of the haemodynamic assessment (left ventricular filling pressure, severity of mitral regurgitation), changes in ventricular structure and prognostic assessment based on systolic and diastolic ventricular function (Nidorf and Marwick 2011). Transthoracic echocardiography (TTE) is relatively accessible, can be brought to the bedside to assess cardiac function and is non-invasive (Nidorf and Marwick 2011).

Transoesophageal echocardiography

Transoesophageal echocardiography (TOE) is not always possible in a critically ill patient due to either obesity or positioning. This is an ultrasound technique that involves introducing a scope-like probe on the end of a flexible gastroscope-like probe, which can be manoeuvred within the oesophagus and stomach, close to the heart (Sturgess and Morgan 2009). TOE is contraindicated in patients with oesophageal stricture, neoplasm or varices, severe coagulopathy and severe congenital spine abnormalities.

SCENARIOS

Scenario 1

Susan, a 45-year-old woman with known gallstones, was admitted to hospital with a history of right upper quadrant pain, pyrexia, vomiting and malaise. Her vital signs were:

BP 115/55 mmHg
Heart rate (HR) 100/min
Respiratory rate 24/min
SpO_2 97% on air
Temperature 37.6°C

A provisional diagnosis of cholecystitis was made and she was commenced on an intravenous (IV) infusion to maintain hydration, an analgesic regimen and cefotaxime 2 g i.v. three times daily and metronidazole 500 mg i.v. three times daily.

On day 2 of her admission Susan's condition deteriorated. She complained of feeling very unwell. On examination she was flushed, warm to the touch with warm peripheries. Her vital signs were:

BP 100/50 mmHg
HR 120/min
Respiratory rate 30/min
SpO_2 93% on air
Temperature 38.5°C

High-flow oxygen was commenced via a non-re-breathe mask and IV fluid increased to 150 ml/h.

Susan continued to deteriorate and was transferred to the ICU for further management. On admission to the ICU Susan was becoming confused and agitated. She was continually trying to remove her oxygen mask and desaturating as a result. The decision was made to electively sedate and ventilate her. On rapid sequence induction Susan developed severe hypotension that required fluid resuscitation and bolus doses of ephedrine. When she had stabilised IV access was established via a quadruple-lumen central venous catheter and an arterial line sited. Susan continued to demonstrate haemodynamic instability and was commenced on an infusion of noradrenaline via the central venous catheter. As a result of her rapid deterioration and suspected

Continued

149

septic shock a PA catheter was inserted and the following readings obtained:

Pulmonary capillary wedge pressure (PCWP) 10 mmHg
Cardiac output (CO) 3.0 l/min
Cardiac Index (CI) 2.1 l/min/m^2
Stroke volume index (SVI) 45 ml/beat per m^2
Systemic vascular resistance (SVR) 1200 dynes s/cm^5
CVP 3 mmHg

The PA catheter results confirmed a reduced cardiac output secondary to septic shock.

Scenario 2

Gordon, a 54-year-old man, presented with a short duration of severe central chest pain with associated nausea and diaphoresis. He was given aspirin 300 mg orally and sublingual glyceryl trinitrate (GTN) before arriving at the emergency department (ED). In the ED he was started on oxygen and given IV morphine 2 mg. Blood was taken for cardiac biomarkers and urea and electrolytes. In the ED 12-lead ECG diagnosis confirmed a non-ST-segment acute coronary syndrome (NSTEAC). As this does not require reperfusion therapy Gordon was immediately transferred to the coronary care unit (CCU).

His observations were within normal limits, he was pain free, warm and well perfused. Shortly after admission he suddenly developed a broad complex tachycardia, rate 180/min. He was conscious, what would you do?

The patient is conscious therefore he must have a pulse (if he was pulseless, CPR and rapid defibrillation would be required). If not already, administer oxygen, secure IV access and establish whether the patient is haemodynamically compromised. Are there any adverse signs (e.g. systolic blood pressure <90 mmHg, chest pain, heart failure, rapid rate >150/min) (Resuscitation Council UK 2010)?

On examination Mr Smith's pulse is weak, rapid (180/min) and thready. His blood pressure has fallen to 70 mmHg systolic, he is cold, pale and clammy, and his conscious level is deteriorating. What would you do?

He is severely haemodynamically compromised and requires urgent treatment, e.g. cardioversion. If the patient had not been compromised, drugs, e.g. amiodarone or lidocaine, would have probably been the first choice of treatment. Any electrolyte imbalance would also need to be treated.

CONCLUSION

Haemodynamic monitoring is central to the care of a critically ill patient. It helps to establish a precise diagnosis, determine appropriate therapy and monitor the response to that therapy. In particular the various methods of haemodynamic monitoring can assist in the early recognition and treatment of shock. Early recognition and prompt treatment of such disorders improves outcomes. It is always preferable to utilise the least invasive, yet most accurate technique available to reduce the risk of complications for the patient. Users of monitoring devices must be familiar with the operation of and how to trouble shoot, which will minimise the risk of erroneous results.

REFERENCES

Adam, S. K. & Osborne, S. (1997) *Critical Care Nursing: Science and practice*. Oxford: Oxford University Press.

Adam, S. K. & Osborne, S. (2005) *Critical Care Nursing: Science and practice*, 2nd edn. Oxford: Oxford University Press.

Bickley, L. & Szilagyi, P. G. (2009) *Bates' Guide to Physical Examination and History Taking*, 10th edn. Philadelphia: PA: Wolters Kluwer Lippincott Williams & Wilkins.

Bridges, E. J. & Dukes, M. S. (2005) Cardiovascular aspects of septic shock. Pathophysiology, monitoring and treatment. *Critical Care Nurse*, **25**(2), 14–40.

British Hypertension Society (2006) Blood Pressure Measurement. Available at: www.bhsoc.org (accessed 16 September 2006).

Cooke, P. A. & Thompson, P. L. (2011) Haemodynamic monitoring. In: Thompson, P. L. (ed.), *Coronary Care Manual*, 2nd edn. Chatswood: NSW: Elsevier.

Diehl-Oplinger, L. & Kaminski, M. F. (2004) Choosing the right fluid to counter hypovolaemic shock. *Nursing* **34**(3), 52–54.

Garretson, S. (2005) Haemodynamic monitoring: arterial catheters. *Nursing Standard*, **19**(31), 55.

Garretson, S. & Malberti, S. (2007) Understanding hypovolaemic, cardiogenic and septic shock. *Nursing Standard*, **21**(50), 46–56.

Giuliano, K. K. (2006) Continuous physiologic monitoring and the identification of sepsis. *AACN Advanced Critical Care*, **17**, 215–223.

Gonce Morton, P. (2009) Anatomy and physiology of the cardiovascular system. In: Gonce Morton, P. & Fontaine, D. K. (eds), *Critical Care Nursing: A holistic approach*, 9th edn. Philadelphia: Wolters Kluwer Lippincott Williams & Wilkins.

Gwinnutt, C. L. (2008) *Clinical Anaesthesia*, 3rd edn. Oxford: Wiley Blackwell.

Harvey, S., Harrison, D. A. & Singer, M. (2005) Assessment of the clinical effect of pulmonary artery catheters in the management of patients in intensive care (PAC-Man): a randomized controlled trial. *The Lancet*, **366**, 472–477.

Heart Foundation (2008) *Guide to Management of Hypertension*. London: Heart Foundation.

Hinds, C. & Watson, D. (2008) *Intensive Care: A concise textbook*, 3rd edn. Philadelphia, PA: Mosby Elsevier.

Jenkins, P. F. & Johnson, P. H. (2010) *Making Sense of Acute Medicine*. London: Hoddeer Arnold.

Kent, B. & Dowd, B. (2007) Assessment, monitoring and diagnostics. In: Elliott, D., Aitken, L. & Chaboyer, W. (eds), *ACCCN's Critical Care Nursing*. Marrickville: Mosby Elsevier.

Leach, R. (2004) *Critical Care Medicine at a Glance*. Oxford: Blackwell Publishing.

McGee, W. T., Headley, J. & Frazier, J. A., eds (2009) *Quick guide to cardiopulmonary care*, 2nd edn. Edwards Critical Care Education.

McLuckie, A. (2009) Shock – an overview. In: Bersten, A. D. & Soni, N. (eds), *Oh's Intensive Care Manual*, 6th edn. Philadelphia, PA: Butterworth Heinemann Elsevier.

Morgan, T. J. & Venkatesh, B. (2009) Monitoring oxygenation. In: Bersten, A. D. & Soni, N. (eds), *Oh's Intensive Care Manual*, 6th edn. Philadelphia: Butterworth Heinemann Elsevier.

Nidorf, S. M. & Marwick, T. H. (2011) Echocardiography. In: Thompson, P. (ed.), *Coronary Care Manual*, 2nd edn. Chatswood, NSW: Elsevier.

Resuscitation Council UK (2006) *Advanced Life Support*, 5th edn. London: Resuscitation Council UK.

Resuscitation Council UK (2010) *Adult Advanced Life Support Algorithm*. London: Resuscitation Council UK.

Scanlon, V. D. & Sanders, T. (2007) *Essentials of Anatomy and Physiology*, 5th edn. Philadelphia, PA: Pennsylvania: F. A. Davis Co.

Snyder, K. A. (2009). Patient assessment: renal system. In P. Gonce Morton & D. Fontaine, K. (eds), *Critical care nursing: a holistic approach*, 9th edn. Philadelphia: Wolters Kluwer Lippincott Williams & Wilkins.

Sturgess, D. J. & Morgan, T. J. (2009) Haemodynamic monitoring. In A. D. Bersten & N. Soni (eds), *Oh's Intensive Care Manual*, 6th edn. Philadelphia: PA: Butterworth Heinemann Elsevier.

Swan, H. J. C. & Ganz, W. (1974) Guidelines for use of balloon-tipped catheters. *American Journal of Cardiology*, **34**, 119–120.

Wallymahmed, M. (2008) Blood pressure measurement. *Nursing Standard*, **2**(19), 45–48.

Walz, J. M., Memtsoudis, S. G. & Heard, S. O. (2010) Analytic reviews: prevention of central venous catheter bloodstream infections. *Journal of Intensive Care Medicine*, **25**, 131–138.

Woodrow, P. (2000) *Intensive Care Nursing, A Framework for Practice.* Routledge, London.

Woodrow, P. (2002) Central venous catheters and central venous pressure. *Nursing Standard*, **16**(26), 45–51.

Woodrow, P. (2008) *Intensive Care Nursin: A framework for practice*, 2nd edn. New York: Routledge.

Monitoring Neurological Function

6

LEARNING OBJECTIVES

At the end of the chapter the reader will be able to:

❑ define *consciousness*
❑ describe the *AVPU* assessment of consciousness
❑ discuss the use of the *Glasgow Coma Scale*
❑ describe *pupillary assessment*
❑ discuss the principles of *intracranial pressure monitoring*
❑ discuss the principles of *jugular venous bulb oxygen saturation monitoring*
❑ outline the monitoring of *sedation*
❑ outline the monitoring of *pain* and *pain relief*

INTRODUCTION

Altered level of consciousness in the critically ill patient is often the first sign of a severe pathological process (Chamberlain and Swope 2007a) therefore, accurate monitoring of neurological status is imperative (Chamberlain and Swope 2007b). In patients with a head injury or other cerebral insult, monitoring neurological function is essential in order to recognise and treat complications promptly and improve prognosis. It can also provide an indication to the function of other systems, e.g. in renal failure confusion could be a sign of rising blood urea levels.

Monitoring neurological function requires accurate assessment and correct interpretation of observed data (Chamberlain and Swope 2007b). It is important to take into account the effects of any administered medications, e.g. sedatives and paralysing agents

Monitoring the Critically Ill Patient, Third Edition.
Philip Jevon, Beverley Ewens.
© 2012 Blackwell Publishing Ltd. Published 2012 by Blackwell Publishing Ltd.

(Woodrow 2008), alcohol consumption, the patient's clinical condition and whether there is a history of head injury.

The aim of this chapter is to understand the principles of monitoring neurological function.

DEFINITION OF CONSCIOUSNESS

The patient's level of consciousness has been described as the degree of their arousal and awareness (Geraghty 2005). It depends on the interaction of the rostral reticular activating system (RAS), located in the upper brain stem, and the cerebral hemispheres (Venkatesh 2009). The area of RAS that is most important in the maintenance of consciousness is located between the rostral pons and the diencephalon (Venkatesh 2009).

The manifestation of impaired or absent consciousness implies an underlying brain dysfunction (Geraghty 2005). Various scales have been designed to describe levels of consciousness (Geraghty 2005); however, the National Institute for Health and Clinical Excellence (NICE 2007) recommends that the Glasgow Coma Scale (GCS) be used to assess all patients with head injuries. Definitions of impaired consciousness are listed in Table 6.1. It is not possible to measure consciousness directly. It can be assessed only by observing the patient's behavioural response to different stimuli (Waterhouse 2005).

AVPU ASSESSMENT

The most important aspect of any neurological assessment is the level of consciousness because this is the most sensitive indicator of neurological deterioration (Waterhouse 2005). A rapid neurological assessment can be carried out using the AVPU method (Resuscitation Council UK 2011). AVPU is a mnemonic for a simple, rapid and effective neurological scoring system that quantifies the response to stimulation and assesses the level of consciousness. It is an ideal tool in the emergency situation when a rapid assessment of conscious level is required. AVPU stands for:

Alert
responsive to **V**erbal stimulation
responsive to **P**ainful stimulation
Unresponsive.

Table 6.1 Definitions of impaired consciousness

Condition	Definition
Consciousness	Awareness of self and environment
Confusion	Reduced awareness, disorientation
Delirium	Disorientation, fear, irritability, misperception, hallucination
Obtundation	Reduced alertness, psychomotor retardation, drowsiness
Stupor	Unresponsiveness with arousal only by vigorous and repeated stimuli
Coma	Unrousable, unresponsiveness
Vegetative state	Prolonged coma (>1 month), some preservation of brain-stem and motor reflexes
Akinetic mutism	Prolonged coma with apparent alertness and flaccid motor tone
Locked-in state	Total paralysis below third cranial nerve nuclei; normal or impaired mental function

Reprinted from *Intensive Care Manual*, 4th edn, T. Oh, © 1997, with permission from Elsevier Inc.

THE GLASGOW COMA SCALE

The Glasgow Coma Scale (GCS) was originally developed to grade the severity and outcome of traumatic head injury (Teasdale and Jennett. 1974). It is used in a wide variety of clinical settings, in particular for patients with head injury (NICE 2007), and has become the standard criterion for the assessment of brain-injured patients (Zuercher et al. 2009). The uniform use of the GCS in clinical practice is essential for diagnostic and therapeutic decision-making, estimation of prognosis, clear communication and clinical research (Zuercher et al. 2009). It provides:

- an objective assessment of neurological function (Chamberlain and Swope 2007b)
- a high level of inter-rater reliability (Rabiu 2011)

- a baseline as to whether the patient is deteriorating
- a guide to the need for airway protection (intubation usually indicated <9/15) (Jenkins and Johnson 2010)
- a prognostic guide for TBI (Rabiu 2011)
- an indication of severity of injury (Zink 2009)

The GSC assesses the two aspects of consciousness:

- *Arousal* or *wakefulness*: being aware of the environment
- *Awareness*: demonstrating an understanding of what the practitioner has said through an ability to perform tasks.

The 15-point scale assesses the patient's level of consciousness by evaluating three behavioural responses: eye opening, verbal response and motor response (Elliott et al. 2007). Within each category, each level of response is allocated a numerical value, on a scale of increasing neurological deterioration (Waterhouse 2005). By assigning a numerical value to the level of response to the individual criteria in each section, three figures are obtained which add up to a maximum score of 15 and a minimum of 3. Patients with a GCS <9/15 require airway intervention and in most cases intubation (Jevon 2008b). A total score of 12 or less should give rise for concern and a reduction in motor score by 1 or an overall deterioration of 2 is significant and should be reported (Jevon 2008b). Although aggregate scores are often documented, the weighting of scores across eye, verbal and motor responses remains untested (Jevon 2008b). Therefore documenting responses individually may provide a clearer indication of remaining functions and deficits (Waterhouse 2005). The neurological observation chart depicted in Fig. 6.1 incorporates the GCS.

The GCS can be used by different observers and still produce a consistent assessment and has been found to be reliable and easy to use (Ciechanowski et al. 2009). However, as with other scoring systems, the GCS should only be used as an aid to patient assessment along with other diagnostic investigations (Zuercher, et al. 2009). Intra-observer differences in measuring the GCS may occur unless training in the use of the tool has been given to prevent inaccurate and inconsistent recordings which could have a detrimental effect on the patient (Mooney and Comerford 2003).

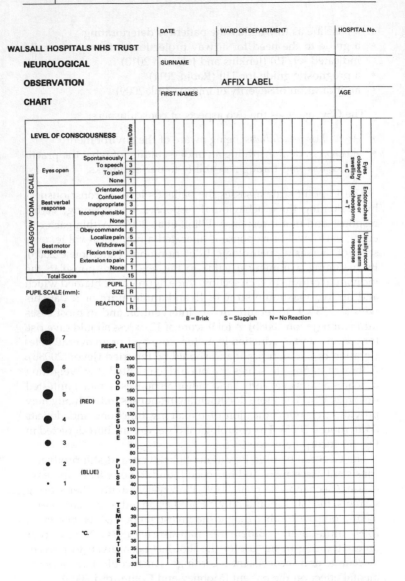

Fig. 6.1 Neurological observation chart incorporating Glasgow Coma Scale (GCS) (Walsall Hospitals NHS Trust).

The frequency of GCS monitoring should depend on the severity of the patient's condition and individual facility guidelines, e.g. after an unwitnessed fall. Instead of stressing the numerical score attached to each response, it is far better to define the responses in descriptive terms.

There are difficulties with using the GCS on an intensive care unit (ICU), particularly in sedated, ventilated, head-injured patients (Ciechanowski et al. 2009). The GCS is not designed to assess sedation levels but how well the brain is functioning (Cree 2003). Differences in scores of two or more have been reported on the same patients by different practitioners (Zuercher et al. 2009), which reiterates the recommendation that clinical decisions should not be based solely on GCS (Holdgate 2006), but that the GCS be used as a component of monitoring neurological function.

Behavioural responses assessed

The three behavioural responses assessed are:

- eye opening
- verbal response
- motor response.

Each is discussed in turn.

Eye opening

Assessment of eye opening involves the evaluation of the arousal mechanism in the brain stem (Zuercher et al. 2009), the first aspect of consciousness. If the patient's eyes are closed, the state of arousal is assessed according to the degree of stimulation required to secure eye opening. If a patient is unable to open their eyes because of swelling or surgery, this is not indicative of falling conscious level (Dawes et al. 2007). The scoring is as follows:

- Score 4 – spontaneously: eyes open without the need for speech or touch (Dawes et al. 2007); optimum response.
- Score 3 – to speech: eyes open in response to a verbal stimulus (usually the patient's name) without touching the patient (Dawes et al. 2007). Begin at normal volume and raise your voice if necessary using clear commands (Fairley 2005).

Table 6.2 Central painful stimuli.

Stimulus	Technique
Trapezium squeeze	Using the thumb and index finger pinch approximately 5 cm of the trapezius muscle (between the head and shoulders) and twist (Woodward 1997)
Suborbital pressure	Running a finger along the supraorbital margin (bony ridge along the top of the eye) it is possible to identify a notch or groove – applying pressure here causes a headache-type pain. Sometimes it may cause the patient to grimace, leading to closing rather than opening of the eyes. Note that should not be used if the patient has facial fractures
Sternal rub	Grinding the sternum with the knuckles. Note alternate with other methods because of marking the skin

- Score 2 – to pain: eyes open in response to central pain only, e.g. trapezium squeeze, suborbital pressure (recommended). Sternal rub (Table 6.2) is no longer recommended. Note that painful stimuli should be employed only if the patient fails to respond to firm and clear commands.
- Score 1 – no response: no eye opening despite verbal and central pain stimulus.

Note, record 'C' if the patient is unable to open the eyes due to swelling, ptosis or a dressing.

Verbal response

Assessment of verbal response involves the evaluation of awareness and the integration of the cerebral cortex and the brain stem (Zuercher et al. 2009), the second aspect of consciousness. Comprehension of what the practitioner has said and functioning areas of the higher centres and ability to articulate and express a reply are being evaluated (Waterhouse 2005). Dysphasia or inability to speak can be caused by any damage to the speech centres, e.g. after intracranial surgery or head injury.

It is important to ascertain the patient's acuity of hearing and understanding of language before assessing this response (Caton-Richards 2010). The lack of speech may not always indicate a falling level of consciousness (Mallett and Dougherty 2000). In addition some patients may require a lot of stimulation to maintain their concentration while answering questions. The scoring is as follows:

- Score 5 – oriented: the patient can tell the practitioner whom they are where they are and the day, the current year and month (avoid using the day of the week or date).
- Score 4 – confused: the patient can hold a conversation with the practitioner, but cannot answer the preceding questions accurately (Fairley 2005).
- Score 3 – inappropriate words: the patient tends to use single words making little sense and being out of context, typically swearing and shouting (Dawes et al. 2007).
- Score 2 – incomprehensible sounds: the patient's response is made up of incomprehensible sounds such as moans or groans (Dawes et al. 2007) but no discernable words. A verbal stimulus together with a pain stimulus may be needed to get a response from the patient. This type of patient is not aware of his or her surroundings (Mooney and Comerford 2003).
- Score 1 – no response: no response from the patient despite both verbal or physical stimuli (Jevon 2008b).

Note, record 'D' if the patient is dysphasic and 'T' if the patient has a tracheal or tracheostomy tube *in situ*.

Motor response

The motor response is designed to ascertain the patient's ability to obey a command and to localise, withdraw or assume abnormal body positions in response to a painful stimulus, and demonstrates the integrity of the brain stem and spinal cord (Zuercher et al. 2009). If the patient does not respond by obeying commands the response to a painful stimulus should then be assessed.

In the past the application of a peripheral painful stimulus (pressure applied to fingernail bed) has been previously advocated (Teasdale and Jennett 1974). However, this can be traumatic and is no longer recommended. It can cause patients to pull the fingers away from the source of pain; only a central painful stimulus will demonstrate localisation to pain (Waterhouse 2005).

A true localising response involves the patient bringing an arm up to chin level, to pull an oxygen mask off, for instance (Waterhouse 2005). To elicit this response the trapezium squeeze, supraorbital ridge pressure or pressure on the jaw margin is recommended. To avoid soft-tissue injury the stimulus should be applied for no more than 10 seconds and released (Waterhouse 2005).

- Score 6 – obeys commands: ask the patient to stick his or her tongue out; never ask a patient just to squeeze your hand because this could elicit a primitive grasp response; ensure that you ask the patient to let go. As it is important to establish that the response is not just a reflex movement, it is important to ask the patient to carry out two different commands (Dawes et al. 2007).
- Score 5 – localises to central pain, if the patient does not respond to verbal stimuli: the patient purposely moves an arm in an attempt to remove the cause of the pain. Supraorbital ridge pressure is considered to be the most reliable technique because this is less likely to be misinterpreted (Fairley 2005).
- Score 4 – withdrawing from pain: the patient flexes or bends arm towards the source of the pain but fails to locate the source of the pain (Waterhouse 2005). There is no wrist rotation.
- Score 3 – flexion to pain: the patient flexes or bends the arm. It is characterised by internal rotation and adduction of the shoulder and flexion of the elbow, and is much slower than normal flexion (Fairley 2005).
- Score 2 – extension to pain: the patient extends the arm by straightening the elbow, sometimes associated with internal shoulder and wrist rotation, sometimes referred to as decerebrate posture (Waterhouse 2005).
- Score 1 – no response: no response to central painful stimuli.

Best practice – application of painful stimuli

Painful stimuli should be employed only if the patient fails to respond to firm and clear commands

To evaluate cerebral function, apply a central not peripheral stimulus, e.g. trapezium squeeze, supraorbital ridge pressure or pressure on the jaw margin

When applying a stimulus, start off with light pressure and increase to elicit a response

To avoid soft-tissue injury no stimulus should be applied for more than 10 seconds

PUPILLARY ASSESSMENT

Although pupillary assessment is not part of the GCS, it is an essential component of neurological assessment, especially when consciousness is impaired (Jevon 2008a). Pupillary reaction is an assessment of the third cranial nerve (oculomotor nerve) which controls constriction of the pupil. Compression of this nerve will result in fixed dilated pupils (Jevon 2008a). GCS may be difficult to assess in sedated ventilated patients, and then the pupillary reaction test indicates much about the patient's neurological status (Dawes et al. 2007). Any changes in pupil reaction, size or shape, together with other neurological signs, are an indication of raised intracranial pressure (ICP) and compression of the optic nerve (Bersten and Soni 2009).

Before undertaking pupillary assessment the following should be noted:

- Any pre-existing irregularity with the pupils, e.g. cataracts, false eye and previous eye injury
- Factors that cause pupillary dilatation, e.g. medications, including tricyclic antidepressants, atropine and sympathomimetics, and traumatic mydriasis (Jevon 2008a)
- Factors that cause pupillary constriction, e.g. medications including opiates (Fairley 2005) and topical beta blockers.

Pupillary assessment should include the following observations:

- *Size* (millimetres): before shining light into the eyes, estimate pupil size using the scale printed on the neurological assessment chart as a comparison. The average size is 2–5 mm (Jevon 2008a). Both pupils should be equal in size.
- *Shape*: should be round; abnormal shapes may indicate cerebral damage; oval shape could indicate intracranial hypertension (Fairley 2005).
- *Reactivity to light*: a bright light source (usually a pen torch) should be moved from the outer aspect of the eye towards the pupil – a brisk pupil constriction should ensue. After removal of the light source the pupil should return to its original size. The procedure should be repeated for the other eye. There should also be a consensual reaction to the light source, i.e.

both eyes constrict when the light source is applied to one. Unreactive pupils can be caused by an expanding mass, e.g. a blood clot exerting pressure on the third cranial nerve; a fixed and dilated pupil may be due to herniation of the medial temporal lobe (Bersten and Soni 2009). The reaction should be documented (see Fig. 6.1) as + or B for brisk, − or 'N' for no reaction and SL or S for some or sluggish reaction (follow local policy). Note that lens implants or cataracts may prevent the pupil from constricting to light (Waterhouse 2005).

- *Equality*: both pupils should be the same shape, size and react equally to light.

Principles of monitoring the patient with seizures

A seizure is an episode of abnormal and excessive discharge of cerebral neurons and varies in severity from being quite mild (partial) to very severe (generalised) (Fitzsimmons and Bohan 2009). During a partial seizure consciousness is impaired and the ability to respond to stimulus is impaired (Considine 2007). A generalised seizure may be non-convulsant (previously referred to as petit mal) or a tonic–clonic seizure characterised by sudden loss of consciousness, stiffening and extension of arms and legs, and forceful clamping of the jaw. This tonic phase usually lasts less than a minute, during which apnoea and cyanosis occur and pupils are dilated and unresponsive (Considine 2007). The tonic phase is followed by the clonic phase in which alternating muscle contraction and relaxation occur along with hyperventilation, eye rolling, excessive salivation, profuse sweating and tachycardia (Considine 2007). Status epilepticus is an emergency situation and requires rapid pharmacological management (Fitzsimmons and Bohan 2009). Psychogenic non-epileptic seizures (pseudo-seizures) may involve asymmetrical motor activity, side-to-side head movements and purposeful movements for many minutes, unlike true epilepsy (Fitzsimmons and Bohan 2009). It is estimated that true epilepsy exists in 20% of cases of pseudo-seizures; however, these patients usually have emotional or psychological disorders and episodes are usually a sign of abnormal coping mechanisms (Fitzsimmons and Bohan 2009). Nursing management of a patient with seizures includes:

- Assessment and thorough history taking are central to accurate diagnosis and management (Fitzsimmons and Bohan 2009)
- Airway protection and prevention of aspiration (lateral positioning) (Considine 2007)
- ABC preservation – lateral position, high-flow oxygen and intravenous (IV) access (Considine 2007)
- Provide support and protection during the seizure activity – remove objects, without applying restraint (Fitzsimmons and Bohan 2009)
- Monitor efficacy of drug therapy
- Document frequency, duration and presentation of seizures.

PRINCIPLES OF INTRACRANIAL PRESSURE MONITORING

Intracranial pressure (ICP) is the pressure exerted by the normal cerebral components (brain tissue, blood and cerebrospinal fluid [CSF]) within the rigid structure of the skull. The Monroe–Kellie hypothesis contends that to maintain a constant ICP any increase in the volume of these three elements, without a compensatory decrease in the other two elements, will lead to raised ICP (Wolfe and Torbey 2009). CSF is the most commonly displaced component and, if ICP remains high after this is displaced, cerebral blood volume is altered. When the maximal volume shift is reached further increases in intracranial volume will significantly increase ICP (Elliott et al. 2007). This can lead to a fall in cerebral perfusion pressure (CPP) resulting in reduced cerebral perfusion and inadequate oxygen delivery to the brain.

Early detection of a raised ICP is therefore essential in order to prevent increasing cerebral damage and death. There is no absolute recommendation for adequate CPP; however, 70–80 mmHg is considered the critical threshold (Elliott et al. 2007). Normal cerebral blood flow (CBF) is estimated to be 50 ml/100 g per min. When this falls below 12 ml/100 g per min, irreversible ischaemic injury occurs (Wolfe and Torbey 2009). CBF and CPP are directly related to mean arterial pressure (MAP) and ICP (Cree 2003):

$$CPP = MAP - ICP$$

MAP is the most crucial factor in maintaining cerebral perfusion (Wolfe and Torbey 2009).

Treatment is aimed at maintaining adequate CPP and oxygenation and the prevention of secondary brain injury (Brain Trauma Foundation 2007).

Vital signs

It is important to monitor the patient's vital signs because they can be dramatically affected by a rise in ICP. The centres controlling heart rate, blood pressure, respiration and temperature are located in the brain stem. Of these four vital signs, the monitoring of respirations provides the clearest indication of cerebral function because respirations are controlled by different areas of the brain (Mallett and Dougherty 2000). The rate, character and pattern of respirations must be noted. Abnormal patterns in respirations were discussed in Chapter 3.

A rising blood pressure and falling heart rate and respiratory rate are signs of raised ICP (Cushing's reflex) (Elliott et al. 2007). A sudden massive rise in ICP, e.g. after a large subarachnoid haemorrhage, can cause a Cheyne–Stokes breathing pattern (Shah 1999). Damage to the hypothalamus can cause changes in temperature.

ICP monitoring Indications

Indications for ICP monitoring include (Wolfe and Torbey 2009):

- All salvageable patients with severe traumatic brain injury (TBI) (GCS 3–8 after resuscitation) and an abnormal CT scan, i.e. haematomas, contusions, swelling, herniation or compressed basal cisterns
- Patients with severe TBI with a normal CT scan but with two of the following: >40 years, unilateral or bilateral motor posturing, or systolic BP <90 mmHg.
- Patients with non-traumatic intracranial hypertension demonstrating clinical deterioration and imaging consistent with mass effect.

METHODS OF ICP MONITORING

Principles of intraventricular catheters

An intraventricular catheter remains the gold standard in ICP monitoring and enables continuous monitoring via a transducer (Padayachy et al. 2010). Intraventricular systems have low infection rates, are considered the most reliable, accurate and inexpensive, and also facilitate drainage of CSF to control ICP (Padayachy et al. 2010). Non-invasive assessment of ICP has been explored but as yet there are no devices accurate enough to be used in clinical practice (Padayachy et al. 2010). ICP is not constant through life and healthy adults and older children have levels of 10–15 mmHg. Evidence suggests that levels persistently >20 mmHg require intervention (Wolfe and Torbey 2009). Non-invasive methods of ICP measurement such as transcranial Doppler sonography and measuring evoked potentials have been explored, but none of these methods has yet reached sufficient accuracy to be used in the clinical setting (Wolfe and Torbey 2009).

Maintaining accuracy

It is important to:

- check all connections and tubing are secure (Woodward et al. 2002)
- maintain the transducer at the same level as the foramen of Monro or at the level of the ear (Littlejohns and Trimble 2005)
- record hourly the amount of CSF drained and empty (Woodward et al. 2002)
- turn off before repositioning the patient and zero balance and recalibrate whenever the patient's position is altered (Woodward et al. 2002)
- ensure that air bubbles do not enter the transducer or tubing because this could dampen the trace and cause inaccurate ICP measurements (Littlejohns and Trimble 2005).

Suspected blockage of the drain must be reported to the neurosurgeon immediately (Woodward et al. 2002).

ICP monitoring should be continued until the ICP has stabilised and cerebral oedema has resolved, which usually occurs within 7 days (Bersten and Soni 2009).

Principles of jugular bulb oximetry monitoring

The measurement of ICP and the evaluation of CPP remains the foundation of current intracranial hypertension management, more complex monitoring such as SjO_2, may help to limit secondary injury (Wolfe and Torbey 2009). This advanced form of monitoring involves the insertion of a fibreoptic catheter into the jugular bulb and provides a continuous estimate of cerebral venous oxygen saturation and therefore an indirect assessment of cerebral perfusion (Bersten and Soni 2009; Wolfe and Torbey 2009).

Jugular venous bulb oxygen saturation monitoring (SjO_2) provides an indication of global cerebral oxygen delivery, but not regional ischaemia (Feldman and Robertson 1997). Normal values for SjO_2 range from 50% to 65% with <55% a possible indication of cerebral hypoperfusion and a high saturation >85% may indicate cerebral hyperaemia or inadequate neuronal metabolism (Bersten and Soni 2009). Both extremes are associated with adverse outcomes (Bersten and Soni 2009).

PRINCIPLES OF MONITORING SEDATION

The purpose of sedation in the critically ill patient is to ensure comfort, reduce anxiety, and facilitate treatment and interventions (Jackson et al. 2009). An appropriate level of sedation produces a calm, cooperative patient who is easier to nurse and treat (Gwinnutt 2006). Where possible the patient should still be able to communicate coherently, though in some situations, e.g. raised ICP, deeper sedation and neuromuscular blockade will be required. Benzodiazepines such as midazolam or lorazepam and the short-acting hypnotic drug propofol are the most commonly used sedative drugs (Wunsch and Kress 2009), although sedation regimens most frequently comprise concurrent infusions of opiates and sedatives.

Effects of over- and under-sedation

Historically patients in ICUs were heavily sedated to reduce movement and invoke amnesia of their ICU experience. However, more recently heavy sedation has been associated with an increase in mortality and morbidity such as delirium and prolonged length of stay (Wunsch and Kress 2009). Sedation regimens should be tailored to individual patient's needs (Aitken et al. 2008) and facilitate comfort, awareness and interaction with their family and carers. Light sedation also enables patients to be assessed for cognitive impairment, i.e. delirium, which is a significant complication of an ICU stay (Wunsch and Kress 2009). Under-sedation may lead to anxiety as well as physical dangers such as accidental extubation and self-harm (Aitken et al. 2008). A relatively new sedative dex-emetomidine provides some analgesia and anxiolysis effects and can be used for up to 24 hours in an ICU patient (Wunsch and Kress 2009). Dexemetomidine is predominantly being used for weaning agitated patients from ventilation and is demonstrating potential benefit in the clinical setting.

Assessment of sedation

There are many different sedation assessment tools currently in use such as Riker Sedation Agitation Scale (SAS), Minnesota Sedation Assessment tool and modified Riker Agitation scale (RAS); the most popular is the Ramsay scale (Jackson et al. 2009). It can be difficult to assess sedation because the needs of patients vary and there are discrepancies between practitioners' assessment (Jackson et al. 2009). Haemodynamic changes are unreliable because most ICU patients are already labile and these changes may not indicate their sedation status. As corneal reflexes remain until the patient is in a deep coma, gently brushing the tips of the patient's eye-lashes as a method of assessing whether the patient is sufficiently sedated to tolerate traumatic interventions, such as intubation, has been suggested (Woodrow 2008).

Over-sedation

Problems associated with over sedation include:

- Hypotension
- Respiratory depression
- Prevention of sleep
- Constipation
- Impaired enteral motility
- Extended weaning times from ventilation
- Ventilator-acquired pneumonia (VAP)
- Delirium
- Amnesia
- Muscle wasting
- Deep vein thrombosis (DVT).

It is also important to be familiar with the specific side effects of the analgesics or hypnotics used for sedation.

Daily sedation interruption

'Ventilator care bundles' is a set of key interventions from evidence-based guidelines which when implemented reduce the incidence of VAP and improve patient outcomes (Rello et al. 2010), including:

- No ventilator circuit change unless indicated
- Strict hand hygiene with alcohol
- Appropriately educated and trained staff
- Sedation vacation and weaning protocol
- Oral care with chlorhexidine
- Cuff pressure control at least every 24 hours
- Unit-specific microbiological surveillance with appropriate control measures
- Non-invasive ventilation preferred
- Follow a restricted transfusion policy
- Avoid stress ulcer prophylaxis
- Heat moisture exchangers (HMEs) preferred
- Use sucralfate where stress ulcer prophylaxis required
- Use of special endotracheal (ET) tubes
- Semi-recumbant positioning (30° head up)
- Selective decontamination of the gut if ventilated >48 hours.

During the process of sedation cessation the patient is allowed to wake up and be assessed for neurological state and readiness for extubation or re-sedated as required (O'Connor et al. 2008). Although some physiological and psychological benefits have been demonstrated, daily sedation interruption requires more investigation to explore the longer-term effects of this practice.

Table 6.3 The Ramsey sedation scale

Awake levels
(1) Patient anxious and agitated or restless or both
(2) Patient cooperative, oriented and tranquil
(3) Patient responds to command only

Asleep levels
(4) Brisk response
(5) Sluggish response
(6) No response

Source: Ramsey et al. (1974).

MONITORING PAIN AND PAIN RELIEF

For the purpose of this book only some basic principles of monitoring pain and pain relief are discussed. Pain management in the critically ill patient is discussed in more detail in Chapter 14.

Causes of pain

The patient may have acute pain, e.g. after surgery, or chronic pain, e.g. osteoarthritis, which makes pain management more complex for such patients. Procedures in the ICU that have been identified to exhibit a pain behavioural response include (Puntillo et al. 2004):

- Removal of femoral sheath
- Central venous catheter insertion
- Tracheal suctioning
- Wound care
- Wound drain removal
- Turning.

Assessing pain

Self-report is considered the most reliable method of pain assessment and patients should be provided with methods and tools to be able to describe the location and intensity of their pain wherever possible, particularly as many patients are unable to self-report pain (Puntillo et al. 2009; Gelinas et al. 2011). When a patient is unable to self-report pain, valid behavioural scales are frequently utilised; however, often patients may not be able to display behavioural signs and when they do they may not be a reliable indicator of pain (Gelinas et al. 2011)

The use of pain assessment tools improves pain control (Puntillo et al. 2009); available tools are discussed in detail in Chapter 14.

Relieving/preventing pain

The pioneering research carried out by Hayward (1975) demonstrated that preparation and honest explanations reduce pain, analgesia requirements and recovery time. Good communication is essential.

Methods of pain relief in the critically ill patient include pharmacological, by a variety of routes: intravenous (e.g. fentanyl, ketamine, morphine), regional (e.g. epidurals), sublingual (e.g.

buprenorphine), transdermal (e.g. fentanyl), oral (e.g. oxycodone) and inhaled (e.g. nitrous oxide). Also non-pharmacological therapies can be utilised (e.g. massage). After administration of the chosen pain relief, it is crucial to evaluate the effectiveness of the intervention (Macintyre and Schug 2007). The use of a pain assessment tool appropriate for the patient and type of pain is essential in the assessment and adequate management of pain (Macintyre and Schug 2007). It is also important to be alert to the possible side effects of pain relief, e.g. respiratory depression following opioid administration.

Epidural analgesia

Epidural analgesia is one of the most effective methods for the management of acute pain (Macintyre and Schug 2007) and is considered to be the gold standard mode of analgesia after major surgery (Chumbley and Thomas 2010). A catheter is inserted into the epidural space and analgesia (e.g. fentanyl) and an anaesthetic (e.g. 0.125% bupivacaine) can be administered either continuously through an infusion in postoperative patients or by bolus injections via nurse or patient-controlled bolus. The insertion site should be checked for leaks, signs of skin irritation and infection (Macintyre and Schug 2007). Close monitoring of the patient is essential to identify any complications which could include:

- respiratory depression
- hypotension due to blockage of sympathetic nerves
- pruritis due to opiates
- urinary retention due to inhibition of the micturition reflex
- bradycardia due to local anaesthetic travelling (Chumbley and Thomas 2010) above T4
- motor block.

Epidural observations are usually recorded on a separate chart from standard observation charts. The following parameters should be monitored and recorded at intervals dictated by local policy:

- Pain score, sedation score and respiratory rate
- BP and heart rate
- Sensory block using the Bromage score
- Motor block.

Scenario

A 25-year-old man is admitted to the emergency department with a head injury after falling off his bicycle. He is fully conscious, talking to you and there are no obvious injuries. What are your initial monitoring priorities?

The airway is clear and the neck is immobilised in a hard collar before cervical spinal injury can be excluded. BP 120/70 mmHg, respiratory rate 15/min, pulse 90/min, SpO_2 98%, GCS 15; pupils are medium and both reacting equally and briskly to light. A CT scan is ordered. What ongoing monitoring will the patient require?

The patient's vital signs, SpO_2, GCS and pupillary assessment continue to be monitored. The patient starts to demonstrate signs of confusion. BP 120/75, pulse 94/min, SpO_2 97%, GCS 13; pupils are medium and both reacting equally and briskly to light. What can be deducted from these observations?

The patient's vital signs are stable, but the slight drop in the GCS is of concern. The patient is taken for a CT scan. During the procedure his conscious level falls dramatically. BP 170/100, pulse 55, respiratory rate 10/min, SpO_2 96%, GCS 9. He is responding and localising to pain and making incomprehensible sounds. His right pupil is dilated and not reacting to light. The left pupil is medium and reacting briskly to light. What can be deducted from these observations?

A right-sided subdural haematoma is confirmed by the CT scan. A rise in BP, fall in heart and respiratory rates, and the deterioration in conscious level are signs consistent with a raised intracranial pressure. The unresponsive right pupil is consistent with third cranial nerve compression secondary to the right-sided subdural lesion. Urgent neurosurgical referral is required. Ongoing monitoring must continue with particular attention to maintenance of a clear airway.

CONCLUSION

Monitoring neurological function is central to the care of all critically ill patients, particularly those with a head injury or other cerebral insult. It enables the early recognition and treatment of complications and can improve prognosis. It can also provide an indication of the function of other major systems in the body. The administration of medications, e.g. sedatives and paralysing agents, and any recent alcohol consumption should be taken into account.

REFERENCES

Aitken, L. M., Marshall, A. P., Elliott, R. & McKinley, S. (2008) Critical care nurses' decision making: sedation assessment and management in intensive care. *Journal of Clinical Nursing*, **18**, 36–45.

Bersten, A. D. & Soni, N., eds (2009) *Oh's Intensive Care Manual*, 6th edn. Philadelphia, PA: Butterworth Heinemann Wlsevier.

Brain Trauma Foundation (2007) Indications for intracranial pressure monitoring. *Journal of Neurotrauma*, **24**(suppl 1), S37–S44.

Caton-Richards, M. (2010) Assessing the neurological status of patients with head injuries: a guide on using the Glasgow Coma Scale in emergency departments to assess patients who have sustained head injuries. (Report) *Emergency Nurse*, **17**(10), 28.

Chamberlain, D. & Swope, W. (2007a) *Support of Neurological Function*. Sydney: Mosby Elsevier.

Chamberlain, D. & Swope, W. (2007b) Support of neurological function. In: Elliott, D., Aitken, L. & Chaboyer, W. (eds), *ACCCN's Critical Care Nursing*. Marrickville, NSW: Mosby Elsevier.

Chumbley, G. & Thomas, S. (2010) Care of the patient receiving epidural analgesia. *Nursing Standard*, **3**(9), 35–40.

Ciechanowski, M., Mower-Wade, D. & McLeskey, S. W. (2009) Anatomy and physiology of the nervous system. In: Gonce Morton, P. & Fontaine, D. K. (eds), *Critical Care Nursing: A holistic approach*, 9th edn. Philadelphia, PA: Wolters Kluwer Lippincott Williams & Wilkins.

Considine, J. (2007) Neurologic emergencies. In: Curtis, K., Ramsden, C. & Friendship, J. (eds), *Emergency and Trauma Nursing*. Marrickville, NSW: Mosby Elsevier.

Cree, C. (2003) Aquired brain injury: acute management. *Nursing Standard*, **18**(11), 45–54.

Dawes, E., Lloyd, H. & Durham, L. (2007) Monitoring and recording patients' neurological observations. *Nursing Standard*, **22**(10), 40–45.

Elliott, D., Aitken, L. & Chaboyer, W., eds (2007) *Critical Care Nursing*. Marrickville, NSW: Mosby Elsevier.

Fairley, D. (2005) Using a coma scale to assess patient consciousness levels. *Nursing Times*, **101**(25), 38–47.

Feldman, Z. & Robertson, C. (1997) Monitoring of cerebral haemodynamics with jugular bulb catheters. *Critical Care Clinics* **13**(1), 51–77.

Fitzsimmons, B. & Bohan, E. (2009) Common neurosurgical and neurological disorders. In: Gonce Morton, P. & Fontaine, D. K. (eds), *Critical Care Nursing: A holistic approach*, 9th edn. Philadelphia, PA: Wolters Kluwr Lippincott Williams & Wilkins.

Gelinas, C., Tousignant-Laflamme, Y., Tanguay, A. & Bourgault, P. (2011) Exploring the validity of the bispectral index, the critical-care pain observation tool and vital signs for the detection of pain in sedated and mechanically ventilated critically ill adults: A pilot study. *Intensive and Critical Care Nursing*, **27**, 46–52.

Geraghty, M. (2005) Nursing the unconscious patient. *Nursing Standard*, **20**(1), 54–64.

Gwinnutt, C. (2006) *Clinical Anaesthesia*, 2nd edn. Oxford: Blackwell Publishing.

Hayward, J. (1975) *Information: A Prescription Against Pain*. London: Royal College of Nursing.

Holdgate, A. (2006) Variability in agreement between physicians and nurses when measuring the Glasgow Coma Scale in the emergency department limits its clinical usefulness. *Emergency Medicine Australasia*, **18**, 379–384.

Jackson, D. L., Proudfoot, C. W., Cann, K. F. & Walsh, T. S. (2009) The incidence of sub-optimal sedation in the ICU: a systematic review. *Critical Care*, **13**(6), R204

Jenkins, P. F. & Johnson, P. H. (2010) *Making sense of Acute Medicine*. London: Hodder Arnold.

Jevon, P. (2008a) Neurological assessment part 2 – Pupillary assessment. *Nursing Times*, **104**(28), 28–29.

Jevon, P. (2008b) Neurological assessment part 4 – Glasgow Coma Scale 2. *Nursing Times*, **104**(30), 24–25.

Littlejohns, L. R. & Trimble, B. (2005) Ask the experts. *Critical Care Nurse*, **25**(3), 57–59.

Macintyre, P. E. & Schug, S. A. (2007) *Acute Pain Management*, 3rd edn. Philadelphia, PA: Saunders Elsevier.

Mallett, J. & Dougherty, L., eds (2000) *The Royal Marsden Hospital Manual of Clinical Nursing Procedures*. Oxford: Blackwell Science.

Mooney, G. P. & Comerford, D. M. (2003) Neurological observations. *Nursing Times*, **99**(17), 24–25.

National Institute fior Health and Clinical Excellence (2007) *Head Injury: Triage, assessment, investigation and early management of head injury in infants, children and adults*. London: NICE.

O'Connor, M., Bucknall, T. & Manias, E. (2008) A critical review of daily sedation interruption in the intensive care unit. *Journal of Clinical Nursing*, **18**.

Padayachy, L. C., Figaji, A. A. & Bullock, M. R. (2010) Intracranial pressure monitoring for traumatic brain injury in the modern era. *Children's Nervous System*, **26**, 441–452.

Puntillo, K., Morris, A. B., Thompson, C., Stanik-Hutt, J., White, C. A. & Wild, L. R. (2004) Pain behaviours observed during six common procedures: Results from Thunder Project II. *Critical Care Medicine*, **32**, 421–427.

Puntillo, K., Pasero, C., Li, D., et al. (2009) Evaluation of pain in ICU patients. *Chest*, **135**, 1069–1074.

Rabiu, T. (2011) Revisiting the eye opening response of the Glasgow Coma Scale (Rapid Communication) (Report). *Indian Journal of Critical Care Medicine*, **15**(1), 58.

Ramsey, M., Savage, T., Simpson, B., et al. (1974) Controlled sedation with alphaxalone and alphadolone. *British Medical Journal*, **ii**, 656–659.

Rello, J., Lode, H., Cornaglia, G. & Masterton, R. (2010) A European care bundle for prevention of ventilator-associated pneumonia. *Intensive Care Medicine*, **36**, 773–780.

Resuscitation Council UK (2011) *Advanced Life Support*, 6th edn. London: Resuscitation Council UK.

Shah, S. (1999) Neurological assessment. *Nursing Standard*, **13**(22), 49–54.

Teasdale, G. & Jennett, B. (1974) Assessment of coma and impaired consciousness: a practical scale. *The Lancet*, **ii**, 81–84.

Venkatesh, B. (2009) *Disorders of Consciousness*, 6th edn. Philadelphia: Butterworth Heinemann.

Waterhouse, C. (2005) The Glasgow Coma Scale and other neurological observations. *Nursing Standard*, **19**(33), 56–64.

Wolfe, T. J. & Torbey, M. T. (2009) Management of intracranial pressure. *Current Neurology and Neuroscince Reports*, **9**, 477–485.

Woodrow, P. (2008) *Intensive Care Nursing a Framework for Practice*, 2nd edn. New York: Routledge.

Woodward, S. (1997) Neurological observations – Glasgow Coma Scale. *Nursing Times*, **93**(45), Suppl 1–2.

Woodward, S., Addison, C., Shah, S. *et al.* (2002) Benchmarking best practice for external ventricular drainage. *British Journal of Nursing*, **11**(1), 47–52.

Wunsch, H. & Kress, J. P. (2009) A new era for sedation in ICU patients. *Journal of the American Medical Association*, **301**, 542–544.

Zink, E. (2009) Traumatic brain injury. In: Gonce Morton, P. & Fontaine, D. K. (eds), *Critical Care Nursing: A holistic approach*, 9th edn. Philadelphia, PA: Wolters Kluwer Lippincott Williams & Wilkins

Zuercher, M., Ummenhofer, W., Baltussen, A. & Walder, B. (2009) The use of Glasgow Coma Scale in injury assessment: A critical review. *Brain Injury*, **23**, 371–384.

Monitoring Renal Function

7

LEARNING OBJECTIVES

At the end of the chapter the reader will be able to:

❑ describe the principles of *urinalysis*
❑ discuss the principles of *urine output monitoring*
❑ outline the key principles of monitoring *fluid balance*
❑ discuss the management of *acute renal failure*
❑ outline the key aspects of *monitoring during renal replacement therapy*

INTRODUCTION

Renal function should be closely monitored in all critically ill patients. First, it can provide an indication of the function of other systems, e.g. the cardiovascular system, where a low cardiac output will result in a diminished urine output. Nurses play a key role in the prevention and early detection of acute renal failure (ARF) (Murphy and Byrne 2010). The early recognition and prompt treatment of ARF are essential if prognosis is to be maximised. Patients receiving renal replacement therapy (RRT) are a frequent occurrence in ICU and these patients should also be closely monitored.

The aim of this chapter is to understand the principles of monitoring renal function.

Monitoring the Critically Ill Patient, Third Edition.
Philip Jevon, Beverley Ewens.
© 2012 Blackwell Publishing Ltd. Published 2012 by Blackwell Publishing Ltd.

PRINCIPLES OF URINALYSIS

Urinalysis can provide the health-care professional with valuable information about health status such as: indications of renal, urological and liver disease, diabetes mellitus, urinary tract infection (UTI) and general hydration (Steggall 2007). This important information ascertained from urinalysis can assist in diagnosis of new disease processes and also in the monitoring of existing conditions. The purpose of urinalysis is threefold:

1. *Screening* for systemic disease, e.g. diabetes mellitus, renal conditions
2. *Diagnosis*: confirm or exclude suspected conditions, e.g. UTIs
3. *Management and planning*: to monitor the progress of an existing condition and/or plan programmes of care (Bishop 2008).

Appearance of urine

Normal urine is clear and yellow to straw coloured, practically odourless but becomes turbid and smells of ammonia if left to stand (Bishop 2008; Snyder 2009b). Variations in the appearance of urine include the following:

- *Pale*: urine is very clear and colourless; causes include diuresis pharmacologically induced or by diabetes insipidus or diabetes mellitus.
- *Dark*: urine is concentrated as seen in fluid depletion or contains conjugated bilirubin in jaundice (Jenkins and Johnson 2010).
- *Orange*: usually caused by specific drugs, e.g. rifampicin (Bishop 2008).
- *Pink/red*: may indicate haematuria, though other causes include ingestion of certain foodstuffs, e.g. beetroot (Bishop 2008).
- *Cloudy*: may indicate the presence of pus, protein or white cells and requires further investigation (Steggall 2007).
- *Sediment:* is particulate material and comprises casts, red cells, white cells, epithelial cells and crystals, which are products of breakdown of cellular materials formed in the collecting tubules. Urinary stasis promotes cast formation which is often present in prerenal disease.
- *Frothy*: may indicate significant proteinuria.

Odour

Normal, freshly voided urine is practically odourless. If left to stand for several hours it acquires a mild smell of ammonia (Bishop 2008). Infected urine has a 'fishy' smell (Bishop 2008). In patients with diabetes who have ketoacidosis or in patients who are anorexic or not eating, acetone is excreted in the urine causing the urine to smell characteristicall'y sweet (Steggall 2007).

Urinary incontinence

Urinary incontinence can occur transiently. Causes include UTIs, delirium, excess urine output, e.g. following diuretics, faecal impaction, immobility (patient unable to reach the toilet or use a urinal) and spinal cord compression (necessitating emergency surgery).

Procedure for dipstick test of urine

A dipstick test of urine can accurately show the presence of a variety of substances, e.g. protein, glucose, ketones and blood, as well as the pH. To ensure reliable results, the following procedure for dipstick urine testing is recommended:

- Check the expiry date on the container, ensuring that the testing strips are in date.
- Remove a testing strip from the container and replace the cap straight away.
- Dip the testing strip into a fresh sample of urine, ensuring that all the reagent pads of the strip are covered. The urine must be fresh because stored urine rapidly deteriorates which can cause false results (Dougherty and Lister 2011).
- Wipe off any excess urine on the rim of the specimen container.
- Place the testing strip flat on a dry surface to prevent the urine from running from square to square resulting in reagents mixing together. This may lead to an inaccurate result.
- Compare the reagent pads with the colour scale at time intervals stipulated by the manufacturer. If the strips are not read at exactly the time intervals specified, the reagents may not have had time to react which could cause inaccurate results (Dougherty and Lister 2011).
- Discard the urine sample and used testing strip.
- Record the results in the patient's notes and report any abnormalities.

It is essential to store and use the reagent strips correctly, following the manufacturer's recommendations, in order to ensure accurate and reliable results. The package insert supplied by the manufacturers will contain detailed instructions which normally include the following general points:

- The reagent strip should be stored in the container supplied by the manufacturer.
- The container cap should be replaced as soon as the reagent strip has been removed.
- The desiccant should never be removed from the bottle – some manufacturers incorporate it into the lid of the container so that it cannot be lost.
- The container should be stored in a cool dry place, but not refrigerated.
- Reagent strips should not be used after the expiry date on the container.

Some drugs can influence urinalysis, e.g. high doses of aspirin or levodopa can cause a false-negative reaction to glycosuria (Wilson 2005). It is therefore paramount to take into account the patient's medication when examining the results of dipstick urinalysis.

Best practice – urinalysis

Always use a fresh sample of urine collected in a clean, dry container
Observe sample for colour, appearance, smell and debris
Ensure that reagent strip is in date
Ensure that whole of reagent strip is immersed in urine sample
Wipe off excess urine, place horizontal and compare reagent pads with colour scale at time intervals stipulated by manufacturer, and document results immediately
Safely discard strip and urine sample
Store reagent strips following manufacturer's recommendations

---

Significance of the results

Glycosuria is not present in the urine under normal conditions (Snyder 2009a). Glucose is present when blood glucose is raised >10 mmol/l (Bishop 2008) and the concentration of glucose in plasma exceeds the renal threshold (Wilson 2005). The most common cause is diabetes mellitus. Glycosuria can also be a sign of physiological stress, when patients are taking corticosteroids and in pregnancy (Steggall 2007). If glycosuria is discovered a fasting blood glucose analysis is recommended (Steggall 2007; Bishop 2008).

Ketones (ketonuria) are byproducts of fat metabolism (Snyder 2009a) and are suggestive of excessive fat breakdown as in starvation, fasting and uncontrolled diabetes mellitus (Steggall 2007).

Proteinuria is the presence of abnormally large quantities of protein, usually albumin (it is sometimes therefore termed albuminuria). Normally, no more than a trace of protein should be found in urine because protein molecules are too large to penetrate Bowman's capsule (Snyder 2009a). Proteinuria is indicative of damage to the capillary structures as in glomerular and intrarenal disease (Snyder 2009a). Persistent proteinuria may indicate infection or advanced diabetic renal disease (Bishop 2008). Protein loss can be increased during febrile illness or after vigorous exercise

Persistent proteinuria is usually a sign of renal disease, e.g. UTI or pyelonephritis, or a renal complication of another disease, e.g. hypertension, congestive cardiac failure and pre-eclampsia. False-positive results can occur with alkaline urine and the use of disinfectants such as chlorhexidine.

The presence of blood (haematuria) is associated with diseases of the kidney or urinary tract, commonly infection, calculi, benign prostatic hypertrophy, coagulopathy, polycystic kidney, trauma, glomerular nephritis and tumours. Haematuria can also be caused by fractures of the pelvis and be present during menstruation (Wilson 2005). Dipstick urinalysis cannot distinguish red blood cells from myoglobin and haemoglobin so microscopic techniques are recommended to confirm the presence of blood cells (McDonald et al. 2006). The presence of haemoglobin (haemoglobinuria) suggests a reaction to a blood transfusion, haemolytic anaemia or severe burns (Dougherty and Lister 2011). Reduction of sensitivity of the agent can occur if the patient is taking ascorbic acid or captopril (Wilson 2005).

Bilirubin is not normally detectable in urine (bilirubinuria) and its presence is usually indicative of liver or gallbladder disease, such as hepatitis, advanced cirrhosis, gallstones or carcinoma of the pancreas (Wilson 2005).

Urobilinogen presence in the urine is related to the production and conversion of bilirubin to urobilinogen in the gastrointestinal tract (Wilson 2005). Traces are normal but elevated levels indicate liver damage or an abnormal breakdown of red blood cells such as in hepatitis, sickle cell disease, thalassaemia, haemolytic or pernicious anaemia, infectious hepatitis, biliary obstruction, jaundice, cirrhosis, congestive cardiac failure or infectious mononucleosis (Tortora and Derrickson 2011).

Nitrite is strongly indicative of infection (Jenkins and Johnson 2010), although a negative result does not rule out infection (Bishop 2008). Nitrites are found in urine only in the presence of infection (Wilson 2005), as infective organisms convert nitrate to nitrite. False-positive results can occur in patients taking vitamin C (Rigby and Gray 2005).

White blood cells in urine (pyuria) usually indicate infection somewhere along the urinary tract (Snyder 2009a) and is an indication for laboratory testing. False-negative results can be caused by glycosuria and drugs such as nitrofurantoin and rifampicin (Rigby and Gray 2005).

The normal range of urine pH is 5–8 (Steggall 2007). Urine pH is an indicator of the degree of hydrogen ion secretion and the reabsorption of bicarbonate ions. Acidic urine (pH < 7.0) is found in patients with diabetic ketoacidosis, starvation, calculi formation, high-protein diet and potassium depletion. Alkaline urine (pH > 7.0) may be indicative of a UTI, or caused by vomiting or excessive intake of antacids (Wilson 2005). Diet has a large influence on the pH of urine; a protein-rich diet may give rise to acidic urine and a diet high in vegetables or dairy may give rise to alkaline urine (Steggall 2007). The specific gravity (SG) of urine is a measure of total solute concentration (Steggall 2007), and an indicator of the kidneys' ability to concentrate and dilute the urine (Snyder 2009a). The normal SG range is 1.001–1.035 (Bishop 2008). Urine of high SG is concentrated and a urine with a low SG is dilute (Bishop 2008). High values are indicative of dehydration and low values are found with high fluid intake, diabetes insipidus, renal failure, hypercalcaemia or hypokalaemia (Wilson 2005).

Other urine tests
Osmolality
The main determinants of osmolality (number of solute particles present in a solution) are sodium, urea and glucose, the normal range being 300–900 mosmol/kg per 24h (Snyder 2009a). As a result of the dynamic interrelationship of sodium, urea and glucose in critical illness a single value of urine osmolality is of little value (Snyder 2009a).

Creatinine clearance
Creatinine clearance is the standard test to assess glomerular function. The principle of clearance is that an estimation of a known substance (which is excreted only in the urine) in the plasma is compared with the amount in the urine. Creatinine is produced by the breakdown of creatinine phosphate, which is manufactured by the muscle mass at a fairly constant rate. It is present in the circulation and is filtered by the glomeruli.

Microscopy and culture
Being the most concentrated, the first voided urine of the day is the best for culture. Ideally the sample should be taken before starting a broad-spectrum antibiotic, which may be given in the interim period before a specific sensitivity is identified.

URINE OUTPUT MONITORING
Although urine output is only an index to renal perfusion, it is frequently used as a guide to the adequacy of cardiac output (renal perfusion amounts to 25% of the cardiac output). However, the use of diuretics, such as frusemide, abolishes its value as a haemodynamic monitor (Gomersall and Oh 1997).

Urine is composed of 95% water and 5% solids, mainly urea and sodium chloride; it is slightly acidic (pH 6.0) and has an SG of 1.010–1.030 (SG of water is 1.000) (Wilson 2005). The average urine output in a healthy adult is 1000–1500ml/day (Snyder 2009a). Listed below are the generally accepted rates of urine production associated with urinary output disorders (Tortora and Derrickson 2011):

- Anuria: <50ml urine in 24h
- Oliguria: <400ml urine in 24h

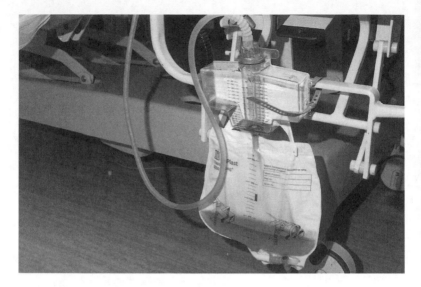

Fig. 7.1 Hourly urine drainage bag.

- Polyuria: >3000 ml urine in 24 h
- Dysuria: painful micturition.

All critically ill patients will require a urinary catheter. If urine output measurements are required the patient should be catheterised and an hourly urine drainage bag attached (Fig. 7.1). The urinary catheter should be closely monitored because it can become blocked, e.g. from a blood clot, or become occluded, e.g. due to kinking. If urine output dramatically falls, always consider mechanical obstruction first. Bladder volume assessment is now readily available via bedside bladder scanners Sometimes bladder washouts are indicated (intermittent or continuous) if difficulties with drainage are encountered, e.g. if there is a lot of debris or blood clots in the urine.

MONITORING FLUID BALANCE
Monitoring fluid balance in critical illness is paramount. Constant monitoring and vigilance by the nurse coupled with an understand-

ing of disease processes are vital because clinical conditions can deteriorate rapidly (Murphy and Byrne 2010). Fluid and electrolyte overload is sometimes difficult to avoid because in critical illness the basic senses such as hunger and thirst are abolished by disease processes or treatments. Therefore survival depends on the appropriate administration of volumes of fluids and appropriate quantities of electrolytes and nutrition to match often excessive losses.

Careful monitoring of the fluid balance chart must be maintained and this should include all input and output. Monitoring the patient for signs of fluid loss/gain should also be undertaken and Table 7.1 provides an overview of this. The importance of monitoring urine output, urine osmolality and specific gravity of urine has already been discussed.

Daily measurement of serum sodium, potassium, urea and creatinine is required to assess fluid and electrolyte balance. In addition, fluid balance charts from the preceding few days should be compared with serum and urine urea and electrolyte values. This will help evaluate the patient's response to fluid administration and guide the fluid regimen over the next 12–24 hours. The nature and volume of any fluid replacement therapy will depend on fluid losses.

MANAGEMENT OF ACUTE RENAL FAILURE

Acute renal failure, or acute kidney injury (AKI) as it is being termed in the literature, is a syndrome characterised by a rapid (hours to days) decrease in the kidneys' ability to eliminate waste products, which results in an accumulation of end-products of nitrogen metabolism (urea and creatinine). It has been reported to occur in up to 20% of the ICU population, with associated high mortality rates of 60–80%, particularly if multiorgan dysfunction syndrome (MODS) coexists.

The kidney is a very vascular organ and acquires about 25% of cardiac output (Murphy and Byrne 2010). Prerenal failure, i.e. when the kidney is affected by systemic factors that cause a reduction in the glomerular filtration rate (GFR), is by far the most common form in critical illness (Bellomo 2009). Inadequate renal perfusion resulting from reduced cardiac output, hypotension or raised intra-abdominal pressure leads to reduced GFR (Bellomo

Table 7.1 Systemic signs and symptoms of fluid loss and gain

System	Signs in fluid loss	Signs in fluid gain	Monitoring and nursing observation
Cardiovascular	Increase heart rate Irregular thready pulse Reduced blood pressure and CVP	Increased heart rate, BP, CVP Neck vein distension may be evident	Pulse Blood pressure CVP
Respiratory	Increased respiratory rate Hyperventilation	Increased rate Dyspnoea and pulmonary oedema may be evident	Nature and frequency of respirations Signs of waterlogging of pulmonary circulation Oxygenation status – skin colour Saturation, i.e. pulse oximetry/blood gases
Urinary system	Urine output decreased, or increased in diabetes insipidus	Output may be increased or decreased depending on the underlying cause and renal function	Volume of urine output/24-hour period
General orientation	Apprehension Restlessness	Confusion Irritability	General orientation status
Skin	Texture is dry and lax, under-perfusion of tissues and reduced vascularity leading to skin colour change, dry mucous membranes and evidence of thirst Excessive perspiration accompanies increased body temperature	Dependent, generalised and/or pitting oedema The skin may be warm, moist and swollen with the appearance of being tight and shiny	General appearance/ hydrational status Colour Temperature Condition of mucous membranes

Reprinted by permission of Baillière Tindall from Sheppard & Wright (2000).

2009). However, around 50–60% of patients who have ARF will revert to normal renal function after treatment (Murphy and Byrne 2010). ARF can be attributed to a multiplicity of different diseases and pathophysiological mechanisms and is classified according to precipitating factors:

- *Prerenal*: caused by inadequate renal perfusion due to (Holcombe and Kern Feeley 2009; Murphy and Byrne 2010):
  - Decreased intravascular volume:
    - Dehydration
    - Haemorrhage
    - Hypovolaemic shock
    - Third-space losses, e.g. burns
  - Cardiovascular failure:
    - Heart failure
    - Myocardial infarction (MI)
    - Cardiogenic shock
    - Valvular heart disease
  - Drugs:
    - Angiotensin-converting enzyme (ACE) inhibitors
    - Non-steroidal anti-inflammatory drugs (NSAIDs)
    - Ciclosporin
    - Radiocontrast dye
    - Ethylene glycol (anti-freeze)
    - anaesthetics
  - Decreased effective renal perfusion:
    - Sepsis
    - Cirrhosis
    - Neurogenic shock
- *Intrinsic (parenchymal)*: occurs when there is structural damage to the renal parenchyma such as acute tubular necrosis (ATN). ATN occurs because of sustained renal hypoperfusion (Perkins and Kisiel 2005). Causes include (Bellomo 2009):
  - Glomerulonephritis
  - Vasculitis
  - Interstitial nephritis
  - Malignant hypertension
  - Pyelonephritis
  - Bilateral cortical necrosis

- Amyloidosis
- Malignancy
- Nephrotoxins
- *Postrenal*: caused by obstruction of urine drainage due to (Holcombe and Kern Feeley 2009):
  - Ureteral obstruction:
    - Intrinsic – stones, carcinoma of the ureter, blood clots, strictures
  - Bladder obstruction:
    - Tumours
    - Blood clots
    - Neurogenic bladder – due to spinal cord injury, diabetes mellitus, ischaemia, drugs
  - Urethral obstruction:
    - Prostate cancer or benign hypertrophy
    - Stones
    - Strictures
    - Blood clots
    - Blocked in-dwelling catheter.

Diagnosis

The clinical presentation of ARF despite adequate resuscitation:

- Anuria or profound oliguria
- Progressive rise in blood creatinine and urea levels
- Developing metabolic acidosis
- Rising serum potassium and phosphate levels
- MODS is common.

Clinical course

The clinical course of ARF can be classified into three distinct phases (Murphy and Byrne 2010):

1. *Initial phase*: this is the phase between the exposure to the insult and a reduction in renal function when renal damage can be reversed
2. *Maintenance phase*: this can last from days to weeks or sporadically up to 2 months; during this time renal damage cannot be reversed. Patients can be anuric, oliguric or non-oliguric during this time.

2. *Recovery phase*: this is marked by a return to normal ranges of urea and creatinine. Patients may experience a polyuric stage when fluid and electrolyte imbalances may occur.

Prevention of ARF

Due to the poor prognosis, prevention of ARF in critical illness is paramount. The fundamental prevention strategy in ARF is to treat the cause (Bellomo 2009). If prerenal factors are likely to contribute they must be identified quickly and resuscitation instigated without delay (Bellomo 2009). Murphy and Byrne (2010) suggest the following to attempt to prevent ARF:

- Early identification of those patients at risk based on pre-existing disease, type of surgery planned and planned use of nephrotoxic substances
- Maintenance of euvolaemia and stable haemodynamics
- Invasive monitoring where indicated and accurate interpretation of results
- Avoidance of hypoxia
- Intravenous acetylcysteine for the prevention of radiocontrast nephropathy
- Monitoring of levels of nephrotoxic drugs and avoidance of using two together.

Complications of ARF

Hyperkalaemia is a serious electrolyte imbalance seen in ARF (Holcombe and Kern Feeley 2009). Characteristic ECG changes include elevated and pointed T waves. Cardiac arrhythmias and cardiac arrest may ensue and active treatment is normally required, e.g. insulin (and dextrose), RRT and in extreme situations intravenous calcium chloride. Continuous cardiac monitoring is essential to ensure early detection of cardiac arrhythmias. Metabolic acidosis is also a serious complication of ARF and may be intensified in critical illness due to the patient's high metabolic rate which releases intracellular acids (Holcombe and Kern Feeley 2009). In severe metabolic acidosis bradycardia and hypotension may manifest due to myocardial suppression. Sodium bicarbonate is reserved for severe metabolic acidosis only, due to complications of extracellular volume increases, metabolic alkalosis and hypokalaemia. Refractory acidosis is an indicator for the commencement of RRT.

Patients with ARF are immunosuppressed and are therefore at greater risk of developing infections such as pneumonia, UTI, wound infection and sepsis, which can be a major cause of mortality (Murphy and Byrne 2010).

Adequate nutritional support is required. Nutrition in critical illness is always preferred by the enteral route; however, patients in ARF may require parenteral nutrition (TPN) because they may have impaired gastrointestinal (GI) function and absorption capacity (Holcombe and Kern Feeley 2009). Patients who are critically ill need their caloric requirements met and adequate protein intake to prevent further catabolism. Protein restriction in ARF is controversial and should not compromise meeting anabolic needs (Holcombe and Kern Feeley 2009). Whichever method of nutrition is instigated regular monitoring of the patient must be undertaken, i.e. serum protein, electrolytes, haemoglobin and urea are essential. Potassium, sodium and fluid intake should be restricted if the patient is not on RRT. Close monitoring of blood glucose levels is essential, particularly if the patient is on dietary supplements.

The patient who is in the oliguric phase of ARF requires careful fluid balance assessment. To prevent volume overload, a general working rule is the previous day's urine output plus 500 ml for insensible loss. Consideration must be given to such variables as pyrexia, diarrhoea and wound drainage.

Serial weights may be more reliable than fluid balance assessment but are not widely used due to technical difficulties; rapid daily gains and losses in weight are usually related to changes in fluid volume. It is also important to observe for signs of fluid overload, e.g. raised central venous pressure (CVP), generalised oedema, pulmonary oedema and dyspnoea.

Clinical features of uraemia include nausea, vomiting, hiccoughs, confusion, irritability, altered conscious level, infection and bleeding. It is important to observe for these complications and treat appropriately.

Criteria for the initiation of RRT:

- Oliguria (urine output: <200 ml/12 h)
- Anuria (urine output 0–50 ml/12 h)
- Urea >35 mmol/l
- Creatinine >400 μmol/l

- K^+ >6.5 mmol/l or rapidly rising
- Pulmonary oedema unresponsive to diuretics
- Uncompensated metabolic acidosis (pH <7.1)
- Na^+ <110 and >160 mmol/l
- Temperature >40°C
- Uraemic complications (encephalopathy, neuropathy, pericarditis)
- Overdose with a dialysable toxin, e.g. lithium.

If two of the above criteria are met, RRT is strongly recommended (Bellomo 2009).

MONITORING DURING RENAL REPLACEMENT THERAPY

Renal replacement therapy in the ICU is usually continuous venovenous haemodiafiltration, which is an extracorporeal venous system whereby blood is driven through a semi-permeable membrane to remove water, electrolytes, and small- and medium-sized molecules from the blood via diffusion, osmosis and convection (Bellomo 2009) (Fig. 7.2). Venous access is via a double lumen

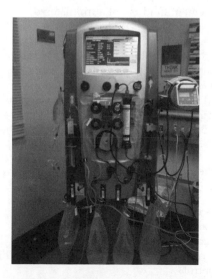

Fig. 7.2 Continuous renal replacement therapy.

venous catheter often in the internal jugular, subclavian or femoral veins. To maximise the removal of solutes dialysate fluid is added to the circuit, which flows in a countercurrent direction to the blood around the fibres of the filter. Modern methods of RRT minimise the risks associated with intermittent haemodialysis, e.g. haemodynamic instability and should be instigated early in ARF in the critically ill patient (Bellomo 2009).

RRT has many modalities:

- *Continuous venovenous haemofiltration (CVVH)*: blood is driven through the semi-permeable membrane filter and replacement fluid is added to prevent excessive loss of fluid. Solutes are mainly removed by convection.
- *Slow continuous ultrafiltration (SCUF)*: blood is driven through the semi-permeable membrane filter but there is no fluid replacement. SCUF is utilised for fluid removal in fluid overload, as solute clearance is very low.
- *Continuous venovenous haemodialysis (CVVHD)*: Blood is driven through the semi-permeable membrane filter with the addition of a countercurrent dialysate solution to improve solute clearance. Replacement fluid is not administered.
- *Continuous venovenous haemodiafiltration (CVVHDF)*: CVVHDF is the same principle as CVVHD but with the addition of replacement fluid to balance fluid losses. This is the most frequently used modality in the ICU patient with ARF.
- *Intermittent haemodialysis (IHD)*: uses high dialysate flows (300–400 ml/min) by mixing purified water and concentrate and treatment can be instituted over 8–10 h. However, CVVHDF is considered physiologically superior to IHD in the correction of metabolic acidosis (Ronco and Ricci 2008).

Whatever the chosen modality of RRT the following outcomes are achievable (Bellomo 2009):

1. Continuous control of fluid status
2. Haemodynamic stability
3. Control of acid–base status
4. Ability to provide protein-rich nutrition while achieving uraemic control

5. Control of electrolyte balance, including phosphate and calcium
6. Prevention of fluctuations in cerebral water
7. Minimal risk of infection
8. High level of biocompatibility.

Blood biochemistry, a full blood count and clotting profile are taken as a screening before the procedure to provide a baseline measurement.

Hypotension will occur if the rate of fluid being removed in the dialyser exceeds the plasma refilling rate in the patient, so haemodynamic measurements are also required. In addition, during the first minutes of starting treatment, a sudden drop in blood pressure can occur and removal rates should be titrated against tolerance, although the most recent machines have a minimal dead space volume in the extracorporeal circuit of around 70 ml, to reduce the risk of haemodynamic instability.

A strict fluid balance must be maintained to prevent accidental hypovolaemia and hypervolaemia, and a careful watch kept on the patient's temperature as circulating the blood outside the body may precipitate hypothermia (Baldwin and Leslie 2007). Patient temperature is often slightly lower because of circulation of blood into the extracorporeal circuit.

Circuit pressure monitoring is also important – a rise may indicate clotting of the line or filter.

Monitoring anticoagulation

As blood comes into contact with plastic and the polymer fibres of the filter, the coagulation cascade is activated and anticoagulation of the extracorporeal circuit is necessary to prevent clotting and maintain the life of the circuit, which is expensive. The anticoagulant is introduced into the circuit before the blood enters the filter (Baldwin and Leslie 2007). Circuits should be routinely changed every 72 hours if they do not clot off before. Heparin is the anticoagulant of choice as it is inexpensive, widely available and reversed by protamine sulphate (Baldwin and Leslie 2007). Low doses of heparin <500 IU/h are usually sufficient to maintain the circuit with minimal effect on the patient's coagulation profile (Bellomo 2009). Prostacyclin and citrate-based solutions are also used for anticoagulation of the circuit; however, if the patient is coagulopathic there may be no need to anticoagulate the circuit to prolong filter life. It is important to remember that it is the circuit that is being anticoagulated not the patient. Close monitoring of the patient's clotting time must be maintained and measured within agreed ranges to prevent haemorrhage.

Scenario

Donald was admitted to the ICU after blunt abdominal trauma sustained in an industrial accident. He was ventilated after a diagnostic laparotomy and repair of mesenteric tear. He was progressing steadily over the next 24 hours when his condition suddenly deteriorated. He developed cardiovascular instability and required inotropic support. He was hyperpyrexic with a white cell blood count of 27.8 cells/l. Intra-abdominal sepsis was suspected.

He was taken to theatre for a further laparotomy to ascertain the focus of the suspected sepsis. At surgery haemorrhagic pancreatitis was diagnosed and several irrigation drains were inserted into the abdomen and saline irrigation started. After return to the unit his condition deteriorated, with inotropic requirements increasing and oliguria developing. It was confirmed that the urinary catheter was not blocked or kinked. Diuretics were administered without effect and anuria developed. The patient's blood chemistry was:

Potassium: 6.8 mmol/l
Serum urea: 29 mg/dl
Creatinine: 420 mg/dl

A diagnosis of acute tubular necrosis (ATN) was made. What is the most appropriate treatment?

Continuous renal replacement therapy is the only treatment suitable for Donald in this scenario.

Haemofiltration was established without complications, removal rate of 120 ml/h, using heparin as the anticoagulant in the circuit. Initially blood was taken twice daily for biochemical analysis to ascertain the efficacy of the RRT in the reduction of serum creatinine and urea, and maintenance of normal potassium levels.

Haemofiltration continued for a further 10 days during which time inotropic requirements reduced and renal function returned to normal. The patient made a full recovery from this episode of ATN secondary to sepsis.

CONCLUSION

Monitoring renal function is central to the care of a critically ill patient. It can provide an indication of the function of the kidneys as well as the performance of other major systems of the body. The early recognition and prompt treatment of acute renal failure are essential if prognosis is to be maximised.

REFERENCES

Baldwin, I. & Leslie, G. (2007) Support of renal function. In: Elliott, D. Aitken, L. & Chaboyer, W. (eds), *ACCCN's Critical Care Nursing*. Marrickville, NSW: Mosby Elsevier.

Bellomo, R. (2009) Acute renal failure. In: Bersten, A. D. & Soni, N. (eds), *Oh's Intensive Care Manual*, 6th edn. Philadelphia, PA: Elsevier.

Bishop, T. (2008) Urine testing: urinalysis (urine testing) can provide valuable information about a patient's condition, allowing the detection of systemic disease and infection.(practice nurse trainer). *Practice Nurse*, **35**(12), 18.

Dougherty, L. & Lister, S., eds (2011) *The Royal Marsden Hospital manual of clinical procedures*, 8th edn. Chichester: West Sussex: Wiley-Blackwell.

Gomersall, C. & Oh, T. (1997) Haemodynamic monitoring. In: T. Oh, ed. *Intensive Care Manual*, 4th edn. Oxford: Butterworth Heinemann.

Holcombe, D. & Kern Feeley, N. (2009) Renal failure. In: Gonce Morton, P. & Fontaine, D. K. (eds), *Critical Care Nursing. A holistic approach*, 9th edn. Philadelphia: Wolters Kluwer Lippincott Williams & Wilkins.

Jenkins, P. F. & Johnson, P. H. (2010) *Making sense of acute medicine*. London: Hoddeer Arnold.

McDonald, M. M., Swagerty, M. D. & Wetzel, L. (2006) Assessment of microscopic haematuria in adults. *American Family Physician*, **73**, 1748–1754.

Murphy, F. & Byrne, G. (2010) The role of the nurse in the management of acute kidney injury. *British Journal of Nursing*, **19**, 146–152.

Perkins, C. & Kisiel, M. (2005) Utilising physiological knowledge to care for acute renal failure. *British Journal of Nursing*, **14**(14), 768–773.

Rigby, D. & Gray, K. (2005) Understanding urine testing. *Nursing Times*, **101**(12), 60–62.

Ronco, C. & Ricci, Z. (2008) Renal replacement therapies: physiological review. *Intensive Care Medicine*, **34**, 2139–2146.

Sheppard, M. & Wright, M. (2000) *High Dependency Nursing*. London: Baillière Tindall, p. 249.

Snyder, K. A. (2009) Anatomy and physiology of the renal system. In: Gonce Morton, P. & Fontaine, D. K. (eds), *Critical Care Nursing. A holistic approach*, 9th edn. Philadelphia, PA: Wolters Kluwer Lippincott Williams & Wilkins.

Snyder, K. A. (2009) Patient assessment: renal system. In: Gonce Morton, P. & Fontaine, D. K. (eds), *Critical Care Nursing. A holistic approach*, 9th edn. Philadelphia: Wolters Kluwer Lippincott Williams & Wilkins.

Steggall, M. (2007) Urine samples and urinalysis. *Nursing Standard*, **22**(14–16), 42–45.

Tortora, G. J. & Derrickson, B. H. (2011) *Principles of anatomy and physiology*, 13th edn. Oxford: Wiley Blackwell.

Wilson, L. A. (2005) Urinalysis. *Nursing Standard*, **19**(35), 51–54.

Monitoring Gastrointestinal Function

8

LEARNING OBJECTIVES
At the end of the chapter the reader will be able to:

- ❐ describe the assessment of *bowel function*
- ❐ discuss the significance of *nausea and vomiting*
- ❐ discuss the monitoring of *stomas and fistulas*
- ❐ outline the causes of acute *upper gastrointestinal bleeding*
- ❐ outline the assessment of *intestinal obstruction*
- ❐ discuss the principles of monitoring *pancreatic function*

INTRODUCTION
The importance of the gastrointestinal (GI) tract as a defence system and an essential resource for other organs is increasingly being recognised. The support of its functions is now considered an essential part of the global treatment of a critically ill patient (Adam and Osborne 2005). It is therefore essential to be able to monitor GI function accurately.

The aim of this chapter is to understand the principles of monitoring GI function.

ASSESSMENT OF BOWEL FUNCTION
Assessing bowel function can provide important information that can assist in diagnosis and can help in the monitoring of a patient's clinical condition. The following should be noted:

Monitoring the Critically Ill Patient, Third Edition.
Philip Jevon, Beverley Ewens.
© 2012 Blackwell Publishing Ltd. Published 2012 by Blackwell
Publishing Ltd.

- *Patient's normal bowel activity*: frequency of bowel movement and any unexplained changes in bowel habit
- *Consistency of stools*: hard, bulky or pellet-like suggestive of constipation; loose, watery and frequent faeces are suggestive of diarrhoea
- *Colour of faeces*: normal faeces should be brown; black, non-sticky stools can be caused by iron tablets
- *Black tarry stools (melaena)*: upper GI haemorrhage, i.e. peptic ulcer, oesophageal varices
- *Presence of fresh blood* is suggestive of bleeding from the lower bowel, rectum or haemorrhoids (Bickley and Szilagyi 2009)
- *Presence of mucus*: normally associated with inflammatory bowel disease
- *Odour*: constipation, malabsorption, diet and bowel infection can cause an offensive odour (pale faeces together with an offensive odour may be suggestive of biliary tract-related problems)
- *Steatorrhoea*: pale, bulky and offensive stools are a sign of malabsorption of fat
- *Pain on defecation or tenesmus (constant need to defecate)*: possible causes include constipation, haemorrhoids and rectal inflammatory disease (Bickley and Szilagyi 2009)
- *Volume of faeces*: particularly if the patient has diarrhoea.

Constipation

Constipation is a subjective and variable symptom but is a common symptom affecting 2–27% of the general population (Nassar et al. 2009). In critically ill patients there are many predisposing factors including enforced bed rest, change in diet, dehydration, medications such as opioids and lack of privacy. Constipation in the critically ill has been associated with organ dysfunction, prolonged length of stay and failure to wean from mechanical ventilation (Nassar et al. 2009).

It is recommended that evidence-based bowel management protocols are implemented to prevent constipation, e.g. Norgine tool (Ritchie et al. 2008).

Diarrhoea

Diarrhoea in critical illness is frequently associated with enteral feeding; however, it is important to consider other interventions before making this assumption (Sabol and Steele 2009). If the patient develops diarrhoea it is important to ascertain the cause, such as infection, medications, e.g. antibiotics, lactose intolerance, medications containing hypertonic sorbitol, magnesium and prokinetics (Sabol and Steele 2009). A sample should be sent for microbial culture and sensitivity, which will identify any pathogens such as *Clostridium difficile* or vancomycin-resistant enterococcus (VRE). Prompt investigation will prevent complications such as dehydration, electrolyte imbalance, and perianal skin excoriation and potential tissue breakdown. A stool chart should be maintained and the patient's hydration and nutrition status should be monitored. Regular monitoring of temperature should be undertaken which may indicate a gut infection.

Significance of nausea and vomiting

There are many causes of nausea and vomiting (Table 8.1). Acute symptoms can be caused by GI tract disorders such as intestinal obstruction, diabetic ketoacidosis, adrenal insufficiency, hypercalcaemia, uraemia, liver disease and adverse drug reactions (Bickley and Szilagyi 2009) or are commonly associated with enteral feeding (Sabol and Steele 2009). The incidence of postoperative nausea and vomiting (PONV) remains significant and can delay postoperative recovery (Macintyre and Schug 2007). Factors that influence PONV include: opiates, inappropriate use of antiemetics, age, gender, type and duration of surgery, history of motion sickness, anaesthetic drugs, phase of menstrual cycle, anxiety and previous PONV (Macintyre and Schug 2007).

The timing of vomiting together with the volume and consistency of the vomit are also helpful.

Timing of vomiting

Vomiting that occurs more than an hour after eating is characteristic of obstruction of the gastric outlet, whereas early morning

Table 8.1 Causes of nausea and/or vomiting

Upper GI causes	Oesophageal reflux
	Hiatus hernia
	Gastritis
	Peptic ulcers
	Tumours
	Oesophagogastric dismotility
	Pyloric stenosis result of chronic peptic ulceration
Biliary tract	Gallstones
	Hepatoma
	Metastic liver disease
Small and large intestine	Crohn's disease
	Irritable bowel syndrome
	Obstruction
Metabolic	Uraemia
	Diabetic ketoacidosis
	Hepatic failure
	Hypercalcaemia
Neurological	Raised intracranial pressure
	Labyrinthine pathology
	Brain-stem pathology
Other	Drugs, e.g. opiates, chemotherapy, sulphonamides
	Hyperemesis gravidarum
	Viral, e.g. norovirus
	Viral hepatitis
	Food or drink infected with organisms, e.g. staphylococci
	Sepsis
	Severe constipation especially in elderly people

Adapted from Bolin (2010) and Jenkins and Johnson (2010).

vomiting is typical of pregnancy, alcoholism and raised intracranial pressure.

Volume of vomit

The volume of the vomit is important: a large volume may be indicative of gastric outflow obstruction. If there are small amounts of vomit it is important to ensure that the patient is actually vomiting and not just expectorating – testing for acidity is recommended.

Consistency of vomit

The consistency is important:

- *'Coffee-grounds'*: old blood clots in vomit; can also be caused by iron tablets, red wine and, of course, coffee ingestion
- *Fresh blood*: the presence of fresh blood is indicative of bleeding from the upper gastrointestinal tract
- *Yellow/green*: presence of bile and upper small bowel contents is suggestive of obstruction
- *Faeculent*: brown offensive material from the small bowel, a late sign of small intestinal obstruction (Bickley and Szilagyi 2009)
- *Projectile*: causes include pyloric stenosis and raised intracranial pressure.

MONITORING STOMAS AND FISTULAS

Stomas

Several factors can influence the characteristics of output from stomas including medication, diet and amount of bowel removed. The position of the stoma is also significant: basically the more proximal the stoma, the more fluid the effluent and the more caustic its effect on the skin, due to the presence of chemical irritants effluent from the stoma (Rolstad and Erwin-Toth 2004). In addition to chemical irritants, other causes of loss of skin integrity include stripping off the ostomy bag adhesive, infection, allergy to the stoma bag adhesive and underlying skin disease, e.g. eczema (Rolstad and Erwin-Toth 2004).

The skin surrounding the stoma should be closely observed for early signs of maceration (Herlufsen et al. 2006). Documentation of the size, length and colour of the stoma should be regularly undertaken as should volume and consistency of the output recorded.

Fistulas

An enterocutaneous fistula is an abnormal communication between a section of the GI tract and the skin (Renton et al. 2006). It usually arises from the small or large intestine, from an underlying area of diseased bowel or as a complication of abdominal surgery (Hollington et al. 2004). These are rare complications but pose serious problems because of the serious underlying gastrointestinal comorbidity, e.g. inflammatory bowel disease, intestinal malignancy, pancreatitis as well as concurrent severe sepsis (Streat 2009). The location of the fistula along the bowel will determine the type of effluent produced, e.g. a small bowel fistula can lead to the leaking of copious volumes of corrosive fluid (Renton et al. 2006). Monitoring priorities include recording the consistency and volume of the effluent and observing the surrounding skin for maceration. Monitoring skin integrity is a key priority (Renton et al. 2006).

ACUTE UPPER GASTROINTESTINAL TRACT BLEEDING

Acute GI bleeding is a common cause for admission to the intensive care unit (ICU) and a major cause of morbidity and mortality (Sung 2009). The mortality rate from upper GI bleeding has remained at 10% for decades (Sung 2009). Peptic ulcer and oesophageal varices are the two most frequent causes of upper GI bleeding (Fiore et al. 2005).

Gastrointestinal bleeding usually manifests itself through haematemesis and melaena or more dangerously through an enlarged abdomen with associated abdominal pain. The vomit may be either bright red or coffee-ground in appearance, depending on the length of time the blood that has been in contact with gastric secretions (gastric acid converts bright red haemoglobin to brown haematin). A history of vomiting and retching preceding the GI bleeding suggests a Mallory–Weiss syndrome – a tear at the junction of the stomach and the oesophagus secondary to forceful vomiting/coughing (Sung 2009).

Although most GI bleeds stop spontaneously, approximately 20% will re-bleed in hospital and many of these will need surgical intervention. Upper GI bleeds are commonly seen in the ICU or high dependency unit (HDU) because of the vast blood supply to the stomach and oesophagus. Bleeding is therefore more likely to be severe causing haemodynamic instability requiring massive fluid resuscitation.

Monitoring priorities include:

- Assessing for signs of hypovolaemia and shock
- Estimating blood loss and accurate maintenance of fluid balance

Table 8.2 Causes of acute upper gastrointestinal (GI) bleeding

Oesophageal	Oesophageal varices
	Coagulopathy
	Oesophagitis
	Tumours
	Mallory–Weiss tear
Gastric	Peptic ulcers
	Gastritis
	Tumours
	Angiodysplasia (arteriovenous malformation of the GI tract)
	Dieulafoy's lesions
Duodenal	Duodenal ulcers
	Angiodysplasia
	Duodenitis
	Crohn's disease
	Meckel's diverticulum

Adapted from Steele and Sabol (2009), Sung (2009) and Jenkins and Johnson (2010).

- Determining the cause of the bleed if possible (Table 8.2)
- Monitoring fluid balance
- Monitoring the function of other major systems
- Laboratory investigations, e.g. full blood count (FBC), prothrombin time, liver function tests (LFTs), platelet count, urea and electrolytes (U&Es)
- Monitoring intra-abdominal pressures for signs of increasing pressure.

If the upper GI bleed is due to persistent bleeding ulcers, haemostasis is recommended by endoscopic and pharmacological means, i.e. endoscopic injection of adrenaline or by clipping with adjunct therapy proton pump inhibitors, e.g. esomeprozole (Sung 2009). Mainstay treatment of bleeding oesophageal varices is endoscopic sclerotherapy. Balloon tamponade, i.e. with a Sengstaken–Blakemore tube, may be helpful to apply pressure on the bleeding points in exceptional cases when other therapies fail to effect control of bleeding (Sung 2009). Balloon tamponade tubes can only remain *in situ* for 24 hours because of the risk of necrosis and close monitoring of tube position, together with the patient's airway and respiratory status is important.

ASSESSMENT OF INTESTINAL OBSTRUCTION

Intestinal obstruction can occur in either the small or the large bowel. It can lead to bowel strangulation, infarction and perforation, resulting in potentially life-threatening peritoneal and systemic infection (Steele and Sabol 2009). It can be classified as mechanical or non-mechanical. Mechanical obstruction results from a physical blockage of the intestinal lumen which may be complete or incomplete. Causes include adhesions, malignancy, hernias, bolus obstruction and bowel strangulation, e.g. volvulus. Non-mechanical obstruction is caused by ineffective intestinal peristalsis (paralytic ileus) which is an ileus without the presence of mechanical obstruction, causes of which include trauma, handling of the bowel during surgery, peritonitis and electrolyte imbalance (Steele and Sabol 2009).

Detailed below are the key monitoring considerations:

- *Blood pressure* and *pulse measurements* to detect early signs of shock
- *Temperature* – pyrexia is usually present
- *Vomiting*: the higher the obstruction, the more profuse the vomit
- *Fluid and electrolyte balance*
- *Abdominal pain and distension*: characteristics and severity
- *Bowel function*: consistency of faeces, regularity, volume.

PRINCIPLES OF MONITORING PANCREATIC FUNCTION

The pancreas secretes water to dilute chyme, bicarbonate to neutralise postgastric chyme and enzymes to help with digestion. Its endocrine function is discussed in Chapter 10.

Severe acute pancreatitis (SAP) is an acute inflammation of the pancreas that can also involve surrounding tissues and/or remote organs (Steele and Sabol 2009). The more severe form of pancreatitis, acute necrotizing pancreatitis (ANP), is mainly responsible for the associated high mortality rates (15%) (Wyncoll 2009). Biliary disease and alcohol remain the causative factors in 70% of cases (Wyncoll 2009). Pancreatitis can compromise most of the major systems in the body. Therefore close monitoring is required. The key priorities are:

- *Fluid and electrolyte monitoring*: fluid and electrolyte imbalances may be present (large volumes of fluid can leak into extravascular spaces).
- *Pulse oximetry and arterial blood gas analysis*: respiratory failure can be a complication.
- *ECG monitoring*: electrolyte imbalances can cause arrhythmias.
- *Blood sugar estimations*: hyperglycaemia may occur as a result of impaired insulin production and increased release of glucagon.
- *Temperature*: the main cause of pyrexia is hypermetabolism, although infection may also be the cause
- *Nutritional status*: may have paralytic ileus patient will be nil by mouth, parenteral nutrition will probably be commenced or enteral feeding to bypass the stomach, i.e. into distal duodenum or jejunum, is considered safe (Steele and Sabol 2009). If there is long-term alcohol abuse, nutrition is an even greater priority.
- *Serum amylase*: peaks at 4–8 hours after onset and returns to baseline within 3–5 days with SAP (Steele and Sabol 2009)
- *Serum lipase:* elevated only in pancreatitis, remains elevated after serum amylase returns to normal (Steele and Sabol 2009)
- *Pain*: the patient may have severe abdominal pain.

Scenario

David a 130-kg 56-year-old welder who presented to the emergency department acutely unwell, with a 5-day history of severe epigastric pain, distension and vomiting. Initial physical assessment was undertaken and bloods taken for a full biochemical and haematological screen. David was given a subcutaneous morphine injection for his pain, which he rated at 7 out of 10, and commenced on intravenous (IV) fluids for hydration.

The initial assessment was:

A – airway was patent and David was speaking in short sentences due to abdominal discomfort

B – respiratory rate (RR) was 30/min, SpO_2 was 91% on room air, and poor bilateral basal air entry was heard on auscultation. Oxygen via a non-re-breather mask was applied at 15 L/min

Continued

C – BP was 88/55 mmHg, heart rate (HR) 125/min regular, core temperature 40°C, peripheries were warm and capillary refill was >3 s. A urinary catheter was inserted and 70 ml of dark urine obtained. The 12-lead ECG was normal

D – pupils were equal and briskly reacting to light. AVPU was A and David was oriented to time and place

E – David's abdomen was moderately distended and tense with Grey–Turners sign (haemorrhagic discoloration).

What would your monitoring priorities be?
A full physical examination and social history was obtained and a working diagnosis of acute pancreatitis was established. A review of blood results demonstrated a serum lipase of 2000 U/l.

In view of the severity of David's condition, the ICU team were consulted and he was transferred to the high dependency unit (HDU).

On arrival in the HDU David was tachypnoeic, hypotensive, tachycardic and diaphoretic. He was attached to the monitor and observations commenced at half-hourly intervals of: heart rate, BP, respiratory rate, SpO_2, AVPU and hourly urine output measurements. A nasogastric tube was also inserted, to decompress his stomach, and placed on free drainage. A right subclavian central line was inserted and fluid resuscitation continued.

After 2 hours in THE HDU David's vital signs were as follows:

HR 110.min
BP 95/60 mmHg
Central venous pressure (CVP) +6 mmHg
RR 26/min
SpO_2 94%
Temperature 37.5°C
Urine output 60 ml/h

It was decided to continue to manage David conservatively and he was booked for an ultrasound scan of his abdomen the following morning.

However, in the early hours David's condition deteriorated and his vital signs were:

HR 125/min
BP 88/55
CVP +3 mmHg
RR 30/min
Temperature 36.8°C
Urine output 20 ml/h

Due to a worsening septic presentation, David was electively venti-lated and transferred to ICU where he was started on a noradrenaline infusion to improve his cardiac output. With continued fluid resuscitation and vasopressor support, David's cardiovascular state improved overnight.

The following morning David was started on parenteral nutrition. He was deemed stable enough to be transferred to the radiology depart-ment and undergo an abdominal CT scan. This demonstrated a large pancreatic pseudocyst and bilateral pleural effusions with consolidation.

David remained in a critical condition for the following 10 days, while he continued to be treated conservatively for his acute pancreatitis. He was extubated at day 10 of his admission after resolution of his sepsis and reduction in the size of his pancreatic pseudocyst.

CONCLUSION

Monitoring GI function is central to the management of a critically ill patient. The principles of monitoring have been discussed and include assessment of bowel function, the significance of nausea and vomiting, and key aspects of monitoring for intestinal obstruc-tion and pancreatitis.

REFERENCES

Adam, S. K. & Osborne, S. (2005) *Critical Care Nursing: Science and practice*, 2nd edn. Oxford: Oxford University Press.

Bickley, L. & Szilagyi, P. G. (2009) *Bates' Guide to Physical Examination and History Taking*, 10th edn. Philadelphia, PA: Wolters Kluwer Lip-pincott Williams & Wilkins.

Bolin, T. (2010) Causes and treatment of nausea. *Australian Journal of Pharmacy*, **91**, 74–75.

Fiore, F., Lecleire, S. & Merle, V. (2005) Changes in characteristics and outcome of acute upper gastrointestinal haemorrhage: a comparison of epidemiology and practices between 1996 and 2000 in a multicen-tre French study. *European Journal of Gastroenterology & Hepatology*, **17**, 641–647.

Herlufsen, P., Olsen, A., Carlsen, B., et al. (2006) Study of peristomal skin disorders in patients with permanent stomas. *British Journal of Nursing*, **15**, 854–862.

Hollington, P., Maudsley, J., Lim, W., et al. (2004) An 11 year experience of enterocutaneous fistula. *British Journal of Surgery*, **91**, 1646–1651.

Jenkins, P. F. & Johnson, P. H. (2010) *Making Sense of Acute Medicine*. London: Hodder Arnold.

Macintyre, P. E. & Schug, S. A. (2007) *Acute Pain Management*, 3rd edn. Philadelphia, PA: Saunders Elsevier.

Nassar, A. P., Queiroz da Silva, F. & de Cleva, R. (2009) Constipation in intensive acre unit: Incidence and risk factors. *Journal of Critical Care*, **24**, 630.e639–630.e612.

Renton, S., Robertson, I. & Speirs, M. (2006) Alternative management of complex wounds and fistulae. *British Journal of Nursing*, **15**, 851–853.

Ritchie, G., Burgess, L., Mostafa, S. & Wenstone, R. (2008) Preventing constipation in critically ill patients. *Nursing Times*, **104**(46), 42–44.

Rolstad, B. & Erwin-Toth, P. (2004) Peristomal skin complications: prevention and management. *Ostomy Wound Management*, **50**(9), 68–77.

Sabol, V. K. & Steele, A. G. (2009) Patient management: gastrointestinal system. In: Gonce Morton, P. & Fontaine, D. K. (eds), *Critical Care Nursing: A holistic approach*, 9th edn. Philadelphia: PA: Wolters Kluwer Lippincott Williams & Wilkins.

Steele, A. G. & Sabol, V. K. (2009) Common gastrointestinal disorders. In: Gonce Morton, P. & Fontaine, D. K. (eds), *Critical Care Nursing: A holistic approach*, 9th edn. Philadelphia: PA: Wolters Kluwer Lippincott Williams & Wilkins.

Streat, S. J. (2009) Abdominal surgical catastrophies. In: Bersten, A. D. & Soni, N. (eds), *Oh's Intensive Care Manual*, 6th edn. Philadelphia: PA: Butterworth Heinemann Elsevier.

Sung, J. J. Y. (2009) Acute gastrointestinal bleeding. In: Bersten, A. D. & Soni, N. (eds), *Oh's Intensive Care Manual*, 6th edn. Philadelphia: PA: Butterworth Heinemann Elsevier.

Wyncoll, D. L. A. (2009) Severe acute pancreatitis. In: Bersten, A. D. & Soni, N. (eds), *Oh's Intensive Care Manual*, 6th edn. Philadelphia: PA: Butterworth Heinemann Elsevier.

Monitoring Hepatic Function

9

LEARNING OBJECTIVES

At the end of the chapter the reader will be able to:

❑ outline the *functions* of the liver
❑ list the causes of *ALF*
❑ discuss the *clinical features of ALF*
❑ discuss how to monitor the specific *complications of ALF*

INTRODUCTION

In the context of critically ill patients, hepatic dysfunction is usually secondary to another disease process, e.g. hypoxia, hypotension (Gwinnutt 2006). Liver dysfunction is a common consequence of critical illness and may be caused by poor perfusion leading to ischaemic injury or as a result of inflammatory response in sepsis or drug toxicity (Mashall and Boyle 2007). Acute liver failure (ALF) is a complex multi-system illness that evolves after significant liver insult (Sizer and Wendon 2009). ALF has a poor prognosis without transplantation with a spontaneous survival rate of <50% (Stravitz 2008). The liver, the largest organ in the body, has three broad functions: *synthesis*, *storage* and *detoxification*. Any hepatic dysfunction can affect most of the other major systems in the body. Patients with ALF frequently develop multiorgan failure and associated complications include encephalopathy, systemic infections, cerebral oedema, haemodynamic instability, coagulopathy, and renal

Monitoring the Critically Ill Patient, Third Edition.
Philip Jevon, Beverley Ewens.
© 2012 Blackwell Publishing Ltd. Published 2012 by Blackwell Publishing Ltd.

and metabolic dysfunction (Stravitz 2008). Close monitoring of hepatic function and complications of ALF is paramount. Treatment is generally supportive for these patients and some will ultimately require liver transplantation.

The aim of this chapter is to understand the principles of monitoring hepatic function, with specific reference to the complications of ALF.

FUNCTIONS OF THE LIVER

The clinical features of ALF are largely attributable to the failure of normal hepatic functions (Steele and Sabol 2009b). Therefore, to appreciate the principles of monitoring hepatic function, it is essential to understand the functions of the liver, which include the following (Steele and Sabol 2009a):

- *Carbohydrate metabolism*: glycogenesis (converts glucose to glycogen), glycogenolysis (breaks down glycogen to glucose), gluconeogenesis (forms glucose from amino acids or fatty acids).
- *Protein metabolism*: synthesis of albumin, transferrin, clotting factors, complement factors and non-essential amino acids.
- *Lipid and lipoprotein metabolism*: synthesis of lipoproteins, fatty acids, formation of ketone bodies, breakdown of triglycerides into fatty acids and glycerol, synthesis and breakdown of cholesterol.
- *Storage*: glucose (as glycogen), vitamins A, D, E, K, B, B_2 and B_{12}, folic acid, fatty acids, minerals, amino acids.
- *Detoxification*: inactivation of drugs and excretion of breakdown products, clearance of procoagulants, activated clotting factors, byproducts of coagulation – *removal of pathogens:* clearance of microorganisms by macrophages.
- Production of heat.
- *Steroid catabolism*: conjugation and excretion of gonadal and adrenal steroids.

CAUSES OF ACUTE LIVER FAILURE

Acute liver failure is subdivided into three different types:

1. *Hyperacute liver failure* – jaundice to encephalopathy interval ≤7 days

2. *Acute liver failure* – jaundice to encephalopathy interval 8–28 days
3. Subacute liver failure – jaundice to encephalopathy > 28 days.

Hyperacute liver failure has the worse prognosis (Stravitz 2008).

Although ALF is relatively rare it occurs mostly in young adults and less so from viral infections than was previously identified. Causes of ALF include the following (Bernal et al. 2010):

- *Viral:* in developing countries viral causes predominate with hepatitis A, B and E accounting for most cases
- *Drugs: non-prescription paracetamol (acetaminophen)* is the most common cause of liver failure in the USA and Europe, anti-infectives, anticonvulsants, anti-inflammatory drugs, herbal or adulterated traditional or complementary medicine in east Asia and recreational drugs rarely, e.g. ecstasy
- *Hyperthermic injury:* from heat shock or protracted seizures
- *Toxic insults:* mushroom poisoning
- *Metabolic disorders:* Wilson's disease
- *Immunological insults:* autoimmune hepatitis
- *Hypotension:* secondary to sepsis, cardiac failure
- *Hepatic venous obstruction:* Budd–Chiari syndrome
- *Pregnancy:* HELLP (*h*aemolysis, *e*levated *l*iver enzymes and *l*ow *p*latelets) syndrome is associated with a good prognosis, fatty liver of pregnancy.

Clinical features of ALF
A patient with ALF will have clinical manifestations that are directly related to the degree of impaired hepatic function.

The effects of ALF on many systems in the body are often catastrophic:

- *Whole body*: systemic inflammatory response, high energy expenditure and catabolism
- *Liver*: loss of metabolic function, hypoglycaemia, lactic acidosis, hyperammonaemia, coagulopathy
- *Lungs*: acute lung injury (ALI), adult respiratory distress syndrome (ARDS)

- *Adrenal glands*: reduced glucocorticoid production, contributing to hypotension
- *Bone marrow*: suppression
- *Circulating leukocytes*: impaired function, increasing risk of sepsis
- *Brain*: hepatic encephalopathy, cerebral oedema, intracranial hypertension
- *Heart*: high output state, myocardial injury
- *Pancreatitis*: particularly in paracetamol-induced ALF
- *Portal hypertension* (Bernal et al. 2010).

MONITORING THE SPECIFIC COMPLICATIONS OF ALF
Encephalopathy
Encephalopathy is a characteristic clinical feature of ALF. The exact cause is unknown, although it is possible that the accumulation of circulating toxic substances such as ammonia plays a key role (Bernal et al. 2010). Encephalopathy encompasses many neuropsychiatric disturbances, ranging from minor confusion and disorientation to coma and cerebral oedema (Bernal et al. 2010). Hepatic encephalopathy can be classified into four grades depending on severity (Table 9.1) and usually progresses over several days, though deep coma can develop in just a few hours (Sizer and Wendon, 2009). In patients with high grades of encephalopathy, the chances of survival are less than 20% with medical management alone (Stravitz 2008).

The neurological status of the patient should be evaluated and closely monitored; in brief, the conscious level, motor movement, sensory pupil size and reaction to light should be examined. In advanced encephalopathy the pupils may become dilated and react sluggishly to light; if they become dilated and unreactive, brain-stem coning is likely (Steele and Sabol 2009a).

Orientation should be monitored together with concentration span, restlessness, personality and behaviour changes, emotional lability, drowsiness, slurred or slow speech, and disturbances in the sleep pattern. A generalised increase in muscle tone is an early sign of progression of encephalopathy. Spontaneous hyperventilation is common so the respiratory rate should be regularly recorded together with blood gas analysis (Table 9.2).

Table 9.1 Modified Parsons–Smith scale of hepatic encephalopathy

Grade	Clinical features	Neurological signs	Glasgow Coma Scale score
0 subclinical	Normal	Only seen on neuropsychometric testing	15
1	Trivial lack of awareness, shortened attention span	Tremor, apraxia, incoordination	15
2	Lethargy, disorientation, personality change	Asterixis, ataxia, dysarthria	11–15
3	Confusion, somnolence to semi-stupor, responsive to stimuli	Asterix, ataxia	8–11
4	Coma	±decerebration	<8

Reprinted from Bersten and Soni (2009), with permission from Butterworth Heinemann Elsevier.

Cerebral oedema

Cerebral oedema is a leading, dramatic cause of death in patients with ALF (Stravitz 2008). Patients with acute and hyperacute ALF are more at risk of grade IV hepatic coma and cerebral oedema (Sizer and Wendon 2009). The clinical signs of cerebral oedema, i.e. systemic hypertension, decerebrate posturing and abnormal pupillary reflexes, are generally attributed to brain-stem compression. Cerebral oedema provokes intracranial hypertension that impairs cerebral perfusion pressure.

Cerebral blood flow correlates to arterial pressure and not cardiac output in patients with ALF; strict cardiovascular control is important when pressure-passive cerebral circulation is present in order to maintain continuous and adequate cerebral oxygenation and avoid the development of cerebral hyperaemia and cerebral oedema (Larsen et al. 2000). Close cardiac and haemodynamic monitoring is therefore imperative.

Intracranial pressure (ICP) monitoring is indicated in patients requiring vasopressor agents to maintain adequate cardiac output (Sizer and Wendon 2009).

Table 9.2 Clinical examination of encephalopathy

Grade of encephalopathy	Tone and reflexes	Response to pain	Pupils
Grade 1	Normal		
Grade 2	Brisk reflexes and increased tone	Obeys	Normal
Grade 3	Upgoing plantar reflexes, clonus, hippus	Localises, flexes	'Hyper-reactive'
Grade 4	Sustained clonus	Extends	Dilated, sluggish
Brain death	Flaccid, absent reflexes	None	Fixed and dilated

Reprinted from Oh (1997), with permission from Elsevier Inc.

The benefits of therapeutic prophylactic hypothermia in this population is currently being evaluated in an international multicentre trial (Bernal et al. 2010).

Coagulopathy and haemorrhaging

Patients with ALF frequently develop severe coagulopathy; the hepatic synthesis of clotting factors is impaired and as a result the clotting times, predominantly prothrombin time and to a lesser extent activated partial thromboplastin ratio (Sizer and Wendon 2009).

The most common site for haemorrhage is the gastrointestinal tract; other sites include the nasopharynx, respiratory tract and skin puncture sites (Stravitz 2008). It is important to monitor for signs of haemorrhage, e.g. in faeces, urine, skin, sputum, endotracheal tube and vomit.

Renal failure

Renal failure is a common complication of ALF with an incidence of about 50% (Sizer and Wendon 2009). Strict control of fluid balance via renal replacement therapy is indicated in established renal failure (Sizer and Wendon 2009).

Sepsis

Bacterial infection is one of the most common causes of death in patients with ALF and commonly precipitates multiorgan dysfunction syndrome (MODS) (Stravitz 2008). Septic patients are more likely to develop renal failure and gastrointestinal haemorrhaging and have a significantly higher mortality risk than non-septic patients (Sizer and Wendon 2009).

The patient's vital signs should be closely monitored, and regular cultures of blood, sputum and urine performed (Stravitz 2008).

Ascites may be associated with ALF, spontaneous bacterial peritonitis is a potential complication (Steele and Sabol 2009b).

Metabolic disturbances

Blood glucose levels should be measured regularly because of the prevalence of hypoglycaemia in these patients. Primary respiratory alkalosis is common in spontaneously breathing patients (see encephalopathy earlier). Impaired hepatic synthesis of urea and hypokalaemia can cause metabolic alkalosis. Electrolyte disturbances are very common.

Scenario

Claire, a 45-year-old woman, was admitted via the emergency department with a history of vomiting and abdominal discomfort. On admission to the ward she was alert but slightly disoriented in time and place. The initial assessment was:

A – airway was patent and she was talking in full sentences

B – respiratory rate was 24/min, SpO_2 was 94%, lung fields clear on auscultation. Oxygen via nasal prongs at 2 l/min applied

C – BP was 95/60, heart rate (HR) 115/min regular, core temperature 35.8°C, peripheries were warm. A urinary catheter was inserted and 100 ml dark urine drained

D – pupils were equal and reacting to light sluggishly. AVPU was A but in view of her disorientation she was started on a Glasgow Coma Scale (GCS) chart

E – Claire's abdomen was moderately distended with spider naevi evident. She was noted to have significant diffuse bruising with slight jaundice. Claire was also found to have muscle wasting possibly due to poor nutrition

Continued

What would your monitoring priorities be?

A full physical examination and social history were obtained and a working diagnosis of chronic liver failure with hepatic encephalopathy was established. Claire exhibited asterix (liver flap) and constructional apraxia (she was unable to draw a five-pointed star). A comprehensive social history indicated that Claire was a heavy alcohol user.

During the course of the day the outreach team was called to review Claire as her conscious level had fallen – her GCS was 10/15. Her supplementary oxygen was increased to 6 l/min via a facemask aiming for a target range of >95%. In view of her worsening conscious level and concerns about protecting her airway, she was transferred to the high dependency unit (HDU) for closer monitoring. She was started on an ECG monitor, with continuous SpO_2, HR, respiratory rate, blood pressure at 30-minute intervals and GCS hourly. Her blood results at that time demonstrated a coagulopathy with a prolonged prothrombin time and a severely reduced platelet count. Her Hb was 9.8 g/dl. The team decided to insert a central venous catheter; however, this was contraindicated with coagulopathy. Therefore Claire was transfused with 4 units of fresh frozen plasma (FFP) and 1 unit of platelets to correct her coagulopathy. Claire was managed conservatively over the next 3 days when her conscious level gradually improved and her coagulopathy did not worsen. She was discharged to the ward 6 days after her admission with outreach team follow-up and a mental health referral for her alcohol abuse.

CONCLUSION

Critically ill patients frequently develop hepatic dysfunction. If ALF develops, widespread hepatocyte necrosis can lead to severely impaired hepatic function and life-threatening complications may result. Close monitoring of hepatic function and complications of ALF is paramount if the patient's prognosis is to improve.

REFERENCES

Bernal, W., Auzinger, G., Dhawan, A. & Wendon, J. (2010) Acute liver failure. *The Lancet*, **376**, 190–201.

Bersten, A. D. & Soni, N., eds (2009) *Oh's Intensive Care Manual*, 6th edn. Philadelphia, PA: Butterworth Heinemann Elsevier.

Budden, L. & Vink, R. (1996) Paracetamol overdose: pathophysiology and nursing management. *British Journal of Nursing*, **5**, 145–152.

Gwinnutt, C. (2006) *Clinical Anaesthesia*, 2nd edn. Oxford: Blackwell Publishing.

Larsen, F., Strauss, G., Knudsen, G., et al. (2000) Cerebral perfusion, cardiac output and arterial pressure in patients with fulminant hepatic failure. *Critical Care Medicine*, **28**, 996–1000.

Mashall, A. & Boyle, M. (2007) Support of metabolic function. In: Elliott, R., Aitken, L. M. & Chaboyer, W. (eds), *ACCCN's Critical Care Nursing*. Marickville, NSW: Mosby Elevier.

Oh, T., ed. (1997) *Intensive Care Manual*, 4th edn. Oxford: Butterworth-Heinemann.

Sizer, E. & Wendon, J. (2009) Acute liver failure. In: Bersten, A. D. & Soni, N. (eds), *Oh's Intensive Care Manual*, 6th edn. Philadelphia, PA: Butterworth Heinemann Elsevier.

Steele, A. G. & Sabol, V. K. (2009a) Common gastrointestinal disorders. In: Gonce Morton, P. & Fontaine, D. K. (eds), *Critical Care Nursing: A holistic approach*, 9th edn. Philadelphia, PA: Wolters Kluwer Lippincott Williams & Wilkins.

Steele, A. G. & Sabol, V. K. (2009b) Anatomy and physiology of the gastrointestinal system. In: Gonce Morton, P. & Fontaine, D. K. (eds), *Critical Care Nursing: A holistic approach*, 9th edn. Philadelphia, PA: Wolters Kluwer Lippincott Williams & Wilkins.

Stravitz, R. T. (2008) Critical management decisions in patients with acute liver failure. *Chest*, **134**, 1092–1102.

Monitoring Endocrine Function

10

LEARNING OBJECTIVES

At the end of the chapter the reader will be able to:

☐ discuss the principles of monitoring *pituitary gland function*
☐ outline the principles of monitoring the *endocrine function of the pancreas*
☐ discuss the principles of monitoring *adrenal gland function*
☐ outline the principles of monitoring *thyroid gland function*
☐ discuss the principles of monitoring *parathyroid gland function*

INTRODUCTION

Monitoring endocrine function is an important aspect of caring for the critically ill patient. Disorders of this function can be life threatening (Savage et al. 2004) and early detection of problems through close monitoring is essential.

For the purpose of this chapter, only the potentially life-threatening disorders of endocrine function are discussed. An understanding of the physiology of the endocrine system is important if the effects of its malfunction are to be appreciated.

The aim of this chapter is to understand the principles of monitoring endocrine function.

PRINCIPLES OF MONITORING PITUITARY GLAND FUNCTION

One of the functions of the pituitary gland is to secrete antidiuretic hormone (ADH). ADH acts on the renal tubules resulting in

Monitoring the Critically Ill Patient, Third Edition.
Philip Jevon, Beverley Ewens.
© 2012 Blackwell Publishing Ltd. Published 2012 by Blackwell Publishing Ltd.

reabsorption of water. Any damage to the posterior pituitary gland or adjacent hypothalamus, e.g. after neurosurgery, head injury, malignancy or drug therapy, e.g. amiodarone, can lead to insufficient or lack of ADH secretion (Adam and Osborne 2005), which can in turn lead to diabetes insipidus.

Diabetes insipidus

Diabetes insipidus is a syndrome that has excessive thirst, polydipsia and polyuria as its hallmarks (Kapustin 2009b). Water loss in extreme cases can be around 20l/day. If untreated, diabetes insipidus can result in severe electrolyte imbalance, i.e. severe hypernatraemia and hyperosmolar states.

Monitoring priorities

Management problems on an intensive care unit (ICU) associated with diabetes insipidus are usually hypovolaemia and polyuria (Vedig 2004). In respect of hypovolaemia, close monitoring of cardiovascular parameters is essential, including pulse, blood pressure and central venous pressure (CVP) monitoring. Maintenance of strict fluid balance and electrolyte monitoring is essential to detect dehydration and electrolyte imbalances (Kapustin 2009b).

As patients with diabetes insipidus have an increased serum osmolarity and reduced urine osmolarity, biochemical investigations of both blood and urine are vital in the accurate monitoring of this syndrome. Specific gravity (SG), a crude measurement, is often ignored on routine ward testing but is invaluable in this scenario: SG <1.010 is indicative of diabetes insipidus. Urine osmolarity is obtained either as a spot specimen or from a 24-hour collection. Normal values are 300–1300 mosmol/kg.

Plasma osmolarity is calculated from the equation of serum sodium, potassium, glucose and urea (normal value 275–295 mosmol/kg). Regular biochemical assessment of urea and electrolytes is essential to monitor the progression of this syndrome.

PRINCIPLES OF MONITORING THE ENDOCRINE FUNCTION OF THE PANCREAS

The pancreas has both exocrine and endocrine functions. The endocrine function is from the islets of Langerhans which secrete the hormones, *insulin* and *glucagon* (Kapustin 2009a). Functions of insulin include lowering blood glucose levels by promoting transport of glucose into the cells, promoting glycogen storage in muscle and hepatic cells, and inhibiting fat metabolism (Adam and Osborne 2005). Glucagon increases blood glucose levels.

Disturbances in pancreatic function that affect insulin production will lead to hyperglycaemia and glycosuria. If left untreated diabetic ketoacidosis will develop.

The normal fasting blood glucose level is 3.9–6.2 mmol/l (Bersten and Soni 2009). When monitoring a critically ill patient it is important to undertake regular bedside blood glucose measurements. These are particularly important if the patient is hypoglycaemic or hyperglycaemic, known to have diabetes, or receiving insulin or nutritional support. Monitoring the patient's blood sugar can, in the short term, prevent hypoglycaemia and ketoacidosis and, in the long term, prevent disorders that affect the vascular and neural pathways (Dougherty and Lister 2011). Blood glucose measurements are more accurate than urinalysis because the results relate to the time of testing.

Procedure for bedside blood glucose measurements

The following is adapted from the Walsall NHS Trust's procedure for 'Blood glucose estimation using the Advantage 11 machine and test strips'.

The procedure for use of the Advantage 11 meter (Fig. 10.1) is as follows:

1. Wash and dry the patient's hands using soap and water.
2. Having ensured that the test strips are in date, remove one from the container and insert it into the test strip slot. Replace the container top.
3. Ensure that the meter and the test strips are calibrated with each other, check test strips' expiry date and load the lancet (Higgins 2008).
4. Once the blood drop symbol flashes on the monitor, prick the side of the patient's finger with a blood lancet as per manufac-

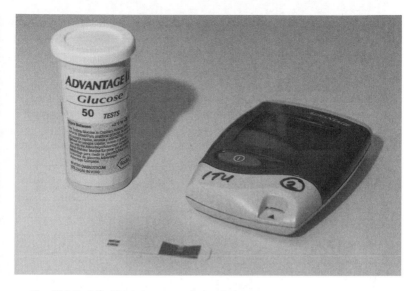

Fig. 10.1 Bedside blood glucose monitoring device.

turer's instructions. The side of the finger is reported to be less painful than the tip. Ensure rotation of sites for comfort and to reduce hardening of the site.

5. After waiting a few seconds to allow the capillaries to relax, squeeze the patient's finger to obtain a small drop of blood, bringing it together with the test strip. The blood will be drawn automatically on to the test strip.
6. Dispose of the lancet in a sharps container.
7. Apply a cotton-wool pad or tissue to the patient's finger.
8. The test result will be displayed in millimoles per litre after a few seconds.
9. Dispose of equipment and wash hands.
10. Document the measurement (Fig. 10.2).

WALSALL HOSPITALS NATIONAL HEATH SERVICE TRUST

BLOOD GLUCOSE MONITORING CHART

Patients Name ....

Hospital No. .... Ward ....

DATE & TIME													
28													
24													
22													
20													
18													
16													
15													
14													
13													
12													
11													
10													
09													
08													
07													
06	This area shaded in light blue to indicate near normal range												
05													
04													
03													
02													
01													
Insulin Given													

BLOOD GLUCOSE MMOLS/L

Fig. 10.2 Blood glucose monitoring chart (Walsall Hospitals NHS Trust).

Best practice – blood glucose measurements

Use soap and water, not alcohol swab, to clean the site

Ensure that test strip is in date, calibrated with the machine and stored following manufacturer's recommendations

Do not use a needle to draw blood

Use side of patient's finger to draw blood, or preferably from an arterial line if in situ

Rotate finger used to avoid multiple stabbing on the same site

Allow blood to be drawn on to test strip

Ensure that sufficient blood has been obtained

Be aware of factors that can affect the result

Ensure that quality control procedures are carried out following local protocols

Sources of blood glucose measurement inaccuracy (Ginsberg 2009):

- *Strip factors:* strips must be in date and not exposed to high temperatures or humidity in an open vial
- *Patient factors:* variations in haematocrit, high levels of triglycerides, high or low oxygen values, uric acid
- *Medications:* L-dopa, tolazamide, ascorbic acid, icodextrin (used in peritoneal dialysis solutions
- *High levels of bilirubin* (>0.43 mmol/l, e.g. in jaundice).

Systems should be in place to ensure that any point-of-care testing devices are subject to rigorous quality control processes and. if any results are incongruent with the patient's physical condition, a laboratory sample should be taken (Higgins 2008).

Newer devices are currently being developed to enable non-invasive methods of monitoring blood glucose (Higgins 2008). Current research into non-invasive testing of blood glucose (using breath analysis) in type 2 diabetes mellitus is currently under way (American Diabetes Association 2010).

Hyperglycaemia and diabetic ketoacidosis

There are many causes of hyperglycaemia including diabetes mellitus, acute pancreatitis, parenteral nutrition and sepsis (Bersten and Soni 2009). Twenty-five per cent of patients who present with acute coronary syndrome have diabetes mellitus which is an independent risk factor with a risk similar to elevated troponin (Aroney 2011). Diabetic ketoacidosis (DKA) results from absolute or relative insulin deficiency (Jerreat 2010). It is a serious life-threatening metabolic complication of diabetes mellitus consisting of three concurrent abnormalities: hyperglycaemia, hyperketonaemia and metabolic acidosis (Savage et al. 2004).

Acute illness, particularly infection, major surgery, myocardial infarction and critical illness, will stimulate the release of stress hormones, including glucagon, which will cause glucose imbalance (Higgins 2008). Criteria for diagnosis of DKA are (Jerreat 2010):

- Blood sugar >11 mmol/l
- Moderate ketonuria or blood ketone levels > 3 mmol/l
- Significant acidosis bicarbonate ≤15 mmol/l or an arterial pH <7.

Signs and symptoms of severe DKA include reduced consciousness, hyperventilation (Kussmaul's respirations) and hypotension (Kapustin 2009b).

Monitoring priorities include the following:

- *Airway patency* (if the patient is semiconscious or in a coma)
- *Arterial blood gas analysis*: indicated if there is altered conscious level or if breathing is compromised (Savage et al. 2004)
- *Pulse oximetry*: breathing may be compromised
- *Pulse, blood pressure and CVP measurements*: hypovolaemia
- *ECG monitoring*: cardiac arrhythmias
- *Blood ketone measurements*: the use of blood ketone tests is preferred to urine ketone tests for diagnosis and monitoring of DKA (American Diabetes Association 2010)
- *Blood glucose measurements*: hourly (Savage et al. 2004) to monitor hyperglycaemia and the effect of prescribed insulin
- *Strict fluid balance*: fluid replacement should be closely monitored
- *Cultures*: blood, urine, throat swab to detect infection
- *Serum potassium measurements*: to detect hypokalaemia or hyperkalaemia (Jerreat 2010).

Hypoglycaemia

Hypoglycaemia is described as a blood glucose level that does not meet metabolic demands (typically <3.9 mmol/L) (Higgins 2008). Causes include hepatic dysfunction, malnutrition, inadequate oral intake and exercise following administration of insulin or oral anti-hypoglycaemic agents, and intentional or accidental overdose (Higgins 2008; Keays 2009). Blood glucose levels <1 mmol/l are a medical emergency (Keays 2009). Regular blood glucose measurements are required.

PRINCIPLES OF MONITORING ADRENAL GLAND FUNCTION

The adrenal glands comprise the medulla and cortex. The adrenal medulla secretes the hormones adrenaline and noradrenaline (catecholamines) in response to sympathetic stimulation. The adrenal cortex secretes three categories of hormones, all of which are steroids.

Phaeochromocytoma

Phaeochromocytoma (tumour of the adrenal medulla) can lead to the secretion of high levels of catecholamines, usually intermittently (Savage et al. 2004). Common symptoms include severe hypertension, headache, tachycardia, hyperglycaemia, bowel disturbances and blurred vision (Adam and Osborne 2005). Hypertension is paroxysmal initially, but later becomes sustained, severe hypertension (Myburgh 2009). Monitoring priorities include:

- *Arterial pressure monitoring*: hypertension
- *ECG monitoring*: cardiac arrhythmias
- *Blood glucose measurements*: to monitor hyperglycaemia and evaluate treatment.

Addisonian crisis

Addisonian crisis results from acute adrenocortisol insufficiency. Acute adrenocortical insufficiency can be caused by a primary failure of the adrenal gland or secondary to the lack of adrenocorticotrophic hormone (ACTH) drive from the pituitary gland (Venkatesh and Cohen 2009). The clinical features, which result mainly from the deficiency of aldosterone, include thirst, polyuria, dehydration, cardiac arrhythmias, electrolyte imbalance and hypotension (Adam and Osborne 2005). Monitoring priorities include:

- *Arterial blood gas analysis*: metabolic and respiratory acidosis may occur
- *ECG monitoring*: cardiac arrhythmias
- *Arterial pressure monitoring*: hypotension
- *CVP monitoring*: hypotension
- *Strict fluid balance*: polyuria
- *Blood glucose measurements*: hypoglycaemia.

PRINCIPLES OF MONITORING THYROID GLAND FUNCTION

The thyroid gland secretes three hormones: *thyroxine* (T_4), *triiodothyronine* (T_3) and *calcitonin*. T_3 and T_4 are responsible for the metabolic rate of all bodily tissues. Calcitonin reduces serum calcium levels. Thyroid crisis and myxoedema coma result from over- and under-secretion of the thyroid gland, respectively. If untreated they have a high mortality rate (Handy 2009).

Thyroid crisis

Hyperthyroidism (also known as thyrotoxicosis) results from oversecretion of T_3 and T_4, leading to hypermetabolism. Thyroid crisis (thyroid storm) is a rare but life-threatening syndrome that often occurs in untreated or undiagnosed hyperthyroidism (Karanikolas et al. 2009).

Thyroid crisis is characterised by fever, tremors, tachycardia, diarrhoea, nausea and vomiting, dehydration, apathy, generalised weakness, seizures, stroke, coma, abdominal pain, liver failure and circulatory instability (Karanikolas et al. 2009). If the patient has underlying cardiac disease or has a compromised cardiovascular system, the risk of serious complications increases. Thyroid crisis carries a relatively high mortality rate, so careful and accurate monitoring is therefore essential. Monitoring priorities include:

- *Respiratory rate, pulse oximetry and arterial blood gas analysis*: patient may develop pulmonary oedema
- *ECG monitoring*: cardiac arrhythmias
- *Arterial blood pressure monitoring*: hypotension may develop
- *CVP monitoring*: patient can develop heart failure; there may also be considerable fluid loss

- *Strict fluid balance*: considerable fluid loss (excessive sweating)
- *Blood glucose measurements*: hypoglycaemia
- *Core temperature measurements*: patient may develop extreme pyrexia (>40°C) (Adam and Osborne 2005)
- *Neurological monitoring*: extreme agitation and coma may develop.

Myxoedema coma

Myxoedema coma results from decreased T_4 production and occurs most commonly in the elderly female population with long-standing or undiagnosed hypothyroidism (Handy 2009). Effects include unconsciousness, hypothermia (as low as 23°C), hypoventilation, hypotension and hypoglycaemia (Handy 2009). Monitoring priorities include:

- *Airway*: unconscious patient
- *Respiratory rate, pulse oximetry and arterial blood gas analysis*: hypoventilation
- *ECG monitoring*: bradycardia
- *Arterial blood pressure monitoring*: hypotension
- *CVP monitoring*: patient may develop heart failure; also there may be considerable fluid gain
- *Strict fluid balance*: there may be considerable fluid gain
- *Blood glucose measurements*: hypoglycaemia
- *Core temperature measurements*: hypothermia
- *Neurological monitoring*: coma.

PRINCIPLES OF MONITORING PARATHYROID GLAND FUNCTION

The parathyroid glands secrete parathyroid hormone, which raises serum calcium levels. Calcium is essential for a variety of bodily functions, including muscle contraction, blood clotting and maintenance of cell membrane integrity. Abnormalities in parathyroid function (hyperparathyroidism and hypoparathyroidism) can lead to calcium disorders which can be life threatening.

Hypercalcaemia

Symptomatic hypercalcaemia requires urgent treatment and if it is severe the patient should be admitted to the ICU (Adam and

Osborne 2005). Severe hypercalcaemia (corrected serum calcium >3.0 mmol/l) requires urgent treatment and is usually caused by malignancy (Muzzy and Adams Snyder 2009). Monitoring priorities include:

- *ECG monitoring*: cardiac arrhythmias
- *Arterial blood pressure monitoring*: hypertension
- *CVP monitoring*: hypovolaemia
- *Strict fluid balance*: dehydration, polyuria and hypovolaemia.

Hypocalcaemia

Hypocalcaemia is present in approximately 70–90% of critically ill patients (Venkatesh 2009). Acute symptomatic hypocalcaemia is a medical emergency, requiring urgent treatment (Venkatesh 2009). Monitoring priorities include:

- *Airway patency*: stridor
- *Respirations, pulse oximetry and arterial blood gas analysis*: respiratory compromise
- *ECG monitoring*: cardiac arrhythmias
- *Arterial blood pressure*: hypotension
- *CVP monitoring*: hypotension
- *Neurological monitoring*: convulsions and altered conscious level.

Scenario

James, a 28-year-old man, was admitted to the high dependency unit (HDU) with a history of weight loss, general malaise, polyuria, polydipsia, lethargy and deep sighing Kussmaul's respirations. He was known to have diabetes but had omitted his insulin injections over the preceding few days and was also complaining of diarrhoea and vomiting. A provisional diagnosis of diabetic ketoacidosis was made. What are the monitoring priorities?

BP 90/60, pulse 125/min, respiratory rate 35/min, temperature 38.5°C, SpO_2 95%, blood glucose 40 mmol/l. The patient's vital signs were consistent with acute circulatory failure secondary to dehydration caused by excessive fluid loss. The pyrexia may be associated with the diarrhoea and vomiting. Blood glucose measurements and urinalysis were undertaken. The presence of hyperglycaemia, glycosuria, ketonuria and ketonaemia helped to confirm the diagnosis of DKA.

Arterial blood gas results are as follows:

pH 7.1
$PaCO_2$ 2.9 kPa (15 mmHg)
PaO_2 11.8 kPa (88.5 mmHg)
HCO_3- 12 mmol/l
BE −13
SaO_2 97%

What do the arterial blood gases show?
The patient has metabolic acidosis with respiratory compensation. He is hyperventilating in order to excrete more carbon dioxide, therefore reducing the level of free hydrogen ions available.

Strict fluid balance monitoring was initiated. Aggressive intravenous fluid replacement was also commenced together with an insulin infusion to treat the hyperglycaemia. ECG monitoring was essential because hypokalaemia (potassium <2.8 mmol/l) was present. Intravenous potassium therapy was also started. Ongoing monitoring priorities include vital signs, arterial blood gases, ECG monitoring, blood glucose measurements, urinalysis, fluid balance and any vomiting/bowel action. In addition it is important to monitor the patient's conscious level because unconsciousness may ensue.

CONCLUSION

Monitoring endocrine function is an important aspect of caring for the critically ill patient. Brief details on normal physiology, in relation to each endocrine gland function, have been provided. The priorities of monitoring endocrine function have been highlighted.

REFERENCES

Adam, S. & Osborne, S. (2005) *Critical Care Nursing: Science and practice*, 2nd edn. Oxford: Oxford Medical Publications.

American Diabetes Association (2010) Clinical practice recommendations 2004. *Diabetes Care*, **27**(suppl 1), S94–S102.

Aroney, C. (2011) Management of non-ST-elevation acute coronary syndromes. In: Thompson, P. L. (ed.), *Coronary Care Manual*, 2nd edn. Chatswood, NSW: Churchill Livingstone Elsevier.

Bersten, A. D. & Soni, N., eds (2009) *Oh's Intensive Care Manual*, 6th edn. Philadelphia, PA: Butterworth Heinemann Wlsevier.

Dougherty, L. & Lister, S., eds (2011) *The Royal Marsden Hospital manual of clinical procedures*, 8th edn. Chichester: Wiley-Blackwell.

Ginsberg, B. H. (2009) Factors affecting blood glucose monitoring: Sources of errors in measurement. *Journal of Diabetes Science and Technology*, **3**(4), 1–11.

Handy, J. (2009) Thyroid emergencies. In: Bersten, A. D. & Soni, N. (eds), *Oh's Intensive Care Manual*, 6th edn. Philadelphia, PA: Butterworth Heinemann Elsevier.

Higgins, D. (2008) Patient assessment. Part 4. Blood glucose testing. *Nursing Times*, **104**(10), 24–25.

Jerreat, L. (2010) Managing diabetic ketoacidosis. *Nursing Standard*, **24**(34), 49–55.

Kapustin, J. (2009a) Anatomy and physiology of the endocrine system. In: Gonce Morton, P. & Fontaine, D. K. (eds), *Critical Care Nursing. A holistic approach*, 9th edn. Philadelphia, PA: Wolters Kluwer Lippincott Williams & Wilkins.

Kapustin, J. (2009b) Common endocrine disorders. In: Gonce Morton, P. & Fontaine, D. K. (eds), *Critical Care Nursing. A holistic approach*, 9th edn. Philadelphia, PA: Wolters Kluwer Lippincott Williams & Wilkins.

Karanikolas, M., Velissaris. D., Karamouzos, V. & Filos, K. S. (2009) Thyroid storm presenting as intra-abdominal sepsis with multiorgan failure requing intensive care. *Anaesthesia and Intensive Care*, **37**, 1005–1007.

Keays, R. T. (2009) Diabetic emergencies. In: Bersten, A. D. & Soni, N. (eds), *Oh's Critical Care Manual*, 6th edn. Philadelphia, PA: Butterworth Heinemann Elsevier.

Muzzy, A. & Adams Snyder, K. (2009) Patient management: Renal system. In: Gonce Morton, P. & Fontaine, D. K. (eds), *Critical Care Nursing. A holistic approach*, 9th edn. Philadelphia, PA: Wolters Kluwers Lippincott Williams & Wilkins.

Myburgh, J. A. (2009) Vasodilators and antihypertensives. In: Bersten, A. D. & Soni, N. (eds), *Oh's Critical Care Manual*, 6th edn. Philadelphia, PA: Butterworth Heinemann Elsevier.

Savage, M., Mah, P., Weetman, A. & Newell-Price, J. (2004) Endocrine emergencies. *Postgraduate Medical Journal*, **80**, 506–551.

Vedig, A. (2004) Diabetes insipidus. In: Bersten, A. D. & Soni, N. (eds), *Intensive Care Manual*, 5th edn. Oxford: Butterworth Heinemann.

Venkatesh, B. (2009) Acute calcium disorders. In: Bersten, A. D. & Soni, N. (eds), *Oh's Intensive Care Manual*, 6th edn. Philadelphia, PA: Butterworth Heinemann Elsevier.

Venkatesh, B. & Cohen, J. (2009) Adrenocortical insufficiency in critical illness. In: Bersten, A. D. & Soni, N. (eds), *Oh's Critical Care Manual*, 6th edn. Philadelphia, PA: Butterworth Heinemann Elsevier.

Monitoring Nutritional Status

11

LEARNING OBJECTIVES

At the end of the chapter the reader will be able to:

❐ discuss the *importance* of assessing nutritional status
❐ outline *how to assess* nutritional status
❐ list the factors that can *affect* nutritional status
❐ discuss the principles of monitoring *enteral feeding*
❐ discuss the principles of monitoring *total parenteral nutrition*

INTRODUCTION

Malnutrition, including the depletion of essential nutrients and erosion of lean body mass, is very common in patients who are critically ill (Ziegler 2009; Joseph et al. 2010).

Malnutrition leads to poor wound healing, complications post-surgery and sepsis (Singer and Webb 2005). Malnourished patients have poorer outcomes after medical treatment or surgery (Leonard 2009). Early nutritional support, preferably within 24 hours of injury or intensive care unit (ICU) admission (Doig et al. 2008), together with ongoing monitoring of nutritional status, should be considered in all critically ill patients (Singer and Webb 2005; Doig and Simpson 2006) and has been demonstrated to positively impact on mortality (Leonard 2009). A nutritional support feeding algorithm improves the nutritional support of intensive care patients and leads to greater consistency in nursing practices with respect to aspiration of gastric contents and monitoring the delivery of nutrients to critically ill patients (Woien and Bjork 2006).

Monitoring the Critically Ill Patient, Third Edition.
Philip Jevon, Beverley Ewens.
© 2012 Blackwell Publishing Ltd. Published 2012 by Blackwell Publishing Ltd.

The aim of this chapter is to understand the principles of monitoring nutritional status.

IMPORTANCE OF ASSESSING NUTRITIONAL STATUS

All critically ill patients have a serious illness, suffered major trauma and/or had major surgery; the stress response to trauma and/or injury results in a striking increase in protein metabolism, leading to a negative nitrogen balance and characteristically significant muscle loss (Joseph et al. 2010).

The consequences of malnutrition in critical illness are: alterations to immune function, decreased respiratory muscle function, increase in infection rates that may lead to increased length of stay, cost, morbidity and mortality (Marshall and Boyle 2007). In particular it is now recognised that maintaining gut integrity is important to help prevent sepsis and to support the immune defence system (Btaiche et al. 2010). Over-feeding can lead to hyperglycaemia and fatty infiltration of the liver (Singer and Webb 2005).

ASSESSMENT OF THE PATIENT'S NUTRITIONAL STATUS

Bedside nutritional assessment should identify patients already suffering from malnutrition and those at risk of malnutrition; early referral for nutritional support together with ongoing monitoring is essential.

Objectives of assessment

The objectives of this assessment are to:

- determine the existing *nutritional status* of the patient
- identify if the patient is *malnourished*
- provide a baseline for *monitoring* nutritional status
- ascertain the patient's *nutritional requirements*.

Assessment

Nutritional assessment in critical illness is difficult because disease processes confound methods used in the general population (Leonard 2009). Indirect calorimetry is the gold standard because it permits measurement of the resting energy expenditure (REE) (Leonard 2009). However, many units do not use calorimetry and other equations to measure basal metabolic rate (BMR), such as the

Harrison–Benedict and Schofield equations, are used (Leonard 2009).

A 24-hour recall of dietary intake, food diaries and taking a dietary history are all frequently used in clinical practice. A diet history can provide information on food frequency, food preferences, food allergies, portion sizes and changes in food intake.

Anthropometric assessment methods such as triceps' skinfold thickness and mid-arm circumference may be obscured by oedema (Leonard 2009).

The measurement of serum albumin levels is not a good indicator of nutritional status, because a fall is more likely to result from albumin's metabolism, reflecting the severity and duration of stress, rather than nutritional status (Leonard 2009).

FACTORS THAT CAN AFFECT NUTRITIONAL STATUS

Common factors that can affect nutritional status in critically ill patients include:

- inability to take oral diet
- vomiting and diarrhoea
- constipation
- glucose intolerance
- renal dysfunction
- pain
- nausea/vomiting
- physical disability
- restricted fluid intake
- delayed gastric emptying
- reduced gut motility
- fasting before procedures/investigations.

PRINCIPLES OF MONITORING ENTERAL FEEDING

If the patient is able to take diet and fluids orally, it is important to monitor intake closely to ensure that hydration and nutritional needs are being met. Sip-feed supplements, which are now produced in many different flavours and consistencies, e.g. Ensure, Sustagen, should be instigated if oral nutritional intake is inadequate.

If oral diet and supplements fail to meet nutritional requirements or if the patient is unable to tolerate oral diet but has a functional gastrointestinal (GI) tract, enteral feeding should be considered as first choice in the critically ill patient (Marshall and Boyle 2007; Sabol and Steele 2009). Enteral feeding, defined as the administration of nutrients via the GI tract, is preferable if it can be given without risk (Wernerman 2005); sometimes optimal nutritional support may necessitate the concomitant administration of enteral nutrition with total parenteral nutrition (TPN) (Woodcock and MacFie 2004).

Benefits of enteral feeding
Benefits of enteral feeding include (Marshall and Boyle, 2007):

- improved function of the gut and liver
- reduced incidence of stress ulceration and GI bleeding (Leach 2009)
- maintenance of gut integrity and preservation of the gut as a barrier thereby reducing translocation of bacteria into systemic circulation (Sabol and Steele 2009)
- enhanced immune function, reduced infection rates and lower sepsis rates compared with parenteral feeding (Leary et al. 2000)
- improved survival rates in critically ill patients (Doig et al. 2008)
- increased gastric mucosal blood flow.

It has been estimated that 85% of critically ill patients can be successfully fed via the enteral route (Btaiche et al. 2010).

Routes of enteral feeding

- *Nasogastric*: tube through the nose into the stomach
- *Nasoduodenal*: tube through the nose into the duodenum
- *Nasojejunal:* tube through the nose into the jejunum (Marshall and Boyle 2007).

Nasogastric feeding
Nasogastric feeding is often started through a wide-bore (12–14 French gauge) tube. This allows aspiration of gastric contents to confirm tube placement and feed tolerance, and facilitates the

administration of medications. Wide-bore tubes are less likely to occlude than fine-bore tubes, but their long-term use is not recommended. Wide-bore tubes should be replaced by fine-bore tubes when feeding is established. Following insertion of a feeding tube, with either a radio-opaque tip or radio-opaque entirety of the tube can be visualised on a chest radiograph, it is important to ensure correct tube placement by observing the following precautions:

- Auscultating over the stomach after injection of air via the tube: no longer recommended because of transferred sounds and subsequent unreliability (Guenter 2010)
- Aspirating gastric contents and testing the pH: if the nasogastric tube is in the stomach and in contact with acidic gastric contents, the aspirate will turn blue litmus paper red. Note that the result may be affected if the patient is taking H_2-receptor agonists or has bile reflux, or if the nasogastric tube is in the duodenum (Sabol and Steele 2009).

Enteral feeds can be delivered by bolus feeds, intermittent, continuous or cyclic. Continuous feeding is best suited in critical illness because of the reduced incidence of gastric distension and risk of aspiration, also acts as protection against stress ulceration and metabolic complications (Sabol and Steele 2009). Aspiration of gastric contents should be undertaken every 4 hours during the first 48 hours of feeding, to assess gastric residual volume and provide an indication to feed tolerance (Guenter 2010). If the patient vomits it is usual practice not to suspend the feed completely but to continue at a reduced rate of 10 ml/h.

The presence or absence of bowel sounds or passing of flatus is not a reliable indicator of absorption of feed in the critically ill population (Guenter 2010). Discarding aspirated volumes may cause an electrolyte imbalance but the definition of high aspirates and the gastric residual volume (GRV) cut-off for returning aspirate differs between 100 and 400 ml depending on varying hospital protocols (Sabol and Steele 2009; Guenter 2010). Delayed gastric emptying is common in critically ill patients, especially in those who are ventilated or who have traumatic brain injury (Btaiche et al. 2010). Complications associated with wide-bore tubes include the following:

- *Erosion of nasal septum, oesophagitis, epistaxis*: small-bore, soft tubes are less likely to cause these complications (Sabol and Steele 2009).
- *Sinusitis.*
- *Regurgitation and aspiration of gastric contents*: particularly in unconscious and ventilated patients. The presence of a nasogastric tube renders the gastro-oesophageal sphincter incompetent, allowing reflux of gastric contents. The nurse should be alert to signs of regurgitation and feed should be immediately ceased.
- *Tube dislodgement*: ensure that the tube is well secured and marked to facilitate the early detection of migration; it should also be regularly monitored; pH testing of gastric aspirate should be undertaken regularly.
- *Risk of nosocomial pneumonia*: wide-bore tubes facilitate the migration of gut commensals into the respiratory tract, particularly if the patient is receiving stress ulcer prophylaxis.
- *Tube blockage.*

Nasoduodenal and nasojejunal feeding

Transpyloric feeding can be given without regard to gastric emptying and reduces the risk of aspiration because the pyloric sphincter provides a barrier to regurgitation (Sabol and Steele 2009). The small bowel is less prone to ileus than the stomach or the colon, and it retains its digestive and absorptive properties, making it a potential feeding modality immediately after trauma or surgery (Sabol and Steele 2009).

Correct tube placement must be confirmed by radiography. Unfortunately, fine-bore tubes can collapse after the application of negative pressure by a syringe, thus making them more difficult to aspirate. This may lead to decreased nursing vigilance in assessing gastric contents (Sabol and Steele 2009).

Complications associated with fine-bore nasogastric tubes include the following:

- *Misplacement into the respiratory tract:* inadvertent bronchial placement including pleural puncture and pneumothorax
- *Tube migration:* coughing and vomiting can dislodge the tube, increasing the risk of aspiration Check the gastric pH if high reflux is present

- *Guidewire-induced trauma*, e.g. oesophageal, gastric and abdominal perforation and a pneumothorax
- Tube blockage.

Complications of enteral feeding

Complications of enteral feeding are more commonly associated with patients requiring intensive care. The most significant ones are:

- *Regurgitation and aspiration of gastric contents*: this is more common in the unconscious patient and supine patient. Nurses need to observe consistency of fluid suctioned from the oropharynx. If possible, the patient's 'head end' should be maintained at 45°.
- *Tube obstruction*: if the feed is stopped or medications are given, the tube should be flushed with 10–20 ml sterile water; if the tube is not in use it should be capped off after flushing in order to trap a column of water in the tube.
- *Diarrhoea*: associated with hyperosmolar feed and antibiotic usage (Marshall and Boyle 2007).
- *Abdominal distension*: if there is poor gastric emptying or rapid infusion of feed. This is also an indication of failure to absorb the feed; careful monitoring is essential in order to prevent perforation of the intestines.
- *Hyperglycaemia*.
- *Mild hepatic dysfunction*.

Best practice – enteral feeding

Adhere to best practice feeding protocols

Commence enteral nutrition within 24 hours of injury or ICU admission

Calculate nutritional needs based on metabolic demand

Use fine-bore tube whenever possible

Always confirm tube position before commencement of feed

Always flush tubes before and after administration of medications

Monitor tube position during feeding regularly

Monitor the patient's vital signs, particularly the airway

Continued

Keep head of the bed elevated to 30–45° while administering feed
Increase feed to meet nutritional requirements following local guidelines
Ensure feed is in date and administered following manufacturer's recommendations
Monitor absorption of feed
Always use clean oral syringes not intravenous syringes and receptacle when aspirating
Maintain fluid balance
Monitor bowel function
Monitor patient's blood chemistry

Percutaneous jejunostomy and percutaneous endoscopic gastrostomy

Percutaneous endoscopic gastrostomy (PEG) is the preferred method for long-term access to the GI tract. Advantages include increased comfort, decreased cost and decreased recovery time (Sabol and Steele 2009). Complications include leaks, wound infection related to bacterial contamination, necrotising fasciitis, aspiration and peritonitis (Sabol and Steele 2009). The insertion site should be closely monitored, particularly as gastric contents can leak around it leading to excoriation, skin breakdown and possible wound dehiscence.

PRINCIPLES OF MONITORING TPN

TPN (Fig. 11.1) involves the intravenous infusion of nutrients, the constituents prescribed based on the patient's calculated BMR (Table 11.1). It can be administered either peripherally via a PICC line or centrally via a CVP line. It should be considered only when enteral nutrition is contraindicated (10-15% of the critically ill population) (Ziegler 2009). Indications include (Gwinnutt 2006):

- ileus
- acute pancreatitis
- inflammatory bowel disease
- short bowel syndrome
- malabsorption syndromes
- multiple organ dysfunction syndrome

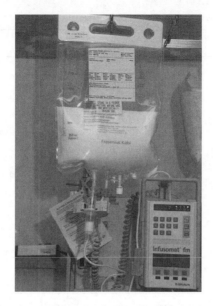

Fig. 11.1 Parenteral nutrition.

Table 11.1 The Harris–Benedict equation for calculating basal metabolic rate

Men	Energy expenditure = 66.5 + (13.7 × weight in kg) + (5 × height in cm) − (6.78 × age in years)
Women	Energy expenditure = 66.5 + (9.56 × weight in kg) + (1.85 × height in cm) − (4.68 × age in years)
Injury factors	Minor operation × 1.2 Trauma × 1.3 Sepsis × 1.6 Severe burns × 2.1

- post-oesophagectomy
- severe catabolic states, e.g. extensive burns, sepsis and trauma.

Table 11.2 provides a comprehensive guide to the relevant monitoring required when a patient is receiving TPN. In particular the nurse should be alert to the possible complications of TPN.

Table 11.2 Parenteral nutrition – relevant monitoring

Monitoring	Specific tasks
Regular clinical	Temperature
	Blood pressure
	Pulse rate
	Respiratory rate
	Fluid balance
	Blood glucose (4-hourly when commencing feed)
Daily (at least)	Fluid balance review
	Nutrient intake review
	Urea, electrolytes and creatinine
	Blood glucose
Weekly (at least)	Full blood count
	Coagulation screen
	Weight
	Liver functions tests
	Serum calcium/magnesium/phosphate
As indicated	Zinc
	Uric acid

Reproduced by permission of Butterworth Heinemann Elsevier, from Bersten and Soni (2009).

During TPN administration, there is a significant risk of morbidity through sepsis, metabolic and mechanical problems (Sabol and Steele 2009; Ziegler 2009). Mechanical complications include: pneumothorax, bleeding, thrombus formation, sepsis; catheter related, metabolic; overfeeding (excess dextrose, fat, calories and re-feeding syndrome (rapid feeding of patients with pre-existing malnutrition) (Ziegler 2009). In addition, rebound hypoglycaemia can occur if the TPN infusions are abruptly stopped. Regular urinalysis and blood glucose monitoring are therefore important.

The function of the gut should be monitored so that conversion to enteral nutrition can be initiated as soon as possible. TPN should be gradually withdrawn in order to avoid complications, e.g. rebound hypoglycaemia. In some instances and enteral and concomitant parenteral feeding may be necessary to meet metabolic demands.

Best practice – parenteral feeding

Only use when enteral route is not possible
Do not use feed bag if there are signs of contamination
Administer feed following local protocols
Ensure that entire infusion line is dedicated to parenteral nutritional use
Ensure that feed and tubing are regularly changed (usually every 24 hours)
Never add anything to a bag of TPN
Monitor patient's blood chemistry
Monitor blood sugar 2-hourly when first initiated
Monitor patient for complications of parenteral nutrition, particularly infection
Regularly flush line when not in use to maintain patency
Avoid breaks in circuit
Monitor gut function so that enteral feeding can be started as soon as possible

Scenario

Mr Brown was admitted to the ICU with an atypical pneumonia. He was sedated and ventilated with midazolam and morphine. A fine-bore nasogastric tube was inserted and the position verified by the litmus paper test and radiography. Enteral feeding was then commenced (standard feed) at 30 ml/h. After 4 hours 100 ml is aspirated. What would you do?

As the aspirate is <200 ml, it is replaced because of its constituents:

- Gastric acid reduces the proliferation of bacteria.
- Gastrin promotes the growth and repair of the gastric mucosa.
- Intrinsic factor facilitates the absorption of vitamin B_{12} from the gut.

The enteral feed was increased to 60 ml/h. After 4 hours 300 ml was aspirated. What would you do?

The 200 ml was replaced whereas 100 ml was discarded and the feed reduced to 30 ml/h. After 4 hours 400 ml was aspirated. Again 200 ml was replaced and the rest discarded. The enteral feed was then re-started at 30 ml/h. Shortly after recommencement of the feed, the patient vomited. What would you do?

Nil was aspirated and the feed was reduced to 10 ml/h continuously and the prokinetic drug metoclopramide 10 mg i.v. prescribed three times daily. The next day the feed was gradually increased following the above process until a desired rate of 90 ml/h was reached. Eight-hourly monitoring of aspirate, urea and electrolytes, fluid balance and bowel movements ensured a successful enteral feeding regimen.

CONCLUSION

Nutritional status should be assessed and monitored in all critically ill patients. The method of nutritional support should also be closely monitored, in particular the patient's tolerance of it. The nurse should also be alert to possible complications.

REFERENCES

Bersten, A. D. & Soni, N., eds (2009) *Oh's Intensive Care Manual*. Philadelphia, PA: Butterworth Heinemann Elsevier.

Btaiche, I. F., Chan, L., Pleva, M., & Kraft, M. D. (2010) Critical illness, gastrointestinal compliactions and medication therapy during enteral feeding in critically ill adult patients. *Nutrition in Clinical Practice*, 25(1), 32–49.

Doig, G. & Simpson, F. (2006) Early enteral nutrition in the critically ill: do we need more evidence or better evidence? *Current Opinion in Critical Care*, 12, 126–130.

Doig, G. S., Simpson, F., Finfer, S., et al. (2008) Effect of evidence-based feeding guidelines on mortality of critically ill adults. *Journal of the American Medical Association*, 300, 2731–2741.

Guenter, P. (2010) Safe practices for enteral nutrition in critically ill patients. *Critical Care Nursing Clinics of North America*, 22, 197–208.

Gwinnutt, C. (2006) *Clinical Anaesthesia* 2nd edn. Oxford: Blackwell Publishing.

Joseph, B., Wynne, J. L., Dudrick, S. J., & Latifi, R. (2010) Nutrition in trauma and critically ill patients. *European Journal of Trauma and Emergency Surgery*, 36, 25–30.

Leach, R. (2009) *Acute and Critical Care Medicine at a Glance*, 2nd edn. Oxford: Wiley Blackwell.

Leary, T., Fellows, I., & Fletcher, S. (2000) Enteral nutrition. *Care of the Critically Ill*, 16(1), 22–27.

Leonard, R. (2009) Enteral and parenteral nutrition. In: Bersten, A. D. & Soni, N. (eds), *Oh's Critical Care Manual*, 6th edn. Philadelphia, PA: Butterworth Heinemann Elsevier.

Marshall, A. & Boyle, M. (2007) Support of metabolic function. In: Elliott, R., Aitken, L. M. & Chaboyer, W. (eds), *ACCCN's Critical Care Nursing*. Marickville, NSW: Mosby Elevier.

Sabol, V. K. & Steele, A. G. (2009) Patient management: gastrointestinal system. In: Gonce Morton, P. & Fontaine, D. K. (eds), *Critical Care Nursing. A holistic approach*, 9th edn. Philadelphia, PA: Wolters Kluwer Lippincott Williams & Wilkins.

Singer, M. & Webb, A. (2005) *Oxford Handbook of Critical Care*, 2nd edn. Oxford: Oxford University Press.

Wernerman, J. (2005) Guidelines for nutritional support in intensive care unit patients: a critical analysis. *Current Opinion in Clinical Nutrition and Metabolic Care*, 8, 171–175.

Woien, H. & Bjork, T. (2006) Nutrition of the critically ill patient and effects of implementing a nutritional support algorithm in ICU. *Journal of Clinical Nursing*, **15**, 168–177.

Woodcock, N. & MacFie, J. (2004) Optimal nutritional support. *Proceedings of the Nutrition Society*, **63**, 451–452.

Ziegler, T. R. (2009) Parenteral nutrition in the critically ill patient. *New England Journal of Medicine*, **361**, 1088–1097.

Monitoring Temperature

12

LEARNING OBJECTIVES

At the end of this chapter the reader will be able to:

- ❏ discuss the factors *influencing* body temperature
- ❏ discuss the methods of *measuring* temperature
- ❏ discuss the physiological effects of *hypothermia*
- ❏ outline the *monitoring priorities* of a patient with *hypothermia*
- ❏ discuss the *physiological effects* of hyperthermia
- ❏ outline the *monitoring priorities* of a patient with *hyperthermia*

INTRODUCTION

The body can only function effectively within a narrow temperature range (Trim 2005). Any significant changes in temperature, either a rise or a fall, can lead to life-threatening complications. As a critically ill patient can experience wide fluctuations in temperature, close temperature monitoring is paramount.

Monitoring the temperature in critically ill patients is a vital yet often neglected part of their management (Andrews and Nolan 2006). As well as depressing organ function, hypothermia causes coagulopathy, increases blood loss and increases adrenergic responses, which can increase morbidity (Andrews and Nolan 2006). Re-warming patients can cause cardiovascular instability.

Close monitoring of the temperature is also important if the patient has a condition that affects basal metabolic rate,

Monitoring the Critically Ill Patient, Third Edition.
Philip Jevon, Beverley Ewens.
© 2012 Blackwell Publishing Ltd. Published 2012 by Blackwell Publishing Ltd.

e.g. thyrotoxicosis, is susceptible to infection, e.g. neutropenic, already has a local or systemic infection, is receiving a blood transfusion, or is in the postoperative phase.

The aim of this chapter is to understand the principles of monitoring temperature.

FACTORS INFLUENCING BODY TEMPERATURE

The normal body temperature is usually between 36 and 37.5°C, regardless of the environmental temperature (Trim 2005). Temperature is regulated by the thermoregulatory centre in the hypothalamus through various physiological mechanisms, e.g. sweating, dilatation/constriction of peripheral blood vessels, and shivering.

The body's core temperature is usually the highest, whereas the skin's is the coolest. Core temperature represents the balance between the heat generated by body tissues during metabolic activity, especially of the liver and muscles, and heat lost during various *mechanisms*.

There are four mechanisms of heat loss (Mains et al. 2008):

1. *Radiation*: flow of heat from a higher temperature (the body) to a lower temperature (environment surrounding the body)
2. *Convection*: heat transfer by flow or movement of air
3. *Conduction*: heat transfer due to direct contact with cooler surfaces
4. *Evaporation*: perspiration, respiration and breaks in skin integrity.

There are several factors that can cause a fluctuation in temperature, including:

- The body's *circadian rhythms*: temperature is higher in the evening than the morning, fluctuations can range between 0.5 and 1.5°C (Mains et al. 2008).
- *Ovulation*
- *Exercise* and *eating* can cause a rise in temperature
- *Old age*: there is an increased sensitivity to the cold and there is generally a lower body temperature
- Illness.

METHODS OF MEASURING TEMPERATURE

The traditional method of using oral/rectal mercury thermometers is now outdated practice because of the risk of mercury poisoning. Mercury is covered by the Control of Substances Hazardous to Health Regulations (COSHH – Department of Health, Social Services and Public Safety 1999) and its vapour is neurotoxic (Woodrow 2000). In addition, although the rectal temperature is close to the core temperature, it is unreliable in the critically ill patient because hypotension and gut ischaemia reduce the blood supply to the rectum and the measurement is influenced by the contents of the rectum. Core temperature should be measured in an internal cavity close to an artery (Mains et al. 2008).

There are, however, several reliable methods of measuring body temperature using electronic devices. These devices are fast and safe, and some can provide continuous measurements of temperature (Tortora and Grabowski 1996). A selection are described in more detail.

Tympanic thermometers

The tympanic membrane is a desirable method of core temperature measurement because of the tympanic membrane's proximity to the hypothalamus (Mains et al. 2008). Measurement of the tympanic membrane temperature should therefore reflect the core temperature (Woodrow 2000).

The tympanic thermometer (Fig. 12.1), which uses infrared light to detect thermal radiation (Bickley and Szilagyi 2009), is designed for intermittent use, offering a 'one-off' digital reading.

Care should be taken when using the tympanic thermometer, because poor technique can render the measurement inaccurate. To ensure that the temperature measurements are accurate, the tympanic thermometer probe should be positioned to fit snugly in the ear canal. This prevents ambient air at the opening of the ear canal from entering it, resulting in a false low temperature measurement (Bickley and Szilagyi 2009). Ear canal size, wax, operator technique and the patient's position can affect the accuracy of the measurements (Knies 2003).

Chemical dot thermometers

Chemical dot thermometers are flexible polystyrene strips with a temperature sensor at one end, designed for single oral/axilla use.

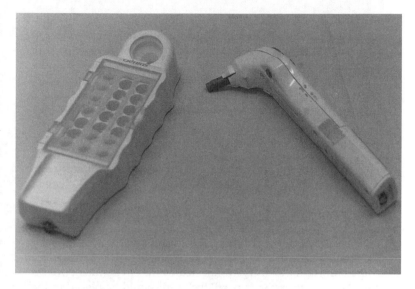

Fig. 12.1 Tympanic thermometer.

These thermometers are unsuitable in patients with hypothermia because their temperature range is restricted to 35.5–40.4°C (Mains et al. 2008).

Best practice – tympanic temperature monitoring

Use the same ear for consecutive measurements

Install a new disposable probe cover for each measurement

Ensure that thermometer probe is positioned snugly in the external auditory meatus

Aim the thermometer towards the tympanic membrane

Measure the patient's temperature following the manufacturer's instructions

Consider the temperature reading alongside other systemic observations and overall condition of the patient

Store the thermometer following manufacturer's instructions

Jevon and Jevon (2001)

If the oral route is used, the strip should be placed in the sublingual pocket of tissue at the base of the tongue, which is close to the thermoreceptors, which respond rapidly to changes in core temperature (Mains et al. 2008). It is important to ensure that the strip is placed in the right or left sublingual pocket (Mains et al. 2008) and not in the area under the front of the tongue because there may be a difference in temperature of up to 1.7°C between the two areas (Dougherty and Lister 2011).

Oral temperature measurements can be affected by the temperature of ingested foods and fluids and by the muscular activity of chewing (Dougherty and Lister 2011). In addition a respiratory rate of >18 breaths/min will reduce core temperature values (Hussein 2009).

The axilla is an alternative route for temperature monitoring if the oral route is unsuitable, e.g. in a convulsive patient. However, it can be difficult to obtain an accurate and reliable measurement because the site is not close to a major blood vessel and the surface temperature of the skin can be affected by the environment (Mains et al. 2008). If the axilla is used, the strip should be placed in the centre of the armpit with the patient's arm positioned firmly against the side of the chest. As the temperature can vary between arms, the same site should be used for serial measurements.

Regardless of what site is used for temperature measurements, the same one should be consistently used, because switching between different sites can produce measurements that are both misleading and difficult to interpret (Dougherty and Lister 2011).

Oesophageal/nasopharyngeal probes

The oesophageal probe should be accurately positioned in the lower quarter of the oesophagus. The nasopharyngeal temperature can be affected by air leaking around the tracheal tube. Both probes can be interfaced with the patient monitoring system, thus offering an accurate and continuous reading.

Bladder probe

Bladder and pulmonary artery temperature correlate well and, as most critically ill patients require a urinary catheter, this method of measuring body temperature avoids additional invasive equipment. A thermocouple attached to the distal end of the catheter can interface with the patient monitoring system and offer continuous temperature measurements. This method of temperature measurement is considered to be very reliable (Lefrant et al. 2003).

Pulmonary artery catheter

Although the pulmonary artery catheter is the gold standard for temperature measurement (Sturgess and Morgan 2009), it is highly invasive and its sole use for temperature measurements cannot be justified. However, if one is inserted, the thermistor sited in the distal end can interface with the patient's monitoring system and provide continuous temperature measurements.

PHYSIOLOGICAL EFFECTS OF HYPOTHERMIA

Hypothermias defined as body temperature <35°C and may be mild (34–35°C), moderate (30–34°C, severe (<30°C) or profound (<20°C) (Farley and McLafferty 2008) can occur when the body loses too much heat or cannot maintain its normothermic state. There are several risk factors (Table 12.1). Table 12.2 shows the various signs and symptoms of hypothermia at different levels of temperature.

Sometimes hypothermia is intentionally induced, e.g. during some cardiac surgery or after a cardiac arrest, either by heat exchange through a heart/lung machine or by surface cooling using ice. Induced hypothermia after a cardiac arrest has been shown to decrease (Morley 2009):

- cerebral oxygen consumption
- free radical formation
- excitatory amino acids
- neuron-specific enolase
- cerebral lactate
- cerebral oedema
- intracranial pressure
- cell destructive enzymes
- neutrophil migration to ischaemic tissue
- ongoing inflammatory response.

When monitoring a patient with hypothermia it is important to understand the physiological effects that it has on the various

Table 12.1 Predisposing factors for hypothermia

Age	Extremes of age
Environmental	Exposure to cold
	Immersion
	Poor living conditions
Drugs	Anaesthetic agents
	Phenothiazines
	Barbiturates
	Alcohol
Central nervous system disorders	Cerebrovascular accident
	Trauma
	Spinal cord transections
	Brain tumours
	Wernicke's encephalopathy
	Alzheimer's and Parkinson's diseases
	Mental illness
Endocrine dysfunction	Hypoglycaemia
	Diabetic ketoacidosis
	Hyperosmolar coma
	Panhypopituitarism
	Hypoadrenalism
	Hypothyroidism
Trauma	Major trauma
Debility	Severe cardiac, renal or hepatic impairment
	Malnutrition, sepsis
Skin disorders	Burns
	Exfoliative dermatitis

Reproduced by kind permission of Butterworth Heinemann Elsevier from Hussein (2009).

systems in the body. The main effects of hypothermia on the bodily systems are detailed below.

Cardiovascular system

Initially there is sympathetic stimulation, which increases heart rate, blood pressure and cardiac output. However, with increasing hypothermia, there is progressive cardiovascular depression lead-

Table 12.2 Signs and symptoms of hypothermia at different levels of temperature

Temperature (°C)	Signs and symptoms
37.6	'Normal' rectal temperature
37	'Normal' oral temperature
36	Increased metabolic rate to attempt to balance heat loss
35	Shivering maximum at this temperature; hyper-reflexia, dysarthria, delayed cerebration
34	Patients usually responsive and with normal blood pressure; lower limit compatible with continued exercise
33–31	Retrograde amnesia, consciousness clouded, blood pressure difficult to obtain, pupils dilated, most shivering ceases
30–28	Progressive loss of consciousness, increased muscular rigidity, slow pulse and respiration, cardiac arrhythmias develop if heart irritated
27	Voluntary motion lost along with pupillary light reflex, deep tendon and skin reflexes; appears dead
26	Victims seldom conscious
25	Ventricular fibrillation may appear spontaneously
24–21	Pulmonary oedema develops (100% mortality rate in shipwreck victims in World War II)
20	Heart standstill
18	Lowest adult accidental hypothermic patient with recovery
17	Isoelectric EEG
15.2	Lowest infant accidental hypothermic patient with recovery
9	Lowest artificially cooled hypothermic patient with recovery
4	Monkeys revived successfully
1–7	Rats and hamsters revived successfully

Reproduced by kind permission of Cambridge University Press from Skinner et al. (1997).

ing to a reduction in tissue perfusion and oxygenation (Hussein 2009), and cardiac arrhythmias, e.g. bradycardia, atrial fibrillation and ventricular fibrillation, can become a problem (Resuscitation Council UK 2010). Rough movement and activity should be avoided because this can precipitate a cardiopulmonary arrest. Sometimes the patient's pulse may be difficult to detect.

Respiratory system

Following an initial reflex stimulation of respiration, there is a progressive decrease in respiratory rate, tidal volume and minute volume (Hussein 2009) leading to hypoxaemia and hypoxia. Sometimes the patient's respirations may be difficult to detect (Resuscitation Council UK 2010).

Neurological system

Cerebral blood flow reduces at a rate of 7% for each 1°C drop in temperature (Hudak et al. 1998) resulting in confusion, decreased reflexes, cranial nerve deficits and lack of voluntary motion. Increased blood viscosity, decreased oxygen availability, lack of shivering and muscle rigidity also develop (Kelly et al. 2001).

Renal system

In mild hypothermia (34–35°C) sympathetic activity leads to an increase in cardiac output, resulting in a 'cold' diuresis. However, with progressive hypothermia, renal blood flow and glomerular filtrate fall. Sodium and water losses may be evident due to metabolic failure of the renal tubules (Morley 2009).

Gastrointestinal system

If the temperature is <34°C, gut motility decreases which can lead to vomiting and malabsorption.

Metabolic system

Metabolic acidosis occurs due to accumulation of lactate and failure to secrete hydrogen ions. Hyperkalaemia resulting from the failure of membrane sodium/potassium pumps and hypoxic liver damage may also occur (Morley 2009).

Endocrine system

Below 30°C pituitary, pancreatic functions and catecholamine secretion are diminished. Increased serum glucose occurs as a result of increased glycogenolysis and insulin resistance (Hussein 2009).

Haematology

Hypothermia increases blood viscosity by 2% and potential complications include thrombocytopenia, leukopenia and coagulopathy (Hussein 2009). In severe hypothermia platelet dysfunction and disseminated intravascular coagulation (DIC) are common (Hussein 2009).

MONITORING PRIORITIES OF A PATIENT WITH HYPOTHERMIA

The monitoring priorities of a patient with hypothermia include the following:

- Regular assessment of vital signs: airway, respirations, blood pressure, pulse and core temperature
- Arterial blood gas analysis
- ECG monitoring to detect cardiac arrhythmias
- Urine output measurements
- Blood sugar measurements to detect hypoglycaemia
- Neurological function observations.

Methods of re-warming should be appropriate to the degree of hypothermia. Methods include warmed fluids, warm blankets. Monitoring during re-warming is also important. A patient warmer (Fig. 12.2) is commonly used for active re-warming, although other methods are available (Farley and McLafferty 2008). Re-warming should not exceed increases of 1–2°C per h (Farley and McLafferty 2008); in cases of mild hypothermia aim for 0.3–1.2°C per h, but rapid re-warming of >3°C per h may be necessary if there are severe hypothermia and cardiovascular instability (Carson 1999).

Peripheral vasodilatation may complicate active re-warming methods. This could induce hypotension and a further drop in core temperature, the latter increasing the risk of arrhythmias (Farley and McLafferty 2008). 'Careful monitoring and supportive therapy during re-warming are mandatory' (Farley and McLafferty 2008).

PHYSIOLOGICAL EFFECTS OF HYPERTHERMIA

Sudden rises in temperature are often caused by infection. However, there are several other causes of hyperthermia, including the following (Hussein 2009):

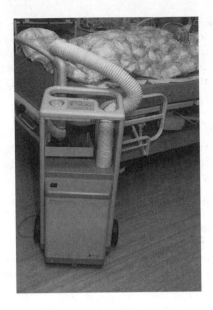

Fig. 12.2 Patient warmer.

- Myocardial infarction
- Deep vein thrombosis (DVT)
- Pericarditis
- Pulmonary emboli
- Inflammatory bowel disease
- Pancreatitis
- Non-viral hepatitis
- Gastrointestinal (GI) haemorrhage
- Cerebral haemorrhage/infarction
- Adrenocortical insufficiency
- Drug and alcohol withdrawal
- Burns
- Drugs
- Transfusion reaction.

Pyrexia in response to infection is a protective mechanism and may lead to enhanced resistance to infection (Hussein 2009). Mild pyrexia is generally not treated.

However, pyrexia and hypermetabolism can cause physiological stress (Woodrow 2000), e.g. a 10% increase in oxygen consumption with each 1°C rise in temperature (Hussein 2009), a rise in intracranial pressure and cerebral damage.

Severe hyperthermia or heat stroke is a core temperature of >42°C (Hussein 2009). It can be caused by MDMA (3,4-methylenedioxymethamphetamine, 'ecstasy'), exposure to high ambient temperatures vigorous activity and certain drugs (malignant hyperthermia) (Hussein 2009). The main effects of severe hyperthermia on the bodily systems include the following (Jones et al. 2003):

- *Cardiovascular system*: tachycardia, ECG changes and cardiac failure
- *Respiratory system*: tachypnoea and respiratory alkalosis
- *Neurological system*: confusion, delirium, convulsions and possibly coma
- *Renal system*: loss of fluid and acute renal failure.

MONITORING PRIORITIES OF A PATIENT WITH HYPERTHERMIA

Monitoring priorities of a patient with hyperthermia include:

- *Regular assessment of vital signs*: airway, respirations, blood pressure, pulse and core temperature
- *Arterial blood gas analysis*: particularly important if the patient has malignant hyperthermia, because acidosis is common
- *ECG monitoring*: to detect arrhythmias
- *Urine output* measurements and strict fluid balance
- *Blood sugar* measurements
- *Neurological function* observations.

In addition it is important to monitor any methods used to cool the patient to ensure that cooling is not too rapid or that the patient becomes hypothermic.

Scenario

A 65-year-old woman was admitted with bronchopneumonia. She looked flushed and was hot to the touch. Her vital signs were BP 130/80 mmHg, pulse 115/min, respiration 25/min, tympanic temperature 34.4°C. The tympanic temperature reading is undoubtedly incorrect. What would you do?

There is probably an error with the equipment or technique. The lens on the thermometer was cleaned with a dry wipe. In addition, the end of the probe was placed in the external auditory meatus, ensuring a snug fit. The tympanic temperature now showed 38.7°C which was more conducive with the patient's clinical condition.

CONCLUSION

A critically ill patient can experience wide fluctuations in body temperature. Severe hypothermia and hyperthermia can be life threatening. Close monitoring of temperature in the critically ill patient is therefore paramount. It is also paramount to understand the principles of monitoring a hypothermic and hyperthermic patient, particularly during re-warming or cooling procedures.

REFERENCES

Andrews, F. & Nolan, J. (2006) Critical care in the emergency department: monitoring the critically ill patient. *Emergency Medicine Journal*, **23**, 561–564.

Bickley, L. & Szilagyi, P. G. (2009) *Bates' Guide to Physical Examination and History Taking*, 10th edn. Philadelphia: PA: Wolters Kluwer Lippincott Williams & Wilkins.

Carson, B. (1999) Successful resuscitation of a 44 year old man with hypothermia. *Journal of Emergency Nursing*, **25**, 356–360.

Department of Health, Social Services and Public Safety (1999) *Control of Substances Hazardous to Health Regulations*. London: The Stationery Office.

Dougherty, L. & Lister, S., eds (2011) *The Royal Marsden Hospital Manual of Clinical Procedures*, 8th edn. Chichester: Wiley-Blackwell.

Farley, A. & McLafferty, E. (2008) Nursing management of the patient with hypothermia. *Nursing Standard*, **22**(17), 43–46.

Hudak, C. M., Gallo, B. M., & Morton, P. G. (1998) *Critical Care Nursing: A holistic approach*, 7th edn. New York: Lippincott.

Hussein. (2009) Thermal disorders. In: Bersten, A. D. & Soni, N. (eds), *Oh's Intensive Care Manual*, 6th edn. Philadelphia, PA: Butterworth Heinemann Elsevier.

Jevon, P. & Jevon, M. (2001) Using a tympanic thermometer. *Nursing Times*, **97**(9), 43–44.

Jones, G., Endacott, R., & Crouch, R. (2003) *Emergency Nursing Care*. London: Greenwich Medical Media Ltd.

Kelly, M., Ewens, B., & Jevon, P. (2001) Hypothermia management. *Nursing Times*, **97**(9), 36–37.

Knies, R. (2003) Temperature Measurement in Acute Care. Available at: www.enw.org/research-Thermometry.htm.

Lefrant, J., Muller, L., Emmanuel Coussaye, J., et al. (2003) Temperature measurement in intensive care patients: comparison of urinary bladder, oesophageal, rectal, axillary and inguinal methods versus pulmonary artery core method. *Intensive Care Medicine*, **29**, 414–418.

Mains, J. A., Coxall, K., & Lloyd, H. (2008) Measuring temperature. *Nursing Standard*, **22**(39), 44-47.

Morley, P. T. (2009) Adult cardiopulmonary resuscitation. In: Bersten, A. D. & Soni, N. (eds), *Oh's Intensive Care Manual*, 6th edn. Philadelphia, PA: Butterworth Heinemann Elsevier.

Resuscitation Council UK (2010) Adult advanced life support, Adult advanced life support algorithm. London.

Skinner, D.V., Swain, A., Robertson, C., & Rodney Peyton, J.W. (1997) *Cambridge Textbook of Accident and Emergency Medicine*. Cambridge: Cambridge University Press.

Sturgess, D. J. & Morgan, T. J. (2009) Haemodynamic monitoring. In: Bersten, A. D. & Soni, N. (eds), *Oh's Intensive Care Manual*, 6th edn. Philadelphia, PA: Butterworth Heinemann Elsevier.

Tortora, G. & Grabowski, S. (1996) *Principles of Anatomy and Physiology*, 8th edn. Boston, MA: Harper Collins.

Trim, J. (2005) Monitoring temperature. *Nursing Times*, **101**(20), 30–31.

Woodrow, P. (2000) *Intensive Care Nursing: A framework for practice*. London: Routledge.

Monitoring Pain

13

LEARNING OBJECTIVES

At the end of this chapter the reader will be able to:

- ❏ discuss the factors *influencing* pain
- ❏ discuss the *methods* of pain assessment
- ❏ discuss the *physiological effects* of unmanaged pain
- ❏ discuss the *modalities of pain management* in this population

INTRODUCTION

The management of pain in the critically ill is an important priority in their care. Critically ill patients often present with painful conditions or have to undergo painful procedures during the course of their intensive care unit (ICU) stay (van Heerden 2009). The adverse consequences of inadequate pain management are complex and both physiological and emotional. These adverse consequences include: anxiety, insomnia, enhancement of the stress response by increasing circulating catecholamines, respiratory complications, and venous and gut stasis (van Heerden 2009). The assessment of pain in the critically ill population is challenging for health-care professionals but it is important that nurses are familiar with the various assessment tools and can monitor the response to pain management strategies.

The aim of this chapter is to understand the principles of monitoring pain.

Monitoring the Critically Ill Patient, Third Edition.
Philip Jevon, Beverley Ewens.
© 2012 Blackwell Publishing Ltd. Published 2012 by Blackwell Publishing Ltd.

FACTORS INFLUENCING PAIN

Pain is a complex subjective phenomenon associated with actual or potential tissue damage (Prevost 2009). The pain in critically ill individuals is classed as acute because it usually has an identified cause, e.g. associated with a procedure either during ICU stay or postoperatively (Prevost 2009). It can be postulated that all patients in an ICU experience acute pain and some, predominantly elderly people, may experience acute and chronic pain associated with pre-existing conditions. Pain is a subjective experience and as such there are many factors that influence the patients' response to and report of pain, such as: previous pain experiences, cultural background, social supports, the meaning and consequence of pain (disease or prognosis), coping styles, degree of control over the pain, anxiety, fear and depression (Macintyre and Schug 2007).

Factors associated with pain in critically ill individuals (Prevost 2009):

- *Symptoms of illness*: e.g. ischaemia, postoperative
- *Sleep disturbance and deprivation*
- *Immobility*: physical constraints due to tubes, etc. or muscle weakness
- *Temperature extremes*: fever
- *Anxiety and depression*
- *Impaired communication*: inability to report pain
- *Fear*: of pain, disability or death
- *Separation*: *from significant others*
- *Boredom*: lack of pleasant distractions
- *Noise overload*: continuous noise from equipment and staff
- *Abnormal light*
- *Disturbance*: awakening and manipulation for re-positioning
- *Procedures*: continuous or intermittent procedures
- *Competing priorities*: life-threatening instability may take precedence over pain management.

Advances in pain management have dramatically altered how pain is effectively managed in the last decade and pain management has become a recognised specialty in itself, with most hospitals implementing acute pain teams because of the detrimental effects that inadequate pain management can have on patients.

Possible barriers to adequate pain relief and the following have been postulated as pain 'myths' (Macintyre and Schug 2007):

- A belief that pain is not harmful but a 'normal' response to surgery
- Concerns that analgesia will obscure a diagnosis, e.g. perforated gut or surgical complication
- Tendency to underestimate pain and not recognise the variability in patients' perceptions of pain
- Lack of regular and frequent assessment of pain and pain-relieving interventions
- Fears that the patients will become addicted to opiates
- Concerns about high risk of respiratory suppression with opiates
- Inadequate patient education
- Patients' reluctance to request analgesia
- Lack of understanding in the variability of patients' opiate requirements
- Lack of recognition that age is a better predictor of opiate requirement than weight in an adult
- Prolonged dosing intervals and a belief that opiates should not be given more frequently than every 4 hours
- Insufficient flexibility in dosing regimens
- Lack of understanding of the need to titrate analgesics to meet individual needs
- Lack of accountability for pain management.

Adverse effects of untreated pain

The adverse effects of untreated pain due to either inaccurate assessment or treatment are well documented and pose considerable risk to the already compromised critically ill patient. Not only does the effect of untreated pain present complications at the time of ICU stay, but it may also contribute to the development of post-traumatic stress disorder (PTSD) or pain syndromes in some ICU survivors (Prevost 2009; van Heerden 2009). The adverse effects of untreated pain can have serious consequences for the already stressed and compromised critically ill patient, and most systems are adversely affected which can lead to inhibition of healing and prolonged recovery (Prevost 2009):

- *Cardiovascular*: tachycardia, hypotension, increased peripheral vascular resistance, increased myocardial oxygen consumption, myocardial ischaemia, DVT, pulmonary embolism
- *Respiratory*: splinting, decreased respiratory effort, sputum retention, atelectasis, pneumonia
- *Gastrointestinal*: decreased gastric emptying and gut motility, leading to ileus and reduced function
- *Genitourinary*: urinary retention
- *Immune system*: suppression of immune function predisposing to infection
- *Metabolic*: increase in catabolic hormones – glucagon, growth hormone, vasopressin, aldosterone. Reduced anabolic hormones, i.e. insulin, testosterone, leading to increased protein breakdown, hyperglycaemia, impaired wound healing and increased muscle breakdown
- *Musculoskeletal*: muscle spasm, immobility, muscle wasting
- *Psychological*: anxiety, fear, helplessness, sleep deprivation, all leading to increased pain
- Central nervous system (CNS): chronic pain due to central sensitisation.

Macintyre and Schug (2007)

METHODS OF ASSESSING PAIN

The inability of health-care professionals to adequately assess pain is one of the primary reasons for inadequate pain management (Prevost 2009). The choice of methods used for assessment are predicted based on our knowledge of what pain is and how pain from an individual is converted to words or expressions perceived by others (Puntillo et al. 2009). Careful consideration needs to be given to the assessment tool chosen for the critically ill population because they are often unable to participate in the assessment process (Puntillo et al. 2009).

Patient's self-report

This is considered the most reliable method of pain assessment (Puntillo et al. 2009). In the ICU population this method is still feasible and offered to patients who are able to communicate, even if not verbally (Puntillo et al. 2009). A numerical rating scale (NRS) with a standard scale of 1–10 can still be utilised if the patient is able to point to the scale or nod to simple commands. It has been reported that even patients with reduced cognitive ability are still able to self-report pain, with the added benefit that this method can be adapted to other variables such as nausea and vomiting (Macintyre and Schug 2007). Laminated charts containing an NRS, as well as an outline of a body that patients can point to locate their pain, are readily available.

Behavioural tools

When the patient is not able to communicate at all, the use of a validated behavioural tool is recommended. Pain assessment using this method is based on behavioural and physiological indicators that guide the practitioner through pain assessment, management and decision-making process (Puntillo et al. 2009). Tools such as the pain assessment, intervention and notation algorithm (PAIN) and critical care pain observation tool (CPOT) prompt the following processes: assessment of pain-related behavioural and physiological indicators, identification of potential risks of opiate administration, and implementation and documentation of analgesic treatment (Puntillo et al. 2009; Gelinas et al. 2011).

Current research

Other methods of pain assessment are currently raising interest and promoting further exploration. The bispectral monitor (BIS) is a non-invasive method using electromyographic (EMG) activity and. in some models. electroencephalographic (EEG) activity to quantify electrophysiological changes in the brain in response to pain (Gelinas et al. 2011).

Pain intervention

The nurse plays a crucial role in the administration of analgesia. Although pharmacological methods are most frequently used, the nurse is uniquely located to give physical and psychological support in the management of pain (Prevost 2009). The mainstay of pharmacological interventions in critically ill patients are opiates, usually intravenous on the ICU (Prevost 2009; van Heerden 2009). Morphine is usually the drug of choice on the ICU because of its efficacy, low cost and availability, although it has some serious side effects in critically ill patients including reduced gut motility and prolonged effect due to its long half-life. Non-steroidal anti-inflammatory drugs (NSAIDs) are not frequently used in the critically ill population because of the potential side effects such as renal dysfunction, gastrointestinal haemorrhage and platelet inhibition leading to increased bleeding tendency (van Heerden 2009).

Monitoring the patient with an epidural

Epidural anaesthesia is viewed as the gold standard in pain relief because it is one of the most effective forms of pain relief (Chumbley and Thomas 2010). A catheter is inserted into the epidural space through the lumbar, thoracic or cervical vertebral processes, facilitating a continuous infusion (Fig 13.1) of opiate (usually fentanyl) and local (anaesthetic, usually bupivacaine), and

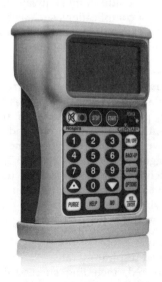

Fig. 13.1 Epidural infusion pump.

facilitating a totally pain-free state (Chumbley and Thomas 2010). Advantages of an epidural include reduction in postoperative complications and reduced cardiovascular stress (Macintyre and Schug 2007).

Monitoring the patient with an epidural

The following should be monitored at regular intervals (Macintyre and Schug 2007):

- Pain score, sedation score and respiratory rate
- BP and heart rate
- Sensory block, testing at the level of block and assessing the sensation of cold and warmth
- Motor block, the ability of the patient to raise the legs. Ideally motor block should not be present, allowing the patient to mobilise freely (Bromage score measures sensory and motor block).

The patient with an epidural must always have patent intravenous access in case of complications such as hypotension and the use of drugs such as naloxone and ephedrine to combat the effects of opiate complications and vasodilatation.

Monitoring the patient with patient-controlled analgesia

Patient-controlled analgesia (PCA) combines the benefits of efficient intravenous pain management with patient control and greater patient satisfaction (Macintyre and Schug 2007). The patients must, however, be able to understand and physically able to operate the trigger on the device (Fig. 13.2) to enable the dose of opiate to be delivered. Most frequently used opiates include morphine, fentanyl and occasionally pethidine.

A patient receiving a PCA should have monitored at regular intervals (Macintyre and Schug 2007):

- Pain score, sedation score
- BP, heart rate and respiratory rate
- The dose delivered, including successful and unsuccessful patient attempts
- Dose of any drug administered for side effects
- Changes that may have been made to the PCA programme.

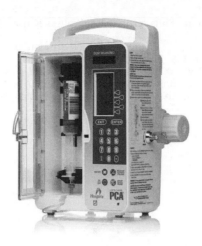

Fig. 13.2 Patient-controlled analgesia (PCA) pump.

CONCLUSION

Effective pain management is an essential component of the nurses' role. The effects of inadequate pain management are significant and can impact on the patient's long- and short-term recovery. The nurse must be proficient in pain assessment techniques and tools, and be able to administer and evaluate pain management methods.

REFERENCES

Chumbley, G. & Thomas, S. (2010) Care of the patient receiving epidural analgesia. *Nursing Standard*, **3**(9), 35–40.

Gelinas, C., Tousignant-Laflamme, Y., Tanguay, A., & Bourgault, P. (2011) Exploring the validity of the bispectral index, the critical-care pain observation tool and vital signs for the detection of pain in sedated and mechanically ventilated critically ill adults: A pilot study. *Intensive and Critical Care Nursing*, **27**, 46–52.

Macintyre, P. E. & Schug, S. A. (2007) *Acute Pain Management*, 3rd edn. Philadelphia, PA: Saunders Elsevier.

Prevost, S. S. (2009) Relieving pain and providing comfort. In: Gonce Morton, P. & Fontaine, D. K. (eds), *Critical Care Nursing. A holistic approach*, 9th edn. Philadelphia, PA: Wolters Kluwer Lippincott Williams & Wilkins.

Puntillo, K., Pasero, C., Li, D., et al. (2009) Evaluation of pain in ICU patients. *Chest*, **135**, 1069–1074.

van Heerden, P. V. (2009) Sedation, analgesia and muscle relaxation in the intensive care unit. In: Bersten, A. D. & Soni, N. (eds), *Oh's Intensive Care Manual*, 6th edn. Philadelphia, PA: Butterworth Heinemann Elsevier.

Monitoring a Patient Receiving a Blood Transfusion

14

LEARNING OBJECTIVES

At the end of the chapter the reader will be able to:

❐ list the *different blood components* and discuss their uses
❐ discuss the importance of *patient identification*
❐ discuss *documentation, traceability and equipment* for a patient receiving a blood transfusion.
❐ discuss *monitoring priorities* in a patient receiving a blood transfusion
❐ outline the *adverse reactions* to a blood transfusion

INTRODUCTION

Blood transfusion is an essential and significant part of modern health-care treatment. It is the ability to transfer blood components from one person to another and can save lives. The process of blood transfusion requires careful preparation and treatment to minimise risks and complications. Most importantly, a patient receiving a transfusion of blood products must be adequately monitored so that any adverse reactions/complications can be recognised promptly and effectively treated and managed.

The aim of this chapter is to understand monitoring of a patient receiving a blood transfusion.

BLOOD COMPONENTS AND THEIR USES

When the National Blood Service centrifuges whole donor blood it can be separated and processed into blood components for transfusion:

Monitoring the Critically Ill Patient, Third Edition.
Philip Jevon, Beverley Ewens.
© 2012 Blackwell Publishing Ltd. Published 2012 by Blackwell Publishing Ltd.

- Red cells (erythrocytes)
- Platelets (thrombocytes)
- Plasma (contains clotting factors).

All donations are tested to detect human immunodeficiency virus (HIV), hepatitis B, hepatitis C, syphilis and human T-cell leukaemia virus (HTLV).

Red cells

Once the plasma and buffy coat (white blood cell and platelets) have been removed from whole blood, the red cells are suspended in an additive solution for preservation purposes during storage. Red cells are stored at 2–6°C in a temperature controlled fridge and have a shelf-life of 35 days from date of donation. Once collected from blood storage, red cells should be transfused within 4 hours.

Red cell transfusions are required to increase the oxygen-carrying capacity of the blood by raising the haemoglobin concentration of patients with acute and chronic anaemia. Experienced clinicians in a suitable setting, such as accident and emergency resuscitation rooms, high dependency (HDU) or intensive care unit (ICU), should ideally manage patients with acute massive blood loss (Blood Committee for Standards in Haematology Blood Transfusion or BSCH 2001). Acute anaemia is often accompanied by the features of hypovolaemic shock such as an increase in pulse and respiration rate. Patients with chronic anaemia should have the cause of the anaemia established and a transfusion should not be given where effective alternatives exist such as treatment of iron deficiency, megaloblastic anaemia and autoimmune haemolytic anaemia. Red cell transfusions for patients with chronic anaemia should be given only to maintain the haemoglobin just above the lowest concentration that is not associated with the symptoms of anaemia. Symptoms may include fatigue, shortness of breath, chest pain and confusion.

There are no reliable parameters to guide the need for red cell transfusion. The decision to transfuse red cells is a complex one and depends on factors such as cause of anaemia, severity, the patient's ability to compensate for the anaemia and the likelihood of further blood loss. The risks of a transfusion need to be balanced against the benefits. Red cell compatibility according to the ABO system is shown in Table 14.1.

Table 14.1 Red cell compatibility

Patient blood group	Red cell antigens	Plasma antibodies	Donor group compatibility
A	A	Anti-B	A and O
B	B	Anti-A	B and O
AB	AB	None	A, B, AB and O
O	O	Anti-A and anti-B	O

Table 14.2 Selection of fresh frozen plasma according to recipient blood group

Recipient group	O	A	B	AB
First choice	O	A	B	AB
Second choice	A	AB	AB	A
Third choice	B	B	A	B
Fourth choice	AB			

Fresh frozen plasma and cryoprecipitate

Standard fresh frozen plasma (FFP) is produced from both UK and non-UK donors; methylene blue FFP is available for children under the age of 16 years. The FFP is sourced from the USA as a precaution against variant Creutzfeldt–Jakob Disease (vCJD). FFP is frozen and stored at −30°C with a shelf-life of 24 months. If required FFP is rapidly thawed at 37°C before being issued. Once thawed, FFP should be transfused within 4 hours. However, if FFP is stored at 4°C after thawing, the transfusion can be completed within 24 hours. FFP may be indicated if the patient has a single factor deficiency for which there is no virus-safe fractioned product, severe bleeding, disseminated intravascular coagulation (DIC) and thrombotic thrombocytopenic purpura (TTP) (BSCH 2004a). Table 14.2 shows the principles of selection of FFP.

Cryoprecipitate is a plasma product that contains clotting factors such as factor VIII, fibrinogen and factor XIII. The most common use for cryoprecipitate is to enhance fibrinogen levels in dysfibrinogenaemia and acquired hypofibrinogenaemia seen in massive transfusion and DIC. Treatment is usually indicated if plasma fibrinogen is less than 1 g/l. Cryoprecipitate once thawed should be transfused immediately. The use of FFP and cryoprecipitate should be guided by monitoring using laboratory coagulation screens.

Platelets
Platelets can be either pooled or apheresis. When pooled platelets are produced from the National Blood Service, donated whole blood is centrifuged to separate the red cells, platelets and plasma. Four donations of platelets are pooled to produce one adult unit of platelets. Apheresis platelets are collected from just the donor who only donates platelets. Red cells are not collected from this donor, although the platelets are in the plasma.

All platelets must be stored on a special agitator rack at 20–24°C to prevent clumping. Each unit of platelets has a shelf-life of 5 days from the date of donation. Platelet transfusions are indicated for the prevention and treatment of haemorrhage in patients with thrombocytopenia (low platelet count) or platelet function defects. The cause of thrombocytopenia should be established before a decision is made for a platelet transfusion (BSCH 2003). Risks associated with platelet transfusions include alloimmunisation, transmission of infection, allergic reactions and transfusion-related lung injury (TRLI).

IMPORTANCE OF PATIENT IDENTIFICATION
Serious hazards of transfusion reports (1996–2008) have identified that a patient identification band missing, defaced or hidden is a significant contributory factor to wrong blood incidents. All patients receiving a blood transfusion must wear a patient identification band (or a risk assessed to be equivalent). The minimum patient identifiers are last name, first name, date of birth and unique patient identification number. The information must be legible and accurate. In emergency situations the patient's core identifiers may be unknown. In this situation, at least one unique identifier, usually a temporary identification number (e.g. accident and emergency number), and the patient's gender (i.e. unknown male/female) must be used.

Patient identification should be checked and confirmed as correct at each stage of the transfusion process. The patient should, whenever possible, be asked to state full name and date of birth. This must match exactly the information on the patient's wristband and any other associated paperwork required at that stage of the blood transfusion process. For patients who are unable to identify themselves, e.g. patients who are unable to respond competently, or are unconscious or confused, verification of the patient's identification should be obtained from a parent or carer if present. If there are patient identification discrepancies at any stage of the transfusion process, the information must be verified and discrepancies investigated and corrected before proceeding to the next stage of the process.

DOCUMENTATION, TRACEABILITY AND EQUIPMENT
Documentation
Full and complete documentation is required at every stage of the blood transfusion process to provide an assured and unambiguous audit trail. Minimum documentation of transfusion episodes in the patient clinical records should include:

Pre-transfusion

- Clinical indication for transfusion
- Pre-transfusion indices (e.g. full blood count, coagulation screen)
- Date of decision
- Date of transfusion (if known)
- Blood component to be transfused and volume
- Rate of transfusion
- Consent from patient (written consent not required)
- Special requirements (e.g. irradiated or cytomegalovirus [CMV]-seronegative components).

Administration

- Date and time component collected
- Date and time transfusion started
- The donation number of component transfused
- Volume administered
- Identification of staff who started the transfusion
- Observations before, during and after transfusion.

Post-transfusion

- Date and time component completed
- Evidence of unit being fated
- An indication of whether transfusion achieved desired effect
- Documentation of any reactions that occurred.

Traceability

To ensure compliance with the Blood Safety and Quality Regulations (MHRA 2005) all blood components should be traceable from the donor to their final destination, whether this be a recipient, manufacturer or disposal. All organisations have a policy on how to achieve this by using electronic or manual methods. This information is then kept for 30 years.

Equipment

Intravenous access

All blood components can be administered through standard peripheral intravenous cannulas according to manufacturer's specifications. The size of the intravenous cannulas depends on the size and integrity of the vein as well as the speed at which the blood component is to be transfused. All blood components can be slowly infused through small-bore cannulas or butterfly needles, e.g. 21 gauge (G). For more rapid infusion, large-bore needles e.g. 14 G, are needed. Peripherally inserted long central catheters (PICC lines) with narrow lumen diameter may lead to slower rates. Many transfused patients have venous access established by the use of short-term or indwelling multi-lumen central lines. These are usually suitable for transfusion of blood components. One lumen should be reserved for administering blood components where possible.

Administration set

Blood components must be administered only using a 'blood administration set' that has an integral 170–200 μm screen filter. It is now deemed unnecessary to prime the blood administration set with saline. The blood administration line should be changed at least every 12 hours and after completion of the prescribed blood transfusion to prevent bacterial growth. Platelets should not be transfused through an administration set that has been previously used for red cells or other components because this may cause aggregation and retention of platelets in the line.

Infusion pumps
Electronic infusion devises may be used for the administration of blood and blood components if they are licensed to do so. Rapid infusion devices may be used when large volumes have to be infused quickly, as in massive haemorrhage. These typically have a range of 6–30 l/h and usually incorporate a blood-warming device. It is important to be familiar with the equipment and use it according to the manufacturer's instructions.

Blood warmers
Rapid infusion of red cells soon after their removal from blood storage refrigeration at 4°C can lead to hypothermia, arrhythmias, cardiac arrest or impaired blood clotting in surgical or trauma patients. This is also of concern when blood is rapidly infused through a central venous catheter terminating in or near the right atrium, or in neonates and small infants undergoing large-volume transfusions (BSCH 2004b). The National Institute for Health and Clinical Excellence (NICE 2008) recommends that, in all adults undergoing elective or emergency surgery under general or regional anaesthesia, all blood components should be warmed to 37°C.

Blood warmers should also be used in the transfusion of patients with clinically significant antibodies. Blood should only be warmed using CE-marked, specifically designed and regularly maintained blood-warming equipment with a visible thermometer and audible warning. Some blood warmers operate up to 43°C but are safe provided that they are used and serviced according to the manufacturer's instructions. Blood must never be warmed in an uncontrolled way, such as in a microwave, in hot water or on a radiator.

MONITORING PRIORITIES IN A PATIENT RECEIVING A BLOOD TRANSFUSION
A blood transfusion should take place only when there are sufficient staff available to observe and monitor the patient. The patient should always be visually observed and monitored throughout the blood transfusion to ensure quick identification of any adverse

reactions. This is particularly necessary if patients are unconscious because they are unable to complain of any transfusion reaction symptoms. A conscious patient should be made aware of the symptoms of a transfusion reaction and advised to inform health-care staff immediately should he or she experience one. Ensure that the patient's 'call bell' is easy to reach.

Pre-transfusion

Transfusion observations must be clearly distinguished from other routine observations and filed in the patient's clinical notes. Immediately before collecting the first unit of blood component record the patient's temperature, pulse rate, blood pressure and respiration rate. These should be taken no more than 60 minutes before the start of the transfusion. This is to provide baseline observations in case of a reaction during the transfusion. It also allows staff to assess the patient's medical condition before starting the transfusion. If there are any concerns raised by the baseline observations, medical advice should be sought before collecting the unit of blood from the transfusion department. Equipment required for the blood transfusion should also be ready because a delay once the blood component has been collected could result in unnecessary wastage.

During transfusion

Many serious reactions occur in within 30 minutes of commencement of the transfusion of a blood component unit (Serious Hazards of Transfusion or SHOT scheme 2006), so close observation during this period is essential. Pulse rate, blood pressure, temperature and respiration rate should be taken and recorded 15 minutes after the start of each component transfusion. For rapid infusion more frequent observations may be required. Assessment should be made for signs of a transfusion reaction, in particular pyrexia, hypo- or hypertension and tachycardia. The National Confidential Enquiry into Patient Outcome and Death (NCEPOD 2005) reported that, in critically ill medical patients, the respiratory rate is an early and important indicator of deterioration. Difficulty in breathing and rapid respiration may both be features of serious transfusion reactions. Possible signs and symptoms of a blood component transfusion reaction include:

- Pyrexia
- Tachycardia
- Change in blood pressure
- Breathlessness or rapid breathing
- Coughing
- Haemoglobinuria
- Nausea
- Vomiting
- Diarrhoea
- Skin flushing/rash
- Rigors
- Collapse
- Chest, abdominal, bone, muscle or loin pain
- Headache
- Restlessness, agitation or confusion.

If a transfusion reaction is suspected, inform the doctor or nurse in charge immediately. Stop the transfusion and check that the correct patient details are on the blood component and the right blood has been given to the right patient. Development of any symptoms suggesting a transfusion reaction should prompt more frequent observations of temperature, pulse, blood pressure, respiratory rate, oxygen saturation levels and urine output. The doctor may request the transfusion to be discontinued due to the transfusion reaction or adverse event. In these cases the blood component, along with the giving set, should be removed and sealed per organisational policy and sent to the hospital transfusion department for further investigations.

Post-transfusion
After each blood component has been transfused, record the post-transfusion pulse rate, blood pressure and temperature. If these measurements have altered significantly from any previous observations, respiratory rate should also be taken. Any routine observations should be continued, particularly if the patient is critically ill.

The SHOT (2008) report emphasises that, on occasion, transfusion reactions can occur many hours after the transfusion is completed and recommends that patients are observed during the subsequent 24 hours. For transfusions administered as day cases, continued direct observation is not possible. Such patients should be counselled about the possibility of late adverse reactions and organisations should ensure that mechanisms are in place that give patients access to clinical advice at all times.

ADVERSE REACTIONS TO A BLOOD TRANSFUSION

It is often difficult to distinguish which type of reaction is taking place because the signs and symptoms of these reactions are very similar and are detailed below. The most important transfusion reactions are:

- Acute haemolytic transfusion reactions
- Infusion of a bacterially contaminated unit
- TRALI
- Severe allergic reaction or anaphylaxis
- Post-transfusion purpura (PTP)
- Transfusion-associated graft-versus-host disease.

In all cases expert medical advice can be sought from a haematologist and the blood transfusion department must be informed as soon as possible, who may need to inform the National Blood Service or the Medicines and Healthcare products Regulatory Agency.

Acute haemolytic transfusion reactions

This often occurs when patients are transfused with incompatible red cells, and is when the patient's own anti-A or anti-B antibodies cause an acute severe clinical reaction. Acute haemolytic transfusion reactions are most commonly due to errors in obtaining or labelling group and antibody screen samples, collecting the wrong blood for the wrong patient, or failure to carry out the required bedside checks before the unit is administered. Signs and symptoms of an acute transfusion reaction are:

- Pain at cannulation site
- Pain in chest, back or abdomen
- Hypotension/Hypertension
- Tachycardia
- Pyrexia
- Bleeding

- Collapse
- Haemoglobinuria.

Acute haemolytic transfusion reactions can lead to acute renal failure and DIC, which can be fatal. Management of haemolytic transfusion reactions would consist of stopping the transfusion immediately but maintaining venous access and seeking more expert advice from a haematologist. Return the blood component to the blood transfusion department with any extra samples requested. Administer intravenous saline via a new giving set. The patient will need to be monitored closely so it is suggested that the patient be admitted onto a critical care unit if possible.

Infusion of a bacterially contaminated unit

The signs and symptoms of this type of reaction may be similar to acute haemolytic reactions or severe acute allergic reactions. Bacterial contamination of blood components are rare, but it is more often reported with infusion of platelets, which are stored at a higher temperature of 22°C than red cells which are stored at 4°C. If a blood component is bacterially contaminated, most probably it will have discoloration, a smell or a Gram stain. The most common signs of infusion of a bacterially contaminated unit are:

- Acute reaction with rigors
- Pyrexia
- Hypo-/hypertension
- Tachycardia
- Collapse.

Suggested treatment would be to stop the transfusion immediately and seek medical advice, and contact a microbiologist for expert advice. Intravenous antibiotics should be administered that cover both Gram-positive and Gram-negative bacteria. Return blood component to the blood transfusion department with any samples requested.

Transfusion-related lung injury

TRALI is mostly associated with transfusion of plasma containing white cell antibodies, which will react with the patient's own white cells. Symptoms usually occur within 6 hours of transfusion, which are:

- Breathlessness
- Non-productive cough
- Loss of circulatory volume
- Hypotension
- Acute dyspnoea
- Hypoxia
- Neutropenia.

The chest radiograph characteristically shows bilateral nodular infiltrates in a batwing pattern, typical of acute respiratory distress syndrome (ARDS). It may be difficult to distinguish TRALI from other non-cardiogenic pulmonary oedema or cardiac failure; therefore it may be necessary to seek advice from a critical care specialist as well as a haematologist. Treatment should be the same as for patients with ARDS. High concentration oxygen or mechanical ventilatory support may be needed.

Allergic reactions or anaphylaxis

Allergic reactions or anaphylaxis to blood units usually occur at the start of transfusion. They are normally associated with rapid transfusion of plasma. Anaphylaxis occurs when a patient who is pre-sensitised to an allergen producing IgE antibodies is again exposed to the antigen. Patients who are deficient in IgA can develop antibodies to IgA and cause anaphylaxis if exposed to IgA in transfusion. Symptoms may include:

- Hypotension
- Bronchospasm
- Chest pain
- Abdominal pain
- Dyspnoea
- Nausea
- Vomiting
- Urticaria
- Periorbital and laryngeal oedema

- Redness of skin
- Conjunctivitis.

In severe anaphylaxis stop transfusion and call for medical advice immediately. Consider giving intravenous chlorpheniramine.

Post-transfusion purpura

This is a rare complication of transfusion that most often occurs in female patients. It is caused by platelet-specific alloantibodies. The main symptoms are an extremely low platelet count typically 5–9 days after transfusion. The patient may also develop bruising or bleeding.

Treatment of post-transfusion purpura is a high-dose intravenous immunoglobulin. Platelet transfusions may be necessary if the patient is at high risk of bleeding.

Transfusion-associated graft-versus-host disease

Transfusion-associated graft-versus-host disease (TA-GvHD) is caused when white cells present in the blood component recognise the recipient's HLA antigens as foreign which leads to engraftment. The skin, gut, liver, spleen and bone marrow are affected, commonly within 2–3 weeks of transfusion, and are usually fatal. There is no effective treatment and expert advise from a haematologist is recommended. High-risk groups, such as patients who are immunocompromised, should be given irradiated blood products only to prevent this from happening. This is when blood components are treated with 25 gray (Gy) gamma irradiation to inactivate lymphocytes that could cause TA-GvHD.

CONCLUSION

Blood transfusions should be carried out only when the risks to the patient are balanced against the benefits. Once a decision has been made to transfuse, full and complete documentation must be completed at every stage of the blood transfusion. Patients should also be monitored throughout their blood transfusion to ensure quick identification of any adverse reactions. All blood components should be traceable from the donor to its final destination.

REFERENCES

British Committee for Standards in Haematology Blood Transfusion (2001) The clinical use of red cell transfusion. *British Journal of Haematology*, **113**, 24–31

British Committee for Standards in Haematology Blood Transfusion (BSCH) (2003) Guideline for the use of platelet transfusions. *British Journal of Haematology*, **122**, 10–23.

British Committee for Standards in Haematology Blood Transfusion (2004a) Guidelines for the use of fresh-frozen plasma, cryoprecipitate and cryosupernatant. *British Society for Haematology*, **126**, 11–28.

British Committee for Standards in Haematology Blood Transfusion (2004b) Transfusion guidelines for neonates and older children. *British Journal of Haematology*, **124**, 433–453.

MHRA (2005) *Statutory Instrument 2005/50*. London: The Stationery Office.

National Confidential Enquiry into Patient Outcome and Death (2005) *An Acute Problem*. London: NCEPOD.

National Institute for Health and Clinical Excellence (2008) *Clinical Practice Guideline: The management of inadvertent perioperative hypothermia in adults*. London: NICE.

Serious Hazards of Transfusion (SHOT) scheme (1996–2008) *SHOT Annual reports 1996–2008*. Manchester: SHOT Office.

Monitoring the Patient with Infection and Related Systemic Inflammatory Response

15

LEARNING OUTCOMES
At the end of the chapter the reader will be able to:

☐ discuss how infection occurs and the relationship between the infectious agent and the host
☐ outline the body's defence mechanisms against infection
☐ describe the systemic inflammatory response syndrome (SIRS)
☐ discuss the monitoring of a patient with SIRS/sepsis

INTRODUCTION
Infection can be defined as a pathological state, the presence of a pathogenic organism, such as a bacterium or virus, in the body. The incidence of infection in the UK is difficult to define because a large proportion of people who develop an infection rarely become sick enough to warrant access to primary and, in particular, secondary health-care services. For any patient accessing health-care institutions, the environment can be considered an excellent culture medium, or breeding ground, for infection; it is an environment in which infected patients meet those susceptible to infection and the transport between these parties, in most cases, are the workers who deliver care and treatment.

If a patient accesses health care with an infection, as a primary or secondary complaint, the term 'community-acquired infection' is used. Other patients develop an infection as a result of exposure

Monitoring the Critically Ill Patient, Third Edition.
Philip Jevon, Beverley Ewens.
© 2012 Blackwell Publishing Ltd. Published 2012 by Blackwell Publishing Ltd.

to organisms while in the health-care setting; this is termed a 'health-care-associated infection' (HCAI). The incidence of HCAIs is thought to be around 9% of patients in hospitals, and has been estimated to cost the NHS £1 billion per year (National Audit Office 2000). HCAIs are considered to be responsible for causing 5000 deaths and being a contributory factor in 15000 deaths per year in the UK (National Audit Office 2004). Not all HCAIs are avoidable; however, a significant proportion can be prevented (Pratt et al. 2007) and this remains one of the greatest challenges to health-care staff. National evidence-based guidelines for preventing HCAIs have been published (Department of Health or DH 2007; Pratt et al. 2007). These guidelines underpin all practice outlined in this chapter; they are, however, not the main focus. Many patients with infections go on to develop sepsis, septic shock and severe sepsis, which carries a mortality rate of more than 25%, the incidence of which appears to be increasing (Dellinger et al., 2008). Evidence suggests that the early recognition and early goal-directed resuscitation of the septic patient during the first 6 hours after recognition can have a beneficial effect on outcome and reduce mortality (Dellinger et al. 2008).

The aim of this chapter is to understand the monitoring of a patient with an infection and related systemic inflammatory response.

HOW INFECTION OCCURS AND THE RELATIONSHIP BETWEEN THE INFECTIOUS AGENT AND HOST

The interrelationship of the infectious agent, host and mechanism through which the microorganism gains access is referred to as the chain of infection (World Health Organization or WHO 2004). The links in this chain can be described as follows:

- The infectious agent – this can be any pathogenic organism
- The host or reservoir – the natural habitat for the organism in which it must propagate
- The portal of exit – the escape route of the pathogen from the reservoir, e.g. body fluids/secretions or breaks in natural barriers such as the skin
- The route of transmission – the transport mechanism of spread, such as direct contact or airborne transmission

- The portal of entry – the route into the new host, such as the respiratory or gastrointestinal system
- The susceptible host – the organism that accepts the pathogen.

Strategies to reduce infection of any origin must be based on breaking the links in the chain of infection transmission. The health-care environment makes this a great challenge because increases in risk, in each link of the chain, are likely to be present.

One of the many ways that infection transmission can be reduced is to identify patients with an infection early and initiate treatment aimed at breaking the transmission chain as early as possible. This will include the application of recognised infection control practices and laboratory testing, with other strategies such as pharmacological treatment, source isolation and organism-specific therapy.

THE BODY'S DEFENCE MECHANISMS AGAINST INFECTION
Physical and chemical barriers to infection (innate defence)

Innate defence consists of physical and chemical barriers as well as an inflammatory response. The skin acts as a physical barrier impermeable to most microorganisms; it is colonised by many commensal organisms. Commensal organisms compete with pathogens for nutrients and inhibit growth by producing lactic acid (Storey and Jordan 2008). Commensal bacteria provide defence in other body systems including the mouth, and gastrointestinal and genitourinary systems.

The respiratory system defences include the ciliated mucosa in its action of propelling secretions out of the respiratory tree and the production of a bactericidal/virucidal mucus; coughing and sneezing accelerate this movement. This process is perhaps best described as a mucociliary escalator (Steen 2009).

Organisms are prevented from entering the lower gastrointestinal system by the bactericidal effects of hydrochloric acid which inactivates ingested microorganisms (Martinsen et al. 2005) Other innate systems include salivary flow and enzyme production in the mouth, and immunoglobulin production in the intestine.

The inflammatory response

When there is either an invasion of foreign material such as bacteria or damage to tissue such as ischaemia, an immune/inflammatory response is provoked (Jenkins et al. 2007). Inflammation is the response of vascularised tissue to local injury, involving white blood cells and inflammatory mediators (Storey and Jordan 2008) The aims of the response are to eliminate the cause of tissue damage, remove any dead cells and restore the constancy of the environment (Montague et al. 2005). Inflammation is usually characterised by four signs/symptoms:

1. Redness (hyperaemia)
2. Pain
3. Localised heat
4. Swelling.

The normal response to infection is illustrated in Fig. 15.1.

Acquired defences

Humoral immunity

Exposure to a certain infectious disease creates a resistance to that disease. Specialised blood proteins called antibodies are produced which bind to the infectious agent or substance (antigen). This binding process destroys the antigen. B lymphocytes processed in the lymphatic tissue, outside the thymus gland, have specific antigen receptors called surface immunoglobulins. The reaction between the immunoglobulin and the antigen causes cell proliferation of the B cells into memory and plasma cells, which secrete large amounts of immunoglobulin molecules

Cell-mediated immunity

Lymphocytes, processed by the thymus (T lymphocytes) carry genetic information to bind with and destroy a multitude of antigens, yet recognise and remain inactive to antigens produced by the body's own cells. T lymphocytes or T cells are classified into certain groups depending on their function, which may include enhancing the effects of other immune responses (T-helper cells) and suppressing or deactivating the response (T-regulator cells).

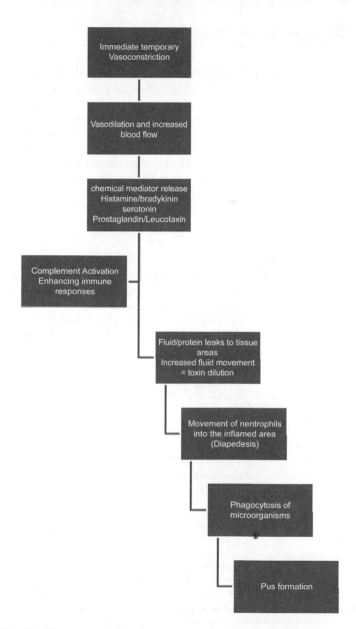

Fig. 15.1 The response to infection.

THE SYSTEMIC INFAMMATORY RESPONSE SYNDROME

The inflammatory process is self-contained by feedback mechanisms that increase and then limit inflammation (Steen 2009). However, the factor that has triggered the inflammation may be overwhelming or not contained, and/or the response itself may not be limited by feedback mechanisms. When this occurs systemic effects are noted which are described as the systemic inflammatory response syndrome (SIRS). This term has been used interchangeably over recent years with terms such as sepsis, septic shock and severe sepsis; there are, however, differences, which are illustrated in Table 15.1.

Patient presentation

A major factor in SIRS is that any organ system in the body can be affected although some, such as the lungs, kidneys or clotting system are more vulnerable (Adam and Osborne, 2005), so presentation may differ. Levy et al. (2003) proposed the variables in Table 15.2 as possible signs of systemic inflammation in response to infection.

Table 15.1 Table of definitions

Term	Definition
Bacteraemia	The presence of viable bacteria in the blood
Septicaemia	The presence of toxins or microorganisms in the blood
Sepsis	Systemic inflammatory response with an infective cause
Systemic inflammatory response	A non-specific inflammatory response of the body to an intrinsic insult (of which infection is only one cause)
Septic shock	Sepsis-induced hypertension (BP < 90 mmHg or reduced by 40 mmHg from baseline without another cause), which is unresponsive to fluid resuscitation with manifestations of hypoperfusion, such as oliguria, altered mental state, etc.
Severe sepsis	Sepsis complicated by organ dysfunction

Adapted from Bone et al. (1992).

Table 15.2 Possible signs of systemic inflammation in response to infection

Infection, documented or suspected, and some of the following:

General variables
Fever (core temperature > 38.3°C)
Hypothermia (core temperature < 36°C)
Heart rate > 90 min
Tachypnoea
Altered mental status
Significant oedema or positive fluid balance (> 20 ml/kg over 24 h)
Hyperglycaemia (plasma glucose >7.7 mmol/l) in the absence of diabetes

Inflammatory variables
Leukocytosis (WBC count >12 000 mm^3)
Leukopenia (WBC count < 400 mm^3)
Normal WBC count with > 10% immature forms
Plasma C-reactive protein > 280 above the normal value

Haemodynamic variables
Arterial hypotension (systolic blood pressure <90 mmHg; mean arterial pressure <70 mmHg or a systolic >40 mmHg
Venous oxygen saturations >70%
Cardiac index >3.5 l/min per m^2

Organ dysfunction variables
Arterial hypoxaemia (arterial oxygen/inspired oxygen ratio <300)
Acute oliguria (urine output < 0.5 ml/kg per h despite adequate fluid resuscitation)
Creatinine increase >0.5 mg/dl
Coagulation abnormalities (INR >1.5 or a PTT >60 s)
Ileus (absent bowel sounds)
Thrombocytopenia (platelet count <100 000)
Hyperbilirubinaemia (plasma total bilirubin >4 mg/dl or 70 mol/l)
Tissue perfusion variables
Hyperlactataemia (>upper limit of lab normal)
Decreased capillary refill or mottling

From Levy et al. (2003).
INR, international normalised ratio; PTT, partial thromboplastin time.

Levy et al. (2003) continue to suggest that SIRS can occur as result of a variety of insults, illustrated in Table 15.3. However, it is usually manifested by two or more of the following conditions:

- Temperature >38°C
- Heart rate >90 beats/min
- Respiratory rate >20 breaths/min or hyperventilation with arterial partial pressure of carbon dioxide (PaO_2) 4.3 kPa

- White cell count >12000 mm^3 or <4000 mm^3 or 10% immature neutrophils.

Table 15.3 Triggers for systemic inflammatory response syndrome (SIRS)

Ischaemic tissue
Haemorrhage
Massive blood transfusion
Organ hypoperfusion followed by reperfusion
Major surgery
Trauma
Pancreatitis
Burns

Levy et al. (2003).

The pathophysiology of SIRS/sepsis

The pathophysiological process of SIRS/sepsis is a result of inappropriate control of the normal responses to inflammation. The normal mechanisms of vasodilatation, leaky capillaries and clot formation are exaggerated (Robson et al. 2005) and may be continually reactivated. This cascade leads to organ dysfunction and failure.

The principal mechanisms of the cascade are as follows:

- Activation of the immune response and inflammatory mediators that activate the complement pathway, enhancing inflammation and phagocytosis. If large amounts of complement activation occur and appear systemically then actions become detrimental (Adam and Osborne 2005).
- The phagocytosis of the pathogenic organism by the white blood cells involves the release of certain proteases and oxygen free radicals which, if they enter the systemic circulation, cause further tissue damage.
- The coagulation pathway is triggered, by either the initial insult or endothelial damage caused predominantly by white blood cell activation. Disseminated intravascular coagulopathy (DIC) can occur if this reaction is not localised. Thrombi caused by DIC can interfere with blood flow to the tissues and organs, and

together with hypotension and hypovolaemia can lead to organ failure (Robson et al. 2005).

- Platelet aggregation (clumping together) is triggered by endothelial damage and this compounds the DIC picture. Normally the body will attempt to break down any blood clots by fibrinolysis and will also release anti-inflammatory mediators to counterbalance the inflammatory mediators.

However, these counter-responses can be inhibited (Robson et al. 2005). The damaged endothelium continues to activate mediator release, which includes powerful vasodilatory substances such as bradykinin and endothelial-derived relaxing factor which, if are not localised, cause systemic vasodilatation with associated increased capillary permeability. This leads to hypotension, intravascular hypovolaemia and further organ hypoperfusion.

Sepsis is associated with systemic, mediator-induced alterations in oxygen utilisation, including increased oxygen demand, altered oxygen extraction and decreased myocardial contractility (Vincent 2008); this may be further influenced by maldistribution of blood flow and impaired oxygen diffusion.

MONITORING A PATIENT WITH SIRS/SEPSIS

Identifying patients with severe sepsis in primary care, emergency departments, wards or admission units is crucial to reducing mortality (Peel 2008). The Resuscitation Council (2006) recommend that clinical staff should follow the ABCDE approach when assessing (and treating) critically ill patients. This will help to ensure that critical illness is promptly identified and appropriately managed (Jevon 2010). The ABCDE framework illustrated throughout this text requires no modification in its application to the patient with SIRS/sepsis. However, its process is demonstrated below to identify key criteria that may lead to early recognition and prompt treatment

Airway

Should the degree of inflammatory response compromise respiratory function, as is common (Adam and Osborne 2005), mechanical ventilatory support may be indicated and an artificial airway will be required. This should be performed by senior anaesthetic staff with skilled assistance.

Breathing

There are many factors in SIRS that could lead towards respiratory compromise. These include:

- Chest infection as a primary cause of SIRS
- Ventilation–perfusion mismatch from maldistribution of blood volume and hypovolaemia
- Pulmonary oedema as a result of fluid shifts, changes in intravascular osmotic pressure and decreased myocardial contractility
- Mediator-induced alterations in oxygen use, including increased oxygen demand and altered oxygen extraction
- Increased respiratory drive due to metabolic acidosis (organ hypoperfusion and hyperlactataemia)
- Acute inflammatory changes in the lungs.

Breathing respiratory assessment should occur as outlined in Chapter 3. Basic assessment should include assessment of general colour, mental state and respiratory rate. Respiratory rhythm, regularity and chest expansion should all be noted (Docherty 2002); increases in respiratory rate may be driven by a metabolic acidosis caused by anaerobic metabolism. Work of breathing may be increased as demonstrated by tachypnoea and the use of accessory muscles. Abnormalities in gas exchange may be evident on arterial blood gas analysis; hypoxia and hypercapnia where present can alter mental state, so confusion/delirium may be present (Higgins and Guest 2008).

Systemic vasodilatation may cause the patient to look flushed, which could mask changes of respiratory failure such as cyanosis. The chest should be auscultated to identify any added sounds, such as wheeze or crepitations which may indicate oedema (Pryor and Prasad 2008).

The volume and characteristics of pulmonary secretions should be assessed (Adam and Osborne 2005); white/pink frothy secretions may indicate pulmonary oedema, whereas green/yellow offensive secretions may indicate an infective process in the chest.

Adam and Osborne (2005) note that, in acute respiratory distress syndrome (ARDS), a common pulmonary presentation of respiratory failure associated with SIRS, secretions may well be loose and white becoming thicker and more profuse as the condition develops.

Pulse oximetry should be instituted, but this must complement basic assessment, not replace it. It must be remembered that pulse oximetry does not provide information on haemoglobin concentration, oxygen delivery to the tissues or ventilatory function, so a patient may have normal oxygen saturations yet still be hypoxic (Higgins 2005).

Arterial blood gas (ABG) analysis provides valuable information about a patient's respiratory and metabolic function (Allen 2005) and is discussed in depth in Chapter 3. Hypoxia/hypercapnia may be present as discussed above, but it must be recalled that the presence of normal arterial blood oxygen content does not always correlate to oxygen delivery to the cells. A compensated or non-compensated metabolic acidosis may be present, which could indicate organ hypoperfusion, particularly when associated with a high lactate (a parameter now measured by most modern blood gas analysers. Lactate is elevated (above 4 mmol/l) in patients with poor tissue perfusion (Peel 2008).

Circulation

Factors that cause circulatory compromise in the patient with SIRS include:

- Distributive shock as a result of vasodilatation and hypovolaemia
- Increased risk of thromboembolus, in particular microemboli, causing microvascular obstruction and end-organ dysfunction
- Increased risk of haemorrhage from clotting factor and platelet consumption
- Decreased myocardial contractility in the presence of increased oxygen consumption (compensatory tachycardia) and decreased oxygen delivery (reduced diastolic time)
- Tissue hypoxia
- Hypo-/hyperthermia
- Electrolyte/acid–base balance.

Circulation assessment should occur as outlined in Chapter 5. Vasodilatation is likely to be present giving the patient a 'flushed' look; vasodilatation in the capillaries may be demonstrated by an increased capillary refill time (CRT) and warm digits.

Hypovolaemia is also likely to be present and a picture of dehydration may be noted including alteration of mental state. Compensatory mechanisms will include an increase in heart rate; pulse should be assessed for rate, volume and regularity; a bounding pulse, with an increased CRT will indicate a hyperdynamic state. A fast, weak volume pulse with decreased CRT could indicate hypovolaemia. Rhythm irregularity indicates arrhythmia. SIRS has been identified as a major trigger for tachyarrhythmias (Vincent 2009) so continual monitoring, and diagnostic 12-lead electrocardiography (ECG) will be required.

Blood pressure monitoring should be haemodynamic, using arterial cannulation with transduced pressures. Blood pressure may well appear normal reflecting compensation; diastolic hypotension may be an indication of reduced venous tone (vasodilatation). Systolic hypertension, particularly over a low diastolic value, may reflect the hyperdynamic state.

Activation of hormonal compensatory mechanisms, including the renin–angiotensin pathway, aldosterone and antidiuretic hormone, cause a decrease in urine output and reabsorption of sodium and water, so observation of urine output is an important indicator of hypoperfusion. A urine output of <0.5 ml/kg of body weight per hour can be used as an indicator of hypoperfusion.

Blood lactate measurement (and its response to treatment) may be a good indicator of organ perfusion (Fischer et al. 2006); however, this should be measured together with monitoring of end-organ function such as diuresis and alterations in mental state.

Disability

Brain dysfunction is often one of the first clinical symptoms in sepsis and may manifest as sepsis-associated delirium in up to 70% of patients (Pytel and Alexander 2009). The causes for neurological dysfunction in sepsis are poorly understood, but are thought to include decreased cerebral perfusion (Burkhart et al., 2010), microcirculatory failure and changes in blood brain barrier permeability (Pytel and Alexander 2009). The sequela of other organ system failure may also carry some responsibility (Burkhart et al. 2010). Assessment should incorporate tools such as AVPU as outlined in Chapter 6 (Resuscitation Council UK 2006) plus pupillary size, and reaction to light. Blood sugar measurement should be performed at the earliest opportunity because imbalance may occur. Hyperglycaemia and insulin resistance as part of a physiological stress response are well documented (Ober 1999; Van Den Berghe 2008) Hypoglycaemia may also occur in non-diabetic and diabetic patients, particularly those with hepatic, renal and/or adrenocortical dysfunction. Capillary sampling in acutely ill patients may provide misleading results, particularly patients with circulatory failure, dehydration, alterations in oxygen tension and extremes of haematocrit, so venous sampling and laboratory analysis are recommended (Medicines and Healthcare products Regulatory Authority or MHRA 2005).

Exposure

Exposure should allow full examination of the patient with respect for dignity and the avoidance of heat loss (Resuscitation Council UK 2006). This will include a full clinical history, a review of notes/charts and any pertinent results. Examination should be comprehensive using a head-to-toe, or body systems, approach. The cause of the inflammatory response may not be known and the patient should be assessed for any possible septic foci.

The abdomen should be assessed and palpated and any guarding, tenderness or distension reported. Gastrointestinal losses should be noted for frequency and characteristics; gut motility tends to be reduced during critical illness, so nausea, vomiting or increased losses from drainage devices may be noted.

Wounds and wound drainage should be examined, with specimens taken for microbiological investigation as required. Further microbiological investigations, such as culture of blood, sputum or urine, will be required. In particular blood cultures should be taken at the earliest opportunity, the guidelines for which are discussed later in this text.

The patient should be examined for signs of fever, or hypothermia; a rise in temperature may indicate inflammation and/or fluctuations in basal metabolic rate. It will also provide a baseline against which to compare further readings.

The patients' fluid balance should be assessed with consideration for insensible losses, which can be significantly increased in the septic patient. Insensible losses from increased respiratory work and excessive diaphoresis must not be overlooked. Oedema may well be noted as a result of intravascular–extravascular fluid shifting and reductions in intravascular osmotic pressure.

Ongoing monitoring

Monitoring and managing the patient with SIRS are complex, requiring a multidisciplinary approach, the use of specialist support services and in most cases admission to a critical care unit for specialist skills and monitoring. This process is outlined from a systems perspective

Airway

The degree of respiratory compromise in SIRS is commonly severe enough to warrant artificial mechanical ventilation, which, in most cases requires airway intubation with an endotracheal tube. If this period of support is prolonged a temporary tracheostomy may be required.

The presence of any artificial airway increases the risks of pulmonary bacterial colonisation, and the likelihood of an HCAI (Newmarch 2006; Higgins 2009)

Respiratory system

As outlined above artificial mechanical ventilation may be required; this predisposes the patient to risks and associated complications, including physiological effects such as compromise to the cardiovascular system. There is also a well-documented association between mechanical ventilation and pneumonia (Henderson 1999; Selvaraj 2010). Monitoring the ventilated patient is beyond the scope of this chapter, but is discussed in Chapter 3.

The relationship between sepsis and ARDS is long established (Fein et al. 1983); the management of this process in itself is complex involving advanced supportive ventilator strategy and techniques. Pulse oximetry will guide therapy as will serial arterial blood gas analysis. Chest radiographs will be required, either as a diagnostic tool or to map inflammatory lung changes. The volume and characteristics of pulmonary secretions should be assessed (Adam and Osborne 2005) and microbiological investigations such as culture and identifying the sensitivity of any cultured organisms to antibacterial agents will be indicated. Some organisations recommend serial analysis, as a form of microbiological surveillance, whereas others perform culture and sensitivity when symptoms are evident. The incidence of ventilator-associated pneumonia (VAP) is again mentioned because patients may present with a septic focus in another organ system, but the ongoing management predisposes the patient to new risks that may further complicate the inflammatory response.

Cardiovascular monitoring

Ongoing ECG monitoring will be required to detect changes in cardiac rhythm; serial diagnostic 12-lead recording may also be required if abnormality is suspected.

Blood pressure monitoring should be haemodynamic, using arterial cannulation with transduced pressures; this is discussed in depth in Chapter 5. Both systolic and diastolic pressures are measured, but frequently the mean arterial pressure (MAP) is used because it can approximate the perfusion of essential organs such as the kidneys (McGhee and Bridges 2002) Hence, MAP is central to goal-related therapy in clinical practice (Dünser et al. 2009).

Central venous pressure (CVP) should be monitored via a central venous catheter; again this is discussed in depth in Chapter 5. The practitioner is reminded that CVP is a reflection of four parameters – intrathoracic pressure, circulating volume, right-sided cardiac function and venous tone – and also to some degree blood viscosity; thus it must not be interpreted as a stand-alone value. Access to the central circulation allows measurement of venous oxygen saturations, which can reflect important pathophysiological changes in oxygen delivery and consumption (Shepherd and Pearse 2009); this can inform clinical practice and guide fluid resuscitation.

More advanced invasive monitoring of cardiac output and other derived values frequently occurs in the critical care unit. Although thermodilution measurement (using a pulmonary artery catheter) remains an established method of determining cardiac output, other techniques such as lithium dilution pulse contour analysis, Doppler ultrasonography offer a less invasive technique (Adam and Osborne 2005)

Serial ABG analysis will be required, not least to inform respiratory/ventilatory support and to provide an indication of tissue hypoperfusion which can be demonstrated by a metabolic acidosis and increased blood lactate

Microbiological monitoring/investigations

The clinical microbiology laboratory plays a fundamental role in the diagnosis of infection (Peterson et al. 2001), ongoing monitoring of the inflammatory response and the management of specific antimicrobial therapies. An appropriate microbiological test is one that is undertaken with the aim of influencing patient treatment (Storr et al. 2005).

In the patient with SIRS/sepsis identification of the causative microorganism is of paramount importance so that bactericidal/virucidal agents can be delivered at the earliest opportunity.

The surviving sepsis campaign (Dellinger et al. 2008) recommends the following:

- Obtaining appropriate cultures (blood) before starting antibiotics provided that this does not significantly delay antimicrobial administration
- Obtaining two or more blood cultures (possibly using a vascular access device) but one should be percutaneous
- Obtaining a blood culture from each vascular access device that has been in place for more than 48h
- The culture of other sites (sputum, urine, etc.) as clinically indicated.

Broad-spectrum antibiotics are indicated in sepsis and these should be administered as early as possible (Dellinger et al. 2008). Liaison with the microbiology team should occur to redirect (if required) therapy once any pathogenic organisms have been identified. Advice may also be required in managing the therapeutic levels of any particular drug therapy, e.g. vancomycin.

Biochemical and haematological monitoring

It is imperative to monitor biochemical markers to identify isolated or multiple organ failure associated with sepsis. Standardised biochemical and haematological profiles should be assessed frequently, as advised by laboratory staff. This will enable organ support to be initiated without delay.

Particular reference is made to indicators of renal function, coagulation profiles/platelet count, liver function tests and serum amylase. The inflammatory process can also be mapped by changes in white blood cell count, which may be raised or lowered A raised white cell count (>11 000/ml) may indicate bacterial infection if associated with a high neutrophil count and increased immature forms. C-reactive protein (CRP) may also be measured but, as with white blood cell count, this is a non-specific marker; it is, however, useful in mapping the inflammatory process. The half-life of CRP is short (5–7 h) and the decline in serum CRP concentration is a sensitive measure of the resolution of infection. Elevations in erythrocyte sedimentation rate and procalcitonin may also be observed. Other specific markers of the immunological response can be measured, including interleukins and specific mediators; these may help identify the specific cause/microorganism of infection.

Track-and-trigger systems

Physiological track and trigger should be used to monitor all adult patients in the acute hospital setting (National Institute for Health and Clinical Excellence or NICE 2007); these are discussed in depth in Chapter 1. Tools such as the modified early warning scoring system are ideal for monitoring the patient with SIRS/sepsis.

Other investigations

A specific anatomical site of infection should be established as rapidly as possible and within first 6 h of presentation (Dellinger et al. 2008).

Diagnostic studies, e.g. ultrasonography, may identify a source of infection leading to early intervention.

SCENARIOS

Scenario 1

You are called to see John, an inpatient who is a 42-year-old man with a surgical wound infection, 2 weeks after a hemicolectomy. The student nurse requesting review says that he looks a bit flushed and she is worried about him; describe your assessment process.

Answer
The assessment process should be structured through the ABCDE framework.

Airway should be assessed using a look, listen and feel approach; any compromise should be treated as an emergency and help summoned as appropriate.

Breathing characteristics should be noted, including respiratory rate, volume and pattern. The patient should be observed for signs of decreased oxygenation and accumulating carbon dioxide. This may be evident in the patient's pallor and mental state. Pulse oximetry is a useful assessment tool but should only complement basic assessment.

Circulation can be assessed by looking at capillary refill time, pulse rate/characteristics and blood pressure. The patient may appear warm and flushed as a result of vasodilatation or cold and peripherally shutdown in an attempt to maintain circulation to major organs. Be aware that blood pressure may be normal through compensatory mechanisms. Heart rate will normally be increased as evidence of this.

Disability should be assessed using the AVPU tool; pupils should be assessed for their size and reaction to light and capillary blood glucose should be sampled.

The patient should be exposed to observe for signs of injury, inflammation or abnormality. Temperature should be recorded and compared against previous values, with cultures sent for microscopy and sensitivity in line with organisational policy. Evidence of inflammation, particularly around surgical sites and sites of line insertion, should be observed and reported as appropriate, with swabs taken as indicated.

Scenario 2

John, the patient described above, has been seen by the surgical and anaesthetic team who suspect intra-abdominal sepsis; he is to be transferred to theatre in 1 hour for exploratory laparotomy. What monitoring will John require before his transfer to theatre?

Answer
John will need to be kept under close observation before transfer. The airway should be monitored observing for signs of distress and failure. Respiratory rate and characteristics should be recorded and any response to oxygen therapy recorded. Pulse oximetry with appropriate set alarms will alert the nurse to any changes in oxygenation.

Blood pressure, pulse and capillary refill should be monitored. In preference a dynamic monitoring system of recording blood pressure, such as intra-arterial invasive pressure monitoring, is desirable. Should this not be the case frequent blood pressure recording should occur and responses to any prescribed therapy such as fluid resuscitation noted. If Intravenous access is not *in situ* this should be performed at the earliest opportunity. Blood sampling may be required for routine biochemical and haematological analysis; cross-match will also be required. Blood glucose monitoring, if not already initiated, should be started alongside a scoring tool to measure level of consciousness. Track-and-trigger systems, with a graded response strategy, such as a modified early warning scoring tool, would be most useful in this situation.

CONCLUSION

The incidence of patients with infection and a related inflammatory response is significant, and is associated with high morbidity/mortality. The monitoring and management of these patients are complex, and require a multidisciplinary, multispecialty approach ideally in a critical care environment. Many patients in the early stages of inflammatory response are cared for in general ward areas. As with all acute illness the ABCDE framework is an ideal assessment tool, which can lead to early identification of these patients, resulting in prompt treatment and management and transfer to a higher level of care.

REFERENCES

Adam, S. & Osborne, S. (2005) *Critical Care Nursing: Science and practice*, 2nd edn. Oxford: Oxford University Press.
Allen. K. (2005) Four-step method of interpreting arterial blood gas analysis. *Nursing Times* **101**(1), 42.

Bone, R. C., Balk, R. A., Cerra, F. B., et al. (1992) Definitions for sepsis and organ failure and guidelines for the use of innovative therapies in sepsis. The ACCP/SCCM Consensus Conference Committee. American College of Chest Physicians/Society of Critical Care Medicine.

Burkhart, C. S., Siegemund, M., & Steiner, L. A. (2010) Cerebral perfusion in sepsis. *Critical Care*, **14**, 215.

Dellinger, R. P., Levy, M. M., Carlet, J. M., et al. (2008) Surviving Sepsis Campaign: International guidelines for management of severe sepsis and septic shock. *Critical Care Medicine*, **36**, 296–327 (published correction appears pp. 1394 –1396).

Department of Health, (2007) *Saving Lives: Reducing infection, delivering clean and safe care*, London: DH.

Docherty, B. (2002) Cardiorespiratory assessment for the acutely ill. *British Journal of Nursing*, **11**, 750–758

Dünser, M. W., Takala, J., Ulmer, H., et al. (2009) Arterial blood pressure during early sepsis and outcome. *Intensive Care Medicine*, **35**, 1225–1233.

Fein, A.M., Lippmann, M., Holtzman, H., Eliraz, A., & Goldberg, S. K. (1983) The risk factors, incidence, and prognosis of ARDS following septicemia. *Chest*, **83**, 40–42.

Fischer, J. E., Bland, K. I., Callery, M. P., & Clagett, G. P. (2006) *Mastery of Surgery*. Baltimore, MA: Lippincot, Williams & Wilkins.

Henderson, N. (1999) Mechanical ventilation. *Nursing Standard*, **13**(44), 49–53.

Higgins, D. (2005) Pulse oximetry. *Nursing Times*, **101**(6), 34–35.

Higgins, D. (2009) Basic nursing principles of caring for patients with a tracheostomy. *Nursing Times*, **105**(3), 14–15.

Higgins, D. & Guest, J. (2008) Acute respiratory failure 1: assessing patients. *Nursing Times*, **104**(36), 24–25.

Jenkins, G. W., Kemnitz, C. P., & Tortora, G. J. (2007) *Anatomy and Physiology: From science to life*. Hoboken, NJ: John Wiley & Sons.

Jevon, P. (2010) How to ensure patient observations lead to prompt identification of tachypnoea. *Nursing Times*, **106**(2), 12–14

Levy, M. M., Fink, M., Marshall, J., et al. (2003) For the international sepsis definitions conference. *Critical Care Medicine*, **31**, 1250–1256

McGhee, B. H. & Bridges, E. J (2002) Monitoring arterial blood pressure: what you may not know. *Critical Care Nurse*, **22**, 60–70

Martinsen, T. C., Bergh, K., & Waldum, H. L. (2005) Gastric juice: a barrier against infectious diseases. *Basic and Clinical Pharmacology and Toxicology*, **96**, 94–102.

Medicines and Healthcare products Regulatory Authority (2005) *Point of Care Testing – Blood Glucose Meters – Advice for health care professionals*. London: DH.

Montague, S. E., Watson. R., & Herbert, R. (2005) *Physiology for Nursing Practice*. Oxford: Baillière Tindall.

National Audit Office (2000) *The Challenge of Hospital Acquired Infection*. London: The Stationary Office.

National Audit Office (2004) *Improving Patient Care by Reducing the Risk of Hospital Acquired Infection : A progress report*. London: The Stationery Office.

National Institute for Health and Clincal Excellence (2007) Acutely ill patients in hospital: Recognition of and response to acute illness in adults in hospital. London: NICE. http://www.nice.org.uk/nicemedia/live/11810/35950/35950.pdf accessed October 2011.

Newmarch, C. (2006) Caring for the mechanically ventilated patient: part two. *Nursing Standard*, **20**(18), 55–64.

Ober, K. P. (1999) *Endocrinology of Critical Disease*. Totowa, NJ: Humana Press.

Peel, M. (2008) Care bundles: resuscitation of patients with severe sepsis. *Nursing Standard*, **23**(11), 41–46.

Peterson, L. R., Hamilton, J. D., Baron, E. J., et al. (2001) The role of clinical microbiology laboratories in the management and control of infectious diseases and the delivery of health care. *Clinical Infectious Aiseases*, **32**, 605–611.

Pratt, R. J., Pellowe, C. M., & Wilson, J. A. (2007) EPIC 2: Evidence based guidelines for preventing healthcare associated infections in NHS hospitals in England. *Journal of Hospital Infection*, **655**, S1–S64.

Pryor, J. A. & Prasad, A. S. (2008) *Physiotherapy for Respiratory and Cardiac Problems: Adults and paediatrics*. Oxford: Churchill Livingstone.

Pytel, P. & Alexander, J. J. (2009) Pathogenesis of septic encephalopathy. *Current Opinion in Neurology*, **22**, 283–287.

Resuscitation Council UK (2006) *Advanced life support*, 5th edn. London: Resuscitation Council UK.

Robson, W., Newell, J., & Beavis, S. (2005) Assessing, treating and managing patients with sepsis. *Nursing Standard*, **19**(50), 56–64.

Selvaraj, N. (2010) Artificial humidification for the mechanically ventilated patient. *Nursing Standard*, **25**(8), 41–46.

Shepherd, S. J. & Pearse, R. (2009) The role of central and mixed venous oxygen saturation measurement in perioperative care. *Anesthesiology*, **111**, 649–656

Steen, C. (2009) Developments in the management of patients with sepsis. *Nursing Standard*, **23**(48), 48–55.

Storey, M. & Jordan, S. (2008) An overview of the immune system. *Nursing Standard*, **23**, 15–17.

Storr, J., Topley, K., & Privett, S. (2005) The ward nurse's role in infection control. *Nursing Standard*, **19**(41), 56–64.

Van Den Berghe, G. (2008) *Acute Endocrinology – From cause to consequence*. Totowa, NJ: Humana Press.

Vincent, J. L., ed. (2008) *Intensive care Medicine: Annual update 2008*. New York: Springer.

Vincent, J. L., ed. (2009) *Intensive Care Medicine: Annual Update 2009*. New York: Springer.

World Health Organization (2004) *Review of Health Impacts from Microbiological Hazards in Health-Care Wastes*. Geneva: WHO.

Monitoring the Critically Ill, Pregnant Patient

16

LEARNING OUTCOMES

At the end of the chapter the reader will be able to:

☐ outline the relevant physiological changes that occur during pregnancy
☐ list acute illnesses and deaths associated with pregnancy
☐ discuss the monitoring of the critically ill pregnant woman

INTRODUCTION

Maternal deaths are extremely rare in the UK. The maternal mortality for 2003–5, calculated from all maternal deaths directly or indirectly due to pregnancy, was 14 per 100000 maternities (Confidential Enquiry into Maternal and Child Health [CEMACH] – Lewis 2007). Studies have shown that the care of critically ill patients in the UK is suboptimal (McQuillan et al. 1998); deficiencies in care are related to the failure to recognise and treat abnormalities in the patient's airway, breathing or circulation, common causes for cardiorespiratory arrest (Resuscitation Council UK 2006). These deficiencies are also present in the care of pregnant patients and a leading factor in maternal deaths (Grady et al. 2007). CEMACH recognises these deficiencies and makes recommendations for the early recognition and management of severely ill pregnant women and impending maternal collapse.

Monitoring the Critically Ill Patient, Third Edition.
Philip Jevon, Beverley Ewens.
© 2012 Blackwell Publishing Ltd. Published 2012 by Blackwell Publishing Ltd.

Assessing and monitoring the critically ill pregnant woman can be challenging. This is, in part, related to the physiological changes that occur during pregnancy and because priorities of care extend not only to the patient but also to the care of the unborn fetus.

The acutely ill pregnant woman must be approached using a systematic ABCDE assessment as outlined in previous chapters, but modifications will be required. These modifications can by made only when the practitioner has a sound understanding of the physiological changes associated with pregnancy.

As with all specialist areas of acute care, expert advice should be summoned at the earliest opportunity. This has been highlighted as a common failure in managing the pregnant patient (Lewis 2007). In many cases effective resuscitation of the mother, which is the leading priority, is often the best way to optimise fetal outcome (Resuscitation Council UK 2006). Early advice and assistance should be summoned from obstetricians, midwives and paediatric staff, in addition to emergency teams. Dynamic and effective communication through these teams is essential in improving outcome.

The aim of this chapter is to understand the monitoring of the critically ill, pregnant woman. Emergency delivery of the child, both perinatal and postnatal, has not been discussed because it is beyond the scope of this chapter and book.

RELEVANT PHYSIOLOGICAL CHANGES THAT OCCUR DURING PREGNANCY

Pregnancy is a period of enormous physiological change mediated by the endocrine and paracrine systems and the physical effects of the uteroplacental unit (Hayes and Arulkumaran 2006).

Airway changes

Increased mucosal oedema may be present in the airways, possibly as a result of increased total body water. Nasal congestion may also occur.

Changes associated with breathing

Functional residual capacity (FRC) is reduced (Adam and Osborne 2005) as a direct result of the gravid uterus, causing displacement of the diaphragm and intra-abdominal organs. FRC reduction may be as much as 20%, reducing significantly further in the supine patient. A decrease in FRC compromises gas exchange and reduces oxygen reserve, meaning that a patient will become hypoxaemic more quickly if breathing becomes compromised.

The basal respiratory rate is usually increased as a compensatory mechanism for a reduction in FRC and as a result of the stimulant effects of increased circulating progesterone (Bayliss and Millhorn 1992). Minute ventilation may increase by up to 50% through a combination of increased respiratory rate and to a lesser extent tidal volume; this results in a respiratory alkalosis. Oxygen consumption will increase because of fetal requirements and the increased work of breathing.

Changes associated with circulation

Circulating volume begins to increase in early pregnancy and can increase by up to 50% approaching term (Silversides and Coleman 2007). This, combined with the metabolic demands of the fetal–placental unit, causes an increase in cardiac output which may also be up to 50% (Adam and Osborne 2005). Hormonal changes influence vascular tone and vascular resistance falls: the increase in cardiac output may not be sufficient to compensate for this decrease, so blood pressure, and in particular diastolic pressure, may be lower than normal. Venous pressure increases as uterine size increases which may cause gravitational oedema (Hayes and Arulkumaran 2006).

Placental blood flow and caval compression

The uteroplacental circulation is a pressure-dependent system with no independent autoregulation (Adam and Osborne 2005). Fetal blood supply can be severely impaired by poor maternal blood flow/pressure. From early pregnancy the gravid uterus can compress the inferior vena cava, with a resultant decrease in right heart preload, reducing cardiac output and placental blood flow. This appears to be particularly evident in the supine position. Aortic compression may also occur but appears to be to a lesser extent.

Haematological changes

Red cell volume increases but this is diluted by the increase in plasma volume creating a dilutional reduction in haemoglobin. The white blood cell count increases, although the platelet count remains fairly constant. An increase in clotting factors creates a hypercoagulable state. The dilution picture also results in a reduced colloid osmotic pressure which contributes further to the development of oedema (Bothamley and Boyle 2009).

Changes associated with disability (neurological function)

Cerebral blood flow remains unchanged during pregnancy (Silversides and Coleman 2007). Hyperglycaemia and glycosuria may occur although this can be related to gestational diabetes which affects 3–10% of pregnancies (Miller et al. 2008)

Changes associated with exposure

There is an obvious increase in body mass index (BMI) in pregnancy. Total body weight may increase by up to 17% (Silversides and Coleman 2007). Breast size increases significantly in preparation for lactation. The accumulation of body water and increases in venous pressure contribute to gravitational oedema.

Gastro-oesophageal reflux is almost universal in pregnancy and gastric and intestinal motility is reduced (Hayes and Arulkumaran 2006).

ACUTE ILLNESSES AND DEATHS ASSOCIATED WITH PREGNANCY

A considerable number of pregnancies are complicated by acute illness processes some of which are related to the physiological changes outlined above. Acute illness can lead to maternal death. CEMACH (Lewis 2007) defines the causes of maternal death as direct, indirect, late or coincidental and this is illustrated in Table 16.1.

Causes of direct maternal death from 1985 to 2005 were related to (in order of prevalence) the following.

Table 16.1 Causes of maternal death in the UK

Maternal deaths	Deaths of women while pregnant or within 42 days of the end of the pregnancy from any cause related to or aggravated by the pregnancy or its management, but not from accidental or incidental causes
Direct	Deaths resulting from obstetric complications of the pregnant state (pregnancy, labour and puerperium), from interventions, omissions, incorrect treatment or a chain of events resulting from any of the above
Indirect	Deaths resulting from previous existing disease, or disease that developed during pregnancy and was not due to direct obstetric causes, but aggravated by the physiological effects of pregnancy
Late	Deaths occurring between 42 days and 1 year after abortion, miscarriage or delivery that are due to *direct* or *indirect* maternal causes
Coincidental (fortuitous)	Deaths from unrelated causes that happen to occur in pregnancy or the puerperium
Pregnancy-related deaths	Deaths occurring in women while pregnant or within 42 days of termination of pregnancy, irrespective of the cause of the death

Reproduced from Lewis (2007), with the permission of the Centre for Maternal and Child Enquiries.

Thrombosis/thromboembolism

Thromboembolic disease is a very common condition in pregnancy, increasing the risk almost sixfold over the non-pregnant patient (Adam and Osborne 2005). It occurs as a result of venous stasis and the haematological changes outlined above. A thrombus may form, commonly in the deep veins of the legs, and emboli from this clot may 'break off' and occlude blood flow to vital areas, in particular the pulmonary circulation, which can cause hypoxia and cardiac arrest. Treatment is preventive; appropriate prophylaxis should be weighed against the risk of complications, and started accordingly (Bourjeily et al. 2010). The National Institute for Health and Clinical Excellence (2010) recommends that pharmacological prophylaxis should be offered to hospitalised women who are pregnant if certain other risk factors are present:

- Expected to have significantly reduced mobility for 3 or more days
- Critical care admission
- Dehydration
- Excess blood loss or blood transfusion
- Obesity (pre-pregnancy or early pregnancy BMI >30)
- One or more significant medical comorbidities
- Pregnancy-related risk factors (such as hyperemesis gravidarum, multiple pregnancy or pre-eclampsia).

It is important to emphasise that pharmacological management of venous thromboembolus should go hand in hand with other preventive measure such as graduated compression stockings and improving mobility.

Pre-eclampsia/eclampsia

Pre-eclampsia can be defined as pregnancy-induced hypertension in association with proteinuria or oedema (Grady et al. 2007). It occurs in 2-8% of pregnancies (Magpie Trial Collaborative Group 2002) and 1 in 10 pregnant women develops partial signs or symptoms, The aetiology of pre-eclampsia is not entirely understood but is thought to be related to placental hypoperfusion and endothelial cell injury. It may present during the latter half of pregnancy, intrapartum or postpartum (Adam and Osborne 2005). Pre-eclampsia is classified as mild or severe and may lead to multiple organ dysfunction if not managed appropriately. Pre-eclampsia is a progressive disorder that can be arrested only by delivery of the fetus (Adam and Osborne 2005); immediate management is based on prompt control of hypertension, meticulous fluid management, seizure prevention and safe delivery of the child.

Eclampsia is defined as the occurrence of one or more convulsions superimposed on pre-eclampsia. The management of both conditions should involve senior multi-specialty, multidisciplinary staff working to a standardised pattern of management guidelines (Grady et al. 2007)

Haemorrhage

Massive blood loss, defined as blood loss of more than 1000–1500 ml, as a leading cause of maternal mortality is usually related to peri-/postpartum loss rather than loss associated with first trimester bleeding (Grady et al. 2007). First trimester bleeding may be related to ectopic pregnancy and this should be considered where vaginal blood loss is observed with associated abdominal pain in early pregnancy. The management of massive haemorrhage is aimed at fluid resuscitation with surgical correction of bleeding. Correction of coagulation will also be required in line with massive blood transfusion protocol.

Amniotic fluid embolism

Amniotic fluid embolism (AFE) occurs when amniotic fluid, normally contained *in utero* enters the maternal circulation. This exposure is not uncommon (De Jong and Fausett 2003), and the maternal predisposition to react to the exposure creates the clinical syndrome (Grady et al. 2007). The response to the exposure is unpredictable and may be related to the constituents or volume of the fluid entering the circulation. Signs and symptoms are related to the respiratory and cardiovascular systems. Clark et al. (1995) contend that AFE closely resembles an anaphylactic reaction in response to fetal debris rather than an embolic event, and propose the term 'anaphylactoid syndrome of pregnancy'.

Ectopic pregnancy

Ectopic pregnancy occurs if a fertilised ovum is implanted outside the uterine cavity (Watkins 2010) because a fallopian tube fails in its normal action of transporting the ovum into the uterus (Alexander et al. 2006). Tubal rupture can occur and the products of conception are expelled into the peritoneal cavity. Haemorrhage occurs from the tubal placental site (Alexander et al. 2006), resulting in hypovolaemic shock. Fluid resuscitation is required with urgent surgical intervention to arrest bleeding.

Miscarriage

Miscarriage is very common, occurring in 25% of pregnancies (Drife and Magowan 2004). Acute illness after a miscarriage may be related to intrauterine haemorrhage or sepsis from retained products of conception.

Liver dysfunction

HELLP syndrome (**h**aemolysis, **e**levated **l**iver enzymes and **l**ow **p**latelets) can occur antenatally and may be related to pre-eclampsia, although pre-eclampsia does not always have to be present for it to occur (Adam and Osborne 2005). It occurs in predominantly white, multiparous women aged >25 and is the most common cause of severe liver disease in pregnancy (Cetin 2006). HELLP syndrome includes the clinical signs outlined above and is considered to be a variant presentation of pre-eclampsia; endothelial cell injury, haemolysis and platelets consumption are thought to be the causative factors. Treatment is aimed at early delivery and supportive care

Acute fatty liver in pregnancy is an uncommon but potentially fatal complication of pregnancy that results in microvesicular fat deposition in the liver, causing severe liver dysfunction (McNulty 2004). The aetiology of the condition is not entirely clear. Supportive care and expeditious delivery are essential to optimal maternal–fetal outcomes and remain as the mainstay treatment (Ko and Yoshida 2006).

Acute illness presentation association with indirect causes

The most common cause for maternal death from indirect causes is related to cardiac disease, either acquired or congenital (Lewis 2007). This includes myocardial infarction, ischaemic heart disease, aortic dissection and pulmonary hypertension. All the above conditions will, in most cases, present physiological indication of deterioration before a terminal event.

MONITORING THE CRITICALLY ILL PREGNANT PATIENT
Assessing and monitoring the acutely unwell pregnant patient

The Resuscitation Council UK (2006) recommend that clinical staff should follow the ABCDE approach when assessing (and treating) critically ill patients. This will help to ensure that critical illness is promptly identified and appropriately managed (Jevon 2010). The fundamental principles of this framework are outlined in Chapter 1. However, the approach should be undertaken with consideration of the physiological changes associated with pregnancy and uteroplacental circulation. The process is outlined below.

Airway

The airway should be assessed using a look-and-listen approach. This includes inspection for signs of obstruction/abnormality. Nasal congestion may affect voice sounds but if a patient is talking the airway is patent. Be aware that the changes in respiratory physiology, in particular diaphragmatic splinting from the gravid uterus, will give rise to an increase in respiratory rate and breathlessness may well occur, particularly on exertion. Airway sounds, such as stridor, wheeze, gurgling or any stertorous breathing, are abnormal signs and require immediate treatment. In any case of partial airway obstruction high-flow oxygen should be delivered at the earliest opportunity; oxygen administration in the acutely unwell patient is discussed in depth in Chapter 1. As with any airway abnormality help should be summoned immediately from those with advanced airway skills. Simple manoeuvres such as head tilt/chin lift and/or jaw thrust are applicable to the pregnant patient; oropharyngeal airways may be of use if the tongue is the cause of obstruction; the use of nasopharyngeal airways may be limited by the presence of nasal congestion. As pregnancy progresses difficulties in endotracheal intubation and bag–valve–mask ventilation should be anticipated (Walls and Murphy 2008), reinforcing the requirement for senior support.

Breathing

Breathing respiratory assessment should occur as outlined in Chapter 3. The patient's general appearance may be one of anxiety or exhaustion, or she may be unresponsive. Hypoxia and hypercapnia can alter mental state, and confusion/delirium may be present (Higgins and Guest 2008). Respiratory rate, pattern and chest excursion should be recorded. Changes in respiratory rate can be the most important early clinical manifestation of critical illness (Goldhill et al. 1999); however, respiratory rate can be altered in pregnancy and should be reviewed in comparison to previous recordings.

The decrease in FRC and increased metabolic demands reduce oxygen reserve, which may herald more rapid respiratory decompensation than observed in the non-pregnant patient. Thus airway and/or breathing problems must be recognised immediately and experienced assistance summoned at the earliest opportunity. High-concentration oxygen supplementation will be indicated, to optimise delivery to the maternal and fetal cells. Able patients with respiratory compromise tend to position themselves to maximise lung expansion, in many cases an orthopnoeic position. This may cause further diaphragmatic splinting in the pregnant patient. Likewise the supine position will further reduce FRC. Patients should be asked what position eases any distress and assisted accordingly. The effects of the right lateral position on caval blood flow and cardiac output must be considered.

Pulse oximetry can aid respiratory assessment; however, this does not provide information on haemoglobin concentration, oxygen delivery to the tissues or ventilatory function, so a patient may have normal oxygen saturations yet still be hypoxic (Higgins 2005). Pulse oximetry can, however, provide a useful 'trend view' of oxygenation, response to therapy and indication of deterioration and is thus indicated in any acutely unwell patient.

Arterial blood gas (ABG) analysis provides valuable information about a patient's respiratory and metabolic function (Allen 2005) and is discussed in depth in Chapter 3. It may be performed as a one-off or serial investigation in monitoring the pregnant patient. Measured values will guide therapy, e.g. oxygen delivery or ventilatory support. Other useful parameters, such as blood acidity/ alkalinity, haemoglobin concentration and electrolyte levels, may also guide other aspects of patient management. In the unstable patient arterial cannulation is of benefit for serial analysis and haemodynamic monitoring (Grady et al. 2007).

Circulation

Assessment of circulation should be performed as outlined in Chapter 1. When assessing circulation note that oedema may be present. The dilutional anaemia of pregnancy may influence the patient's colour, giving a paler look than normal; however, this should be considered against other vital signs.

Capillary refill time (CRT) may be normal or increased due to a decrease in vascular resistance and increase in circulating volume. The fingers and the lower limbs may be oedematous, the soft tissues may become tense and the digital vessels may throb (Nihoyannopoulus 2007).

As a result of increases in circulating volume and cardiac output fluid loss may be difficult to detect until a significant amount of fluid has been lost. Insensible fluid losses may increase and certain specific complications of pregnancy such as hyperemesis gravidarum (severe vomiting during pregnancy) may influence hydration state. Thus, the practitioner must be aware that dehydration may be evident despite clinical presentation suggesting otherwise. Jugular venous pressure may be increased (Nihoyannopoulus 2007) but may be related to increases in intrathoracic pressure rather than circulatory overload.

Bleeding during pregnancy is common and loss may be obvious or concealed; per vagina losses should be assessed and the duration of any bleeding noted.

Pulse rates may be higher than those of non-pregnant patients yet persistent tachycardia is an abnormal sign and warrants further investigation. Pulse rate irregularity is again an abnormal sign and may indicate underlying cardiac dysfunction or electrolyte imbalance. In both cases, electrocardiogram rhythm analysis and diagnostic 12-lead ECG are required. Many pregnant patients experience palpitations, and premature atrial and ventricular contractions, and these are usually benign (Nihoyannopoulus 2007). However, any arrhythmias together with adverse signs, such as changes in blood pressure, changes in level of consciousness, chest pain or signs of heart failure, warrant urgent medical assessment.

Blood pressure should be recorded using appropriate cuff size; the increase in BMI associated with pregnancy may mean that a larger cuff should be used. Quinn (1994) suggests that automated blood pressure machines may underestimate pregnant women's blood pressure by as much as 30 mmHg. Manual aneroid machines are recommended as a non-invasive technique in any acutely unwell patient. Blood pressure changes that occur during pregnancy are generally monitored throughout gestation, so 'normal pregnant values' should be available for the particular patient to allow comparison. Hypertension in pregnancy may be related to pre-eclampsia and, although certain definitions exist with regard to elevated blood pressure levels (Magpie Trial Collaborative Group 2003), any hypertension or episodes must be reported to senior specialist staff at the earliest opportunity.

Venous blood analysis should occur in any acute illness presentation; standard haematological and biochemical profiles should be requested. Liver function tests and clotting profiles are also indicated to identify any liver dysfunction.

Many cardiovascular problems are related to caval compression (Resuscitation Council UK 2006) and certain treatments may reduce this. The patient should be placed in the left lateral position and/or have gentle manual displacement of the gravid uterus to the left. This should be performed together with supportive measures such as high-flow oxygen delivery and fluid resuscitation (Resuscitation Council UK 2006)

Disability

The AVPU assessment tool (outlined in Chapter 6) provides a rapid assessment of the patient's level of consciousness, and this should precede any more formalised tools such as the Glasgow Coma Scale. Blood glucose assessment should be undertaken at an early opportunity, not only to exclude hypoglycaemia but also to detect any gestational diabetes. Pupillary response to light and accommodation should also be assessed as outlined in Chapter 6. Alterations in levels of consciousness are an ominous sign; in particular if a score of P or U on the AVPU scale is evident, expert help should be summoned immediately. Confusion may be encephalopathic in origin and should alert the practitioner to liver dysfunction. The unconscious patient will normally need to be nursed in the lateral position to minimise the risk of soiling to the airway, particularly as gastro-oesophageal reflux is common; however, positioning the patient in the right lateral position may cause caval compression and should be avoided. The cause for any change in conscious level should be explored and history/charts noted to detect any reversible conditions. Convulsions, should they occur, may indicate eclampsia and immediate, expert assistance should be sought without delay.

Exposure

Exposure and overall assessment of the patient should occur as outlined in Chapter 1. Oedema may be noted throughout. Lower limbs must be assessed for any indication of thrombosis, redness, swelling or localised heat plus any pain/tenderness around the calf area should be noted. The patient should be assessed for signs of bleeding or fluid loss which will include concealed/obvious loss. 'Dipstick' urine analysis may indicate the presence of blood in the urine, indicating genitourinary trauma (Higgins 2008) or uterine blood loss. Glycosuria in pregnancy may indicate gestational diabetes, one of the most common medical conditions complicating pregnancy (Meltzer 2010), and blood glucose assessment should follow if glycosuria present. Proteinuria may indicate pre-eclampsia and should be reported immediately. The patient should be assessed for signs of liver dysfunction including jaundice, epigastric, right upper quadrant pain and evidence of ascites.

Cardiac arrest during pregnancy

Specific causes for cardiac arrest during pregnancy are outlined in Table 16.2; however, most are caused by the conditions outlined

Table 16.2 Specific causes for cardiac arrest during pregnancy

Haemorrhage	As outlined above – can occur during any stage of pregnancy. Drugs may be indicated postpartum to cause uterine contraction but in most cases surgical intervention is required. Ectopic pregnancy must be considered
Toxicity	Magnesium overdose may occur in pre-eclamptic/eclamptic patients receiving the drug as anticonvulsant therapy – calcium is the agent of choice in magnesium toxicity
Cardiovascular disease	As outlined above. Pulmonary hypertension and peripartum cardiomyopathy are key causes. Thrombolysis is relatively contraindicated as a treatment for myocardial infarction during pregnancy
Pre-eclampsia/ eclampsia	As outlined above
Amniotic fluid embolism	As outlined above

Adapted from Resuscitation Council UK (2006).

above, although many cardiovascular problems are caused by caval compression. In cardiac arrest standard principles of basic and advanced life support apply (Resuscitation Council UK 2006). However, obstetric and paediatric/neonatology staff should be summoned immediately as part of the emergency response team. During cardiac compressions a left lateral tilt >15° will relieve caval compression (Resuscitation Council UK 2006) improving right-sided venous return and optimising compressions. The patient will, however, require physical support in this position to maximise the efficacy of compressions, so wedges (e.g. Cardiff wedge) or firm pillows/spinal boards may be necessary. Left displacement of the uterus should also be performed and will be required together with lateral tilting. Cardiac compressions should be performed with a hand positioned one hand higher than normal to account for elevation of the diaphragm. Early endotracheal intubation is indicated to prevent aspiration.

Caesarean section is indicated when initial resuscitation attempts fail because delivery of the fetus may improve maternal and fetal chances of survival (Resuscitation Council UK 2006), although this may be influenced by gestational age. This should occur within 5 minutes of the maternal cardiac arrest. This process requires considerable multidisciplinary and multi-specialty collaboration.

SCENARIOS

Scenario 1

Sarah, a 24-year-old woman, presents to A&E with abdominal and back pain and has experienced recent blood loss per vagina.
  Your findings are as follows:

- A – Airway is clear, Sarah is talking clearly and in sentences although very worried
- B – Respiratory rate is 23, she looks rather pale and oxygen saturations are not picking up correctly
- C – Sarah looks pale, CRT is 4 s, BP 100/70, pulse rate 115
- D – Alert, but worried

Continued

E – Some lower abdominal tenderness. Sarah also states that she lost 'quite a lot of blood' from her vagina

What Is Your Course of Action?

Help should be summoned with some urgency; ideally this would be the medical emergency team, but surgical staff will also be needed. Tachycardia and decreased CRT with a slightly compromised blood pressure may well be a compensation for hypovolaemic shock as a result of blood loss. Sarah should be observed/monitored closely.

Oxygen therapy should be administered to maintain saturations of 96–98%; as Sarah is conscious she will probably determine her most comfortable position.

Respiratory rate should be recorded, alongside oxygen saturations. The failure of the machine to pick up saturations may be related to decreased peripheral perfusion; this may improve with volume repletion.

Volume resuscitation will be required immediately; intravenous cannulation should not be delayed, and preferably two large-bore devices should be inserted into large veins. Volume should be administered with dynamic blood pressure and heart rate monitoring. Warmed fluids may prevent hypothermia. Crystalloid/colloid should be used in the first instance until blood values are available Once access is obtained blood should be taken for 'routine' haematological and biochemical analysis. An arterial or venous sample may be processed through a department-based blood gas analyse; co-oximetry values can be relied on in the first instance to detect any anaemia/decrease in haematocrit. Blood should also be 'emergency' cross-matched for use in volume resuscitation. If blood loss and anaemia are severe universal donor blood may be required. Conscious level should be monitored using AVPU/Glasgow Coma Scale (GCS), and blood glucose should be checked.

A full history should be taken from Sarah including sexual history: Has she been sexually active recently? Is it possible that she is pregnant? Has she missed any periods lately? A pregnancy test may be of use but resuscitation should not be delayed by performing this.

Although this presentation could be of other gynaecological cause, it is likely that a ruptured ectopic pregnancy may have occurred. Surgical gynaecological staff should be summoned at the earliest opportunity because surgical intervention may be required alongside fluid resuscitation.

Scenario 2

You are called as part of the cardiac arrest team to the maternity ward, where basic life support is in progress on a heavily pregnant woman. Describe how initial cardiac arrest management will differ from that for a non-pregnant patient.

What Is Your Course of Action?
Experienced help should be summoned immediately; this should include an obstetrician and a neonatologist.

Basic life support is already in progress; this in itself will require some modification, but all the principles of basic and advanced life support apply. Caval compression can complicate the effectiveness of basic life support in the pregnant patient after 20 weeks' gestation/ The uterus should be manually displaced to the left to reduce caval compression; a wedge may also be used to create a left-sided lateral tilt of between 15 and 30°. However, this needs to be performed so that cardiac compressions are effective, so sand bags or purpose-made Cardiff wedges may be used; alternatively the knees of rescuers may be used.

Airway management may well be difficult, so expert help will be required. There is a high risk of pulmonary aspiration of gastric contents, so early tracheal intubation will be required.

Preparations should be made for emergency caesarean section because this will be required if initial attempts at resuscitation fail. This ideally should occur at about 4 minutes after cardiac arrest.

CONCLUSION

Assessing and monitoring the critically ill pregnant woman is a challenge, notably because of the physiological changes that occur during pregnancy. The ABCDE approach to assessing the acutely unwell patient is recommended in assessment but requires the practitioner to possess essential knowledge of these physiological changes to ensure that its application meets the needs of the patient. The onus is on the individual practitioner to ensure that this process occurs.

As with any acutely unwell patient, a multidisciplinary approach and senior assistance are required at the earliest opportunity. This approach is extended in treating the pregnant patient to include groups of staff not frequently called upon in other situations, e.g. obstetricians/neonatologists and midwifery staff. Collaborative working among these professional groups/staff is the key to optimising maternal and fetal outcome. There is an urgent need for the routine use of a national obstetric early warning chart, similar to that in use in other areas of clinical practice, which can be used for all obstetric women, helping the more timely recognition, treatment and referral of women who have, or are developing, a critical illness (Lewis 2007).

REFERENCES

Adam, S. & Osborne, S. (2005) *Critical Care Nursing: Science and practice*, 2nd edn. Oxford: Oxford University Press.

Allen, K. (2005) Four-step method of interpreting arterial blood gas analysis. *Nursing Times*, **101**(1), 42.

Alexander, M. F., Fawcett. J. N., & Runciman, P. J. (2006) *Nursing Practice: Hospital and home – the adult*. Oxford: Churchill Livingstone.

Bayliss, D. A. & Millhorn, D. E. (1992) Central neural mechanisms of progesterone action: application to the respiratory system. *Journal of Applied Physiology*, **73**, 393–404.

Bothamley, J. & Boyle, M. (2009) *Medical Conditions Affecting Pregnancy and Childbirth*. Oxford: Radcliffe Publishing.

Bourjeily, G., Paidas, M., Khalil, H., et al. (2010) Pulmonary embolism in pregnancy. *The Lancet*, **375**, 500–512.

Cetin, A. (2006) Cited in Mohler, E. R., and Townsen R. R., (2006) *Advanced therapy in hypertension and vascular disease*. Peoples Medical Publishing House, USA http://www.amazon.co.uk/Advanced-Therapy-Hypertension-Vascular-Disease/dp/1550093185/ref=sr_1_1?s=books&ie=UTF8&qid=1318937701&sr=1-1

Clark, S. L., Hankins, G .D. V., Dudley, D. A., et al. (1995) Amniotic fluid embolism: analysis of the national registry. *American Journal of Obstetrics and Gynecology*, **172**, 1158–1169.

De Jong, M. J. & Fausett, M. (2003) Anaphylactoid syndrome of pregnancy: A devastating complication requiring intensive care. *Critical Care Nurse*, **23**, 42–48.

Drife, J. & Magowan, B. A. (2004) *Clinical Obstetrics and Gynecology*. Oxford: Baillière Tindall.

Goldhill, D.R., White, S.A., & Sumner, A. (1999) Physiological values and procedures in the 24 h before ICU admission from the ward. *Anaesthesia*, **54**, 529–534.

Grady, K., Howell, C., Cox, C., eds (2007) *The MOET Course Manual, Managing obstetric emergencies and trauma*, 2nd edn. London: Advanced Life Support Group/RCOG Press.

Hayes, K. & Arulkumaran, S. (2006) Chapter 1 In: Arulkumaram, S. (ed.), *Emergencies in Obstetrics and Gynaecology*. Oxford: Oxford University Press.

Higgins, D. (2005) Pulse oximetry. *Nursing Times*, **101**(6), 34–35.

Higgins, D. (2008) Specimen collection. Part six: Urinalysis. *Nursing Times*, **104**(18), 26–27.

Higgins, D. & Guest, J. (2008) Acute respiratory failure 1: assessing patients. *Nursing Times*, **104**(36), 24–25.

Jevon, P. (2010) How to ensure patient observations lead to prompt identification of tachypnoea. *Nursing Times*, **106**(2), 12–14.

Ko, H. H. & Yoshida, E. (2006) Acute fatty liver of pregnancy. *Canadian Journal of Gastroenterology*, **20**, 25–30.

Lewis, G., ed. (2007) The Confidential Enquiry into Maternal and Child Health (CEMACH). Saving MothersLives: Reviewing maternal deaths to make motherhood safer – 2003–2005. The Seventh Report on Confidential Enquiries into Maternal Deaths in the United Kingdom, London.

Magpie Trial Collaborative Group (2002) Do women with pre-eclampsia, and their babies, benefit from magnesium sulphate? The Magpie Trial: a randomised placebo controlled trial. *The Lancet*, **359**, 1877–1890.

McNulty, J. (2004) Acute fatty liver of pregnancy. In: Foley M. R., Strong T. H., & Garite T. J. (eds), *Obstetric Intensive Care Manual*. New York: McGraw-Hill Medical.

McQuillan, P., Pilkington, S., Allan, A., et al., (1998) Confidential Enquiry into quality of care before admission to intensive care. *British Medical Journal*, **316**, 1853–1858.

Meltzer, S. (2010) Treatment of gestational diabetes: The question is not whether to treat, but how and who? *British Medical Journal*, **340**, 1708.

Miller, F.P., Vandome. A.F., & McBrewster. J (2008) *Gestational Diabetes*. Mauritius: VDM Publishing.

National Institute for Health and Clinical Evidence (2010) *Venous Thromboembolism: Reducing the risk of venous thromboembolism (deep vein thrombosis and pulmonary embolism) in patients admitted to hospital*, London: NICE. Available at: www.nice.org.uk/nicemedia/live/12695/47195/47195.pdf (accessed August 2010).

Nihoyannopoulus, P. (2007) Cardiovascular examination in pregnancy and the approach to the diagnosis of cardiac disorder. In: Oakley, C. & Warnes, C.A. (eds), *Heart Disease in Pregnancy*. Oxford: BMJ Publishing/Blackwell.

Quinn, M. (1994) Automated blood pressure measurement devices: a potential source of morbidity in pre-eclampsia? *American Journal of Obstetrics and Gynaecology*, **107**, 1303–1307.

Resuscitation Council UK (2006) *Advanced Life Support*, 5th edn. London: Resuscitation Council, UK.

Silversides, C.K. & Coleman, J.M. (2007) Physiological changes in pregnancy. In: Oakley, C. & Warnes, C.A. (eds), *Heart Disease in Pregnancy*. Oxford: BMJ Publishing/Blackwell.

Walls, R. & Murphy, R. M. (2008) *Manual of Emergency Airway Management*. London: Lippincott Williams & Wilkins.

Watkins, J. (2010) Ectopic pregnancy. *Practice Nursing*, **21**(2). Available at: www.amazon.co.uk/Heart-Disease-Pregnancy-Celia-Oakley/dp/1405134887/ref=sr_1_1?s=books&ie=UTF8&qid=1281624819&sr=1-1.

Monitoring the Critically Ill Child $\quad$ **17**

LEARNING OUTCOMES

At the end of the chapter the reader will be able to:

☐ discuss the aetiology of cardiorespiratory arrests in children
☐ discuss the importance of treating children differently to adults
☐ outline the ABCDE approach

INTRODUCTION

Children are a diverse group of the population. They vary dramatically in weight, size, shape, intellectual ability and emotional responses. At birth a child is, on average, 3.5 kg with a small respiratory and cardiovascular reserve and an immature immune system. They are capable of limited movement, exhibit limited emotional responses and are dependent on adults for their needs. Fourteen or more years later at the other end of childhood, the adolescent is a 50-kg, 160-cm tall person who looks like an adult. Therefore competent management of the critically ill child who may fall anywhere between these two extremes requires a knowledge of these anatomical, physiological and emotional differences (Advanced Life Support Group 2011).

Use of the structured ABCDE approach (Box 17.1) helps to ensure that potentially life-threatening problems are identified and dealt with in order of priority: the early recognition and effective management of respiratory and/or circulatory failure will

Monitoring the Critically Ill Patient, Third Edition.
Philip Jevon, Beverley Ewens.
© 2012 Blackwell Publishing Ltd. Published 2012 by Blackwell Publishing Ltd.

Box 17.1 ABCDE approach to assess and treat the critically ill child (Resuscitation Council UK 2010)

Airway
Breathing
Circulation
Disability
Exposure

---

hopefully prevent deterioration to cardiorespiratory arrests (Resuscitation Council UK 2010).

The aim of this chapter is to understand the principles of monitoring the critically ill child following the ABCDE approach.

AETIOLOGY OF CARDIORESPIRATORY ARREST IN CHILDREN

The aetiology of cardiorespiratory arrest in children usually differs greatly to that in adults, due to the anatomical, physiological and pathological differences that change throughout childhood.

In adults, cardiorespiratory arrests are commonly due to cardiac arrhythmia, relating to underlying ischaemic heart disease; such an arrest is an acute event and can occur without warning.

In children, however, cardiorespiratory arrest is rarely a sudden event, but a progressive deterioration as respiratory failure and circulatory failure worsen. In children, cardiorespiratory arrest is usually due to hypoxia, reflecting the end of the body's ability to compensate for the effects of underlying illness or injury (Resuscitation Council UK 2010). Some of the causes of respiratory failure and circulatory failure are listed in Box 17.2.

IMPORTANCE OF TREATING CHILDREN DIFFERENTLY

The key differences to consider are weight, anatomical (size and shape), physiological (cardiovascular, respiratory, immune function) and psychological (intellectual ability and emotional response).

Box 17.2 Causes of respiratory failure and circulatory failure in children (Advanced Life Support Group 2011) (not an exhaustive list)

Respiratory failure
Asthma
Bronchiolitis
Foreign body airway obstruction
Medications
Head injury
Anaphylaxis
Seizures

Circulatory failure
Severe diarrhoea and vomiting
Meningococcal septicaemia
Anaphylaxis
Trauma and blood loss

Weight

The most dramatic changes in a child's weight occur during the first year of life; an average birthweight of 3.5 kg will increase to 10 kg by the child's first birthday. After this time weight increases more slowly until puberty. In paediatric resuscitation most drugs and fluids are given per kilogram of body weight so it is important to determine a child's weight as soon as possible.

The most accurate method is to weigh the child but this may not always be possible; in this situation a child's weight can be estimated by a number of methods. Examples of these are the Broselow tape, which relates the length of the child to the body weight, or centile charts that estimate weight against age. If a child's age is between 1 and 10 years the following is the most commonly used formula (Resuscitation Council UK 2010):

$$\text{Weight (in kg)} = [\text{Age (in years)} + 4] \times 2.$$

This formula is not suitable, however, for use in a child aged <1 year; although a term newborn infant averages 3.5 kg, by 6 months the birthweight has usually doubled and at 1 year trebled.

Whichever method has been used to establish body weight, it is essential that health-care professionals are familiar and competent in its use (Resuscitation Council UK 2010).

Anatomical

A child's airway goes through many changes; in the younger child the head is large and the neck short, which causes neck flexion and airway narrowing. The face and mandible are small and the tongue is relatively large and can obstruct the airway easily. Also the floor of the mouth is easily compressible and can be obstructed by positioning of the fingers during airway manoeuvres

The anatomy of the airway itself changes with age. Infants aged <6 months are nose breathers and, as upper respiratory tract infections are common in this age group, their airways are commonly obstructed by mucous secretions.

In all young children the epiglottis is horse-shoe shaped and the larynx high and anterior, making tracheal intubation much more difficult.

Physiological

There are many differences in the respiratory and cardiovascular systems of infants and adults. The infant has a greater metabolic rate and oxygen consumption, which is the reason for their increased respiratory rates, Stroke volume is also relatively small in infancy and increases with heart size. However, the cardiac output is the product of stroke volume and heart rate, so high cardiac outputs in infants and young children are achieved by rapid heart rates. Tables 17.1–17.3 give some of the respiratory indices.

Table 17.1 Normal respiratory rate according to age

Age (years)	Respiratory rate (breaths/min)
<1	30–40
1–2	26–34
2–5	24–30
5–12	20–24
>12	12–20

Table 17.2 Normal heart rate according to age

Age	Mean (beats/min)	Awake (beats/min)	Deep sleep (beats/min)
Newborn to 3 months	140	85–205	80–140
3 months to 2 years	130	100–180	75–160
2–10 years	80	60–140	60–90
>10 years	75	60–100	50–90

Table 17.3 Normal blood pressure according to age

Age	Normal (mmHg)	Lower limit (mmHg)
0–1 month	>60	50–60
1–12 months	80	70
1–10 years	90 + 2 × age in years	70 + 2 × age in years
>10 years	120	90

Immune function

At birth the immune system is immature so babies are much more susceptible to illness.

Psychological

Children vary greatly in their intellectual ability and emotional response. Knowledge of the child's developmental structure is of great benefit. Infants and young children find it very difficult to communicate and the importance of non-verbal communication and fear must be thought about.

ABCDE APPROACH

The ABCDE approach (see Box 17.1), as for in adults (see Chapter 2), can be used when assessing and treating a critically ill child; the underlying principles of assessment, initial management and ongoing reassessments are the same. The general principles are as follows (Resuscitation Council UK 2007):

- Observe the child generally to determine the overall level of illness (i.e. Does the child look seriously unwell? Is he or she interacting with parents).
- Speak to the child and assess the appropriateness of their response; ask the parents about the child's 'usual' behaviour.
- If the child is unconscious and unresponsive to your voice, administer tactile stimulation (gently shake the arm or leg). If the child responds by speaking or crying, this indicates that he or she has a patent airway, is breathing and has brain perfusion. Regardless of the child's response to initial stimulation, move on rapidly to full assessment of ABCDE.
- Appropriate high-flow oxygen delivery should be started immediately.
- Vital sign monitoring should be requested early.
- Circulatory access should be achieved as soon as possible. Bloods for laboratory investigations and a bedside glucose should be obtained.
- Ensure personal safety.

Initial approach to the child

- Ensure that it is safe to approach the child; check the environment and remove any hazards.
- On approach to the child and before touching him or her, rapidly look around for any clues to what may have caused the emergency because this may influence the way the child is managed (e.g. any suspicion of any head or neck injury).
- Determine the responsiveness of the child; an appropriate way of doing this is calling the child's name and telling him or her to 'wake up'. For an infant it is appropriate to 'flick the feet' or pick him or her up if no trauma is suspected. A normal response implies that the child has a patent airway, is breathing and has cerebral perfusion. An inappropriate response or no response indicates that the child may be critically ill and help needs to be summoned immediately.

Assessment of airway

If the child is talking or crying he or she will have a patent airway. In a conscious child it is important to establish airway patency: Is the airway at risk or obstructed? Airway obstruction can be partial or complete; the airway may be restricted by mucus or vomit and simple actions such as repositioning or suction may be required. A foreign body could be present; in unconscious children the tongue may fall backwards and occlude the airway. Airway obstruction may be demonstrated by difficulty in breathing and/ or increased respiratory rate; if the obstruction is partial there may be 'gurgling' or 'stridor'. It is important to note that, when assessing airway patency, chest movement does not guarantee that the airway is clear.

Causes of airway obstruction include (Resuscitation Council UK 2007):

- foreign body
- tongue
- secretions – vomit/blood
- respiratory tract infections
- altered level of consciousness
- pharyngeal swelling
- epiglottitis
- laryngo-/bronchospasm
- trauma – face/throat
- congenital abnormality

The repositioning of an airway is simply overcome using the head-tilt and chin-lift manoeuvre: place one hand on the child's forehead and gently tilt the head back; in the infant (<1 year of age) this is the neutral position. For the child this is the 'sniffing' position with some extension of the head and neck required. If this position is not possible or any trauma is suspected, a jaw thrust manoeuvre can be performed, which is achieved by placing two or three fingers under the angle of the mandible bilaterally and lifting the jaw upwards.

In children with airway obstruction it is important to deliver supplemental oxygen as soon as possible to minimise the effects of hypoxia. If there is a reduced level of consciousness, airway compromise must be assumed; the familiar look, listen and feel approach can easily detect if an airway is obstructed.

Look

Look for chest and abdominal movements. If the airway is obstructed paradoxical chest movements (see-saw respirations) and the use of accessory muscles can be seen.

Listen

Listen for breathing: normal respirations are quiet, partial obstructed breathing is usually noisy whereas complete obstruction will be silent.

Feel

Feel for signs of airway obstruction: place your face in front of the child's mouth to determine whether there is movement of air.

Treatment of airway obstruction

Once airway obstruction has been identified, treat appropriately. Simple methods such as suction, airway positioning, or insertion of oropharyngeal or nasopharyngeal airways are often very effective. As described earlier administer high-flow oxygen as soon as possible.

Assessment of breathing

Once the airway is open it is important to assess for effective, spontaneous breathing. Appropriate management of airway and breathing is the priority in all seriously ill children. This is also achieved by the look, listen and feel approach.

Look

Look for general signs of respiratory distress; look at the respiratory rate, the work of breathing, tidal volume. Is there tachypnoea, central cyanosis, chest expansion, use of accessory muscles?

In children recognition of respiratory failure is based on full assessment of respiratory effort and efficacy, and the inadequacy on major organs (Resuscitation Council UK 2007).

Tachypnoea is usually the first sign of respiratory insufficiency (Smith 2003). As discussed earlier, normal respiratory ranges vary with age and it is important to consider this (see Table 17.1). Remember also that fever, pain and anxiety will alter the respiratory rate so it is more important to monitor the trend in the rate rather than rely on an absolute value (Resuscitation Council UK 2007).

Recession in the sick child is common and shows the effort of breathing; this may be sternal, subcostal or intercostal. The degree of recession gives an indication of the severity of respiratory distress. Infants and younger children can exhibit significant recession with relatively mild-to-moderate respiratory compromise, due to their highly compliant chest wall. However, in children over about 5 years of age recession is a sign of significant respiratory compromise (Resuscitation Council UK 2007).

The use of accessory muscles is also a common sign when the work of breathing is increased. The sternocleidomastoid muscle in the neck is often used as an accessory respiratory muscle (Resuscitation Council UK 2007). In infants this can cause the head to bob up and down with each breath – known as 'head bobbing'.

Another common breathing pattern seen in severe respiratory distress is 'see-saw' breathing; this is the paradoxical movement of the abdomen during inspiration. It is a very inefficient respiration because the tidal volume is greatly reduced. Nostril flaring can also be seen in infants and young children.

Assess the depth of breathing. Ascertain whether chest movement is equal on both sides. Unilateral chest movement may be a sign of pneumothorax, pneumonia or pleural effusion (Smith 2003).

Children in respiratory compromise will usually adopt a position that helps their respiratory capacity. This position must be supported to maximise comfort and prevent further upset which may result in further deterioration.

The degree of increased work of breathing generally provides clinical evidence of the severity of respiratory insufficiency; however, there are exceptions to this (Resuscitation Council UK 2007):

- *Exhaustion*: children who have had severe respiratory compromise for some time may have progressed to decompensation and no longer show signs of increased work of breathing; exhaustion is a pre-terminal event.
- *Neuromuscular diseases*, e.g. muscular dystrophy.

- *Central respiratory depression*: reduced respiratory drive results in respiratory inadequacy, e.g. encephalopathy and medications such as morphine.

Pulse oximetry should be used on any child showing signs of respiratory distress and at risk of respiratory failure. An arterial oxygen saturation (SaO_2) of <90 % in air or <95% in supplemental oxygen indicates respiratory failure. It should be noted that SaO_2 measurements are unreliable when a child has poor peripheral circulation. When SaO_2 is <70%, pulse oximetry is inaccurate (Resuscitation Council UK 2007).

Listen

Listen to the child's breath sounds a short distance from the face. Normal breathing is quiet. Noisy breathing indicates the presence of airway obstruction (Resuscitation Council UK 2007):

- Stridor: associated with partial upper airway obstruction, wheezing is generally an expiratory noise
- *Wheeze*: may be heard audibly or on chest auscultation with a stethoscope; it indicates narrowing of the lower airways, e.g. bronchospasm.
- *Grunting*: mainly heard in young babies, but can occur in small children. It is the result of exhaling against a partially closed glottis, and is an attempt to generate a positive end-expiratory pressure, thus preventing airway collapse at the end of expiration. Grunting is usually associated with 'stiff' lungs and is an indication of severe respiratory compromise.

If possible, auscultate the chest. Air entry should be heard in all areas of the lungs. The depth and equality of breath sounds on both sides of the chest should be evaluated. Any additional sounds, e.g. crackles or wheeze, should be noted and it is often useful to compare one side of the chest with the other. A silent chest indicates a dangerously reduced tidal volume and is an ominous sign.

Feel

If possible palpate and percuss the chest wall. Palpation may identify deformities, surgical emphysema or crepitus (suggesting pneumothorax until proven otherwise) (Smith 2003).

Percussion of the chest wall can demonstrate areas of collapse (dullness) or hyper-resonance (e.g. in pneumothorax).

Respiratory compromise also affects other systems of the body, including heart rate, skin perfusion and conscious level.

Management of respiratory compromise

The treatment of breathing problems depends on achieving a patent airway and effective delivery of oxygen. This will vary depending on the child's clinical condition and age. Children who do have adequate spontaneous breathing should have high-flow oxygen delivered in a manner that is non-threatening and best tolerated by them, e.g. from a non-re-breathing facemask or nasal cannulas.

When breathing is not adequate (or absent) high-flow oxygen should be delivered by ventilation with a bag–valve–mask system. In situations where the child is exhausted and likely to require ongoing respiratory support (or is in imminent cardiorespiratory arrest), tracheal intubation may be indicated (Resuscitation Council UK 2007).

Assessment of circulation

Appropriate management of the airway and breathing is the priority in all sick children, and should be assessed before moving on to circulatory status.

Circulatory failure is the clinical state where the flow of blood (and associated delivery of nutrients, e.g. oxygen and glucose) to the body tissues is inadequate for metabolic demand (Resuscitation Council UK 2007).

In children most cases of circulatory failure are a result of hypovolaemia, sepsis or anaphylaxis. Other uncommon causes include obstruction of blood flow, e.g. tension pneumothorax, or anaemia or carbon monoxide poisoning in which the oxygen-carrying capacity of the blood is reduced.

Initially children are compromised for reduced tissue perfusion so it is essential to promptly recognise and treat any child with compensated circulatory failure to prevent deterioration to a decompensated state. The familiar look, listen and feel approach can be used for the assessment of the circulation.

Look

Look at the skin temperature and colour, heart rate, capillary refill time (CRT) and conscious level.

The skin of a healthy child is pink and warms to touch. Signs of cardiovascular compromise include cool, pale, mottled peripheries.

Measure CRT; a normal capillary refill is <2 seconds but when there is reduced skin perfusion this is prolonged. In children with pyrexias or cool peripheries a central CRT (e.g. chest or forehead) is much more reliable.

Demarcation lines are also seen in very sick children – this is peripheral vasoconstriction and decreased perfusion which leaves a line between warm and cold skin.

Look for other signs of a poor cardiac output, e.g. reduced conscious level, or poor urine output, Parents of young children will be very aware of how many wet nappies their child has had that day. Normal urine output is 0.5 ml/kg per h (Smith 2003).

Listen

Measure the child's blood pressure. In most forms of shock a child's blood pressure (BP) is maintained within the normal ranges (see Table 17.3) for a long time; only when compensation is no longer possible will hypotension occur. In hypovolaemia, hypotension occurs only after approximately 40% of the child's circulatory volume has been lost, so it is essential that compensated circulatory failure be detected and managed early before decompensation occurs.

Another important point is that the appropriate cuff size be used. The cuff width should be >80% of the child's upper arm length (Resuscitation Council UK 2007).

Hypotension is a sign of physiological decompensation and indicates imminent cardiorespiratory arrest.

Feel

Feel the central pulse; the heart rate initially rises to maintain cardiac output. Heart rates vary with age (see Table 17.2), but are also altered by fever, pain and anxiety, so other signs of circulatory function must be observed.

When the heart rate is unable to maintain tissue perfusion, the tissue hypoxia and acidosis result in bradycardia. The presence of bradycardia is a pre-terminal sign.

The pulse volume gives a subjective indication of stroke volume. Is the pulse strong or weak, thready or bounding or is there a difference when comparing central and peripheral pulses? Is a pulse present at all?

Circulatory compromise also affects other systems of the body including respiratory function and conscious level.

Management of circulatory compromise

The treatment of circulatory problems depends on achieving a patent airway and effectively managing ventilation with delivery of high-flow oxygen before turning attention to circulatory procedures (Resuscitation Council UK 2007).

Immediate life-threatening causes of circulatory failure must be sought and urgently treated.

Insertion of, ideally, two large-bore vascular cannula should be performed rapidly; if after three attempts or 90 seconds this is unsuccessful, then the intraosseous (IO) route should be used. Placement of an IO cannula involves insertion of a needle through the skin, periosteum and cortex of the bone, into the medullary cavity (Resuscitation Council UK 2007). The preferred sights are the anteromedial surface or the lower end of the tibia so as to avoid the growth plates. This route, once inserted, can be used to deliver all resuscitation fluids, medications and blood-derived products.

Unless contraindicated (e.g. cardiac failure) volume replacement should be initiated as soon as possible. A 20 ml/kg bolus of crystalloid solution, usually 0.9% saline, should be given as soon and as quickly as possible. The child's circulatory status should then be reassessed and, if signs of failure are still present, this should be repeated. A further infusion, making three in total, is also available if required while the underlying cause is sought. If the cause of the circulatory failure is identified as haemorrhage, blood products must be considered. Glucose-containing solutions should never be used for volume replacement because they can be dangerous, causing hyponatraemia and hyperglycaemia (Resuscitation Council UK 2007).

Assessment of disability

After appropriate management of the child's circulatory airway, breathing and circulation, an evaluation of the neurological status should be made.

Causes of altered conscious levels include hypoxia, hypoglycaemia and medications (e.g. for status epilepticus) so it is very important to:

- review ABC to exclude anything previously missed
- check the medication already received for drug-induced causes
- undertake a bedside glucose measurement to exclude hypoglycaemia.

A rapid assessment of conscious level can be carried out by using the AVPU score.

A – Alert
V – responds to Voice
P – responds to Pain
U – Unresponsive to painful stimuli.

The Glasgow Coma Scale (GCS) is another common scale used to assess level of consciousness and a child who is unresponsive to painful stimuli is equivalent to a GCS score of "8.

Interaction is also a good sign of disability assessment: how is the child interacting with the parents and surroundings? A young child who is lying very still letting staff perform examinations and investigations is a worrying sign.

Look at a child's posture: Is the infant floppy, the young child drowsy? Is he or she stiff which may be the sign of a serious brain dysfunction?

Look at the pupil reactions: size, equality and reaction to light – brisk or sluggish?

Management of altered conscious level

The first priority is to reassess ABC to make sure that nothing has recurred or been missed. If hypoglycaemia is confirmed, administer glucose to treat. If drug-induced altered conscious level is suspected and the effects are reversible, administer antidote if available.

Exposure

Full exposure of the child is necessary in order to undertake a thorough examination and ensure that important details are not overlooked (Smith 2003)

Appropriate measures to minimise heat loss (especially in infants) and respect dignity must be adopted at all times.

Look for evidence of blood loss, skin lesions, wounds, rashes – blanching, petechia; are there bruises that show evidence of non-accidental injury, etc.?

Check the child's core temperature: is he or she pyrexial or hypothermic?

Control any bleeding found; reconsider fluid management as directed by loss. Dictate treatment to any rashes found, e.g. petechial rashes are a sign of meningococcal septicaemia and need antibiotics. Investigate any bruises for signs of malignancy, e.g. leukaemia, or of non-accidental injury – which need referral to safeguarding team for further investigation. Consider appropriate temperature measures, e.g. antipyretics or blankets or warm fluids.

In addition:

- Undertake a full clinical history
- Review the child's case notes, observation chart and prescription chart
- Ensure that prescribed medications and fluids are being administered
- Review laboratory and radiology results once available
- Consider the level of care that the child requires, e.g. ward, high dependency unit, paediatric intensive care unit
- Provide effective communication to the child and parents/carers at all times.

CONCLUSION

Early recognition and treatment of the critically ill child are paramount. Research has shown that early recognition prevents most cardiorespiratory arrests. The use of the structured ABCDE in assessing the critically ill child has been described and the importance of calling for expert help early on has been emphasized.

REFERENCES

Advanced Life Support Group (2011) *Advanced Paediatric Life Support,* 5th edn. Oxford: Wiley.

Resuscitation Council UK (2007) *Paediatric Immediate Life Support.* London: Resuscitation Council UK.

Resuscitation Council UK (2010) *Guidelines 2010.* London: Resuscitation Council UK. Available at: www.resus.org.uk (accessed 8 April 2011).

Smith, G. (2003) *ALERT – Acute Life-threatening Events Recognition and Treatment,* 2nd edn. Portsmouth: University of Portsmouth.

Monitoring During Transport

18

LEARNING OBJECTIVES

At the end of the chapter the reader will be able to:

☐ list the possible *reasons* for transporting a critically ill patient, both within a hospital and from one hospital to another
☐ discuss the potential *problems* and *hazards* associated with transport
☐ discuss what *monitoring equipment* is required for transport
☐ discuss *what should be monitored* during transport

INTRODUCTION

Moving an intensive care unit (ICU) patient is a high-risk procedure, which requires detailed planning and preparation in order to minimise risk to the patient (Everest and Munford 2009). The main reasons for inter-hospital or intra-hospital transport include local ICU bed shortages, access to specialist services, diagnostic tools such as computed tomography (CT) or magnetic resonance imaging (MRI), and specialised operative procedures (Everest and Munford 2009).

Inter-hospital transport imposes essential risk for critically ill patients (Markakis et al. 2006). All patient movement is associated with an increase in morbidity and mortality, and poses significant risks to patient safety and should not be undertaken without full consideration of the risk benefits to the patient (Everest and Munford 2009; Jarden and Quirke 2010). The quality and outcome

Monitoring the Critically Ill Patient, Third Edition.
Philip Jevon, Beverley Ewens.
© 2012 Blackwell Publishing Ltd. Published 2012 by Blackwell Publishing Ltd.

of the transfer depend on the experience of the transfer team, meticulous clinical preparation and adequate monitoring facilities (Everest and Munford 2009). This same level of supervision and preparation is also required for intra-hospital transfer of critically ill patients (Intensive Care Society 2011). *Transport of the Critically Ill Adult Patient* (3rd edition), published by the Intensive Care Society (2011), makes recommendations for the organisation and clinical provision of transfers.

The aim of this chapter is to understand the principles of monitoring a critically ill patient during transport.

REASONS FOR TRANSPORT

Possible reasons for *intra-hospital* transport of critically ill patients include the following:

- Diagnostic and therapeutic procedures that can not be undertaken at the bedside, e.g. CT scan
- The need for surgery
- Transfer to ICU/high dependency unit (HDU)/coronary care unit (CCU)

Possible reasons for *inter-hospital* transport of critically ill patients include the following:

- Non-clinical need, e.g. ICU bed shortages
- Requirement for specialist services, e.g. spinal unit
- Requirement for specialist investigations, e.g. radiologically guided services such as vascular embolisation or angioplasty (Everest and Munford 2009b)
- Requirement for specialist surgery, e.g. neurosurgery, cardiac surgery
- Complex organ support, e.g. extracorporeal membrane oxygenation (ECMO)
- Social reasons, e.g. transfer to a hospital nearer to the patient's home.

POTENTIAL PROBLEMS AND HAZARDS ASSOCIATED WITH TRANSPORT

Mortality rates during transport are low but adverse events have been stated to be as high as 30% (Jarden and Quirke 2010). However, it is still potentially hazardous to transport a critically ill patient, particularly if intensive haemodynamic and respiratory support is required or if it is undertaken by unqualified or inexperienced staff (Everest and Munford 2009; Jarden and Quirke 2010).

The transport of critically ill patients can result in physiological deterioration (Jarden and Quirke 2010). The patient may be unable to tolerate lifting, tipping, abrupt movements, vibration and acceleration/deceleration (Lawler 2000). Accelerational forces and vertical movements can cause cardiovascular instability, particularly in patients who are hypovolaemic or vasodilated due to sepsis, drugs or sedation (Hinds and Watson 1996).

Significant changes in intracranial pressure can be induced by transport, e.g. placing a patient in the head-down position when loading on to the ambulance can exacerbate intracranial hypertension (Hinds and Watson 1996).

An ambulance is probably the worst environment to care for a critically ill patient (Figs 18.1 and 18.2). Space limitations,

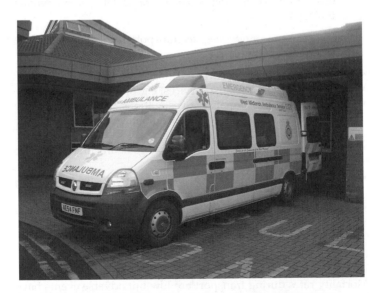

Fig. 18.1 Paramedic ambulance: the most common means of land transport.

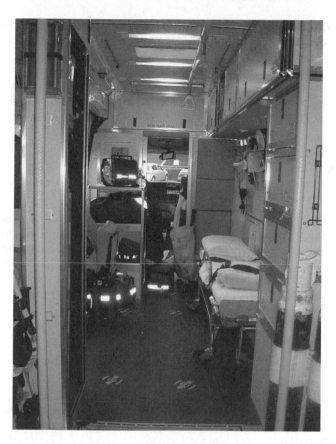

Fig. 18.2 Inside a paramedic ambulance.

movement, noise, power sources and lighting can all impose restrictions. Movement of the vehicle can make the performance of even the most routine medical and nursing procedures difficult. A particularly common problem is motion sickness, for both the patient and the staff.

Noise and daylight may render monitors and their alarms unreadable and inaudible. Ambulances rely on battery sources for electrical power. Consequently hospital-based equipment that needs alternating current (AC) can be used only with its own power source or an AC/DC converter.

Untoward occurrences do occur in up to 70% of transfers and are associated with equipment failure; acute deterioration of PaO_2/FiO_2 ratio is common and ventilator-associated pneumonia (VAP) is significantly increased (Everest and Munford 2009).

Hazards associated with air transport

The hazards encountered with air transport depend to a degree on the mode of transport (helicopter or aeroplane) and can be summarised as follows:

- *Expansion of gas in closed cavities*: as atmospheric pressure falls with increasing altitude, the volume occupied by gas rises; clinically this results in expansion of trapped gases. This exacerbates a pneumothorax. In addition air in a tracheal tube cuff is susceptible to these changes; either gently fill the cuff with physiological (0.9%) saline or continuously monitor the cuff pressure during altitude changes.
- *Fluid loss*: a fall in atmospheric pressure can cause fluid to extravasate from the intravascular to the interstitial space, resulting in oedema, hypotension and tachycardia; in addition, the effects of dehydration can be exacerbated (Hinds and Watson 1996).
- *Increased altitude:* associated with a fall in temperature.
- *Hypoxia*: increasing altitude causes a fall in the partial pressure of oxygen, which can lead to a fall in alveolar oxygen and hypoxia.
- *Temperature control*: heating in helicopters can be particularly difficult. In addition the patient may be exposed to the environment when being transferred to and from the aircraft.
- *Noise and vibration*: may cause nausea, pain and motor dysfunction (Intensive Care Society 2011).
- *Visibility*: may be limited; this together with the high ambient noise levels can make monitoring even more difficult; the patient visual alarms may be obscured (Intensive Care Society 2011).
- *Unfamiliar environment*: can be stressful for the patient and staff.

PATIENT MONITORING EQUIPMENT REQUIRED
FOR TRANSPORT

Determining what monitoring equipment should be taken will depend on the condition of the patient and the available resources on the mode of transport. Any equipment taken should be (Intensive Care Society 2011):

- lightweight, yet durable and robust
- mounted at or below the level of the patient
- restrained, yet easily accessible
- regularly checked
- battery powered if electrical (with battery life display).

Ideally equipment should be standardised across critical care networks and have both audible and visual alarms. A small versatile portable monitor such as a Propaq (Fig. 18.3) is invaluable.

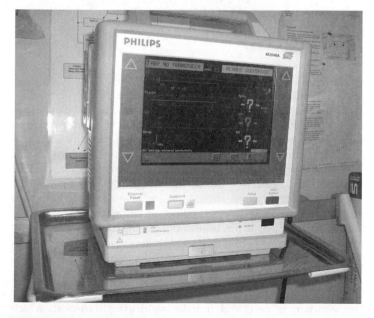

Fig. 18.3 Propaq portable monitor.

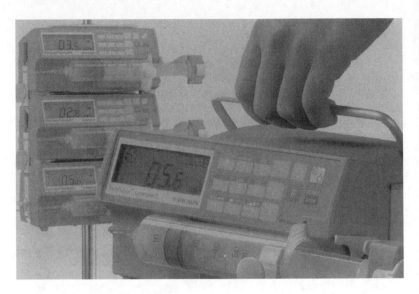

Fig. 18.4 Infusion pumps.

Depending on what is required, recordings of ECG, oxygen saturation, non-invasive blood pressure, temperature, invasive pressures and capnography can be taken. Capnography is recommended as a mandatory requirement by the Intensive Care Society (2011).

Infusion pumps (Fig. 18.4) and appropriate medications should be available. In particular it is important to ensure that essential infusions, e.g. vasoactive drugs, do not run out during transfer. Although a mobile phone should ideally be available to help with communications, any possible effect on monitoring equipment should be checked. If air transport is being undertaken, *always* check with the pilot before using a mobile phone, because mobiles can interfere with aircraft navigation and avionics.

MONITORING DURING TRANSFER

The standard of care and monitoring during transport, which will depend on the individual needs of the patient, should be maintained at the same level as on the ICU. The Intensive Care Society (2011) makes the following recommendations:

- *Arterial oxygenation, ECG and arterial pressure* should be monitored in every patient.
- *Invasive arterial monitoring* is preferable to non-invasive because the latter is sensitive to motion.
- *Central venous pressure, pulmonary artery wedge pressure or intracranial pressure* may be required in some patients; interpretation may, however, be difficult in a moving ambulance and treatment is therefore difficult to control.
- If the patient is being *mechanically ventilated* the oxygen supply and airway pressure should be monitored; a means for detecting disconnection should be established
- *End-tidal CO_2 measurement* is desirable in all patients.
- *Temperature* should be monitored if it is abnormal, during long journeys or in cold weather.

Assessment of adequacy of ventilation is notoriously inaccurate in an ambulance (Knowles et al. 1999). There are now sophisticated portable ventilators that can maintain the most dependent patient, without compromising the respiratory rate, for limited periods of time (Fig. 18.5). These offer different modes and run on a battery, requiring only an oxygen cylinder source.

If parenteral nutrition is halted it is recommended to administer 10% glucose to avoid rebound hypoglycaemia (Gilligan 1997). The blood glucose should be closely monitored during transfer.

As well as monitoring the patient, it is also important to monitor the equipment continuously, particularly alarms. Intravenous infusions should be closely monitored to ensure that the prescribed dose is being administered and that they have not run out.

Unskilled or inexperienced staff may not recognise or rectify problems. Experienced staff should be in attendance, e.g. a senior ICU nurse and an anaesthetist, who should have the necessary skills to manage any sudden and unexpected outcome (Intensive Care Society 2011).

CONCLUSION

Transporting a critically ill patient can be fraught with difficulties and is potentially hazardous. Therefore it is important to justify

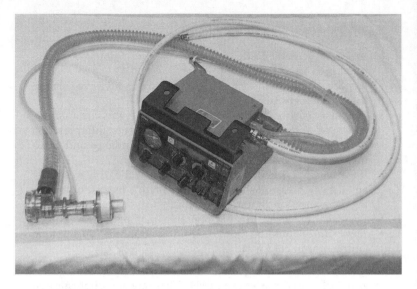

Fig. 18.5 Transport ventilator.

any transport whether it is intra-hospital or inter-hospital. Knowledge of potential problems and hazards associated with transport is essential if patient monitoring during transport is to be undertaken accurately and effectively, thus minimising morbidity and mortality.

Risks are reduced when there is meticulous clinical preparation and appropriate equipment available for use, and when transfer is undertaken by experienced staff familiar with the transfer environment. The same level of supervision and preparation is also important when critically ill patients are transferred between departments within a hospital.

ACKNOWLEDGEMENT
Some text in this chapter has been reproduced, with kind permission, from Jevon and Ewens (2001).

REFERENCES

Everest, E. & Munford, B. (2009) Transport of the critically ill. In: *Bersten*, A. D. & Soni, N. (eds), *Oh's Intensive Care Manual*, 6th edn. Philadelphia, PA: Butterworth Heinemann Elsevier.

Gilligan, J. (1997) Transport of the critically ill. In: Oh, T. (ed.), *Intensive Care Manual*, 4th edn. Oxford: Butterworth-Heinemann.

Hinds, C. J. & Watson, D. (1996) *Intensive Care, A concise textbook*, 2nd edn. London: W.B. Saunders.

Intensive Care Society (2011) *Guidelines for the transport of the critically ill adult*. 3rd edn. London: Intensive Care Society.

Jarden, R. J. & Quirke, S. (2010) Improving patienty safety and documentation in intrahospital transport: Development of an intrahospaital transport tool for critically ill patients. *Intensive and Critical Care Nursing*, **26**, 101–107.

Jevon, P. & Ewens, B. (2001) Care of patients on the move. *Nursing Times*, **97**, 35–36.

Knowles, P. R., Bryden, P. C., Kishen, R., & Gwinnutt, C. L. (1999) Meeting the standards for interhospital transfer of adults with severe head injury in the United Kingdom. *Anaesthesia*, **54**, 283–288.

Lawler, P.G. (2000) Transfer of critically ill patients: Part 1 – Physiological concepts. *Care of the Critically Ill*, **16**(2), 61–65.

Markakis, C., Dalezios, M., Chatzicostas, C., et al. (2006) Evaluation of a risk score for interhospital transport of critically ill patients. *Emergency Medicine Journal*, **23**, 313–317.

Record Keeping

19

LEARNING OBJECTIVES
At the end of the chapter the reader will be able to:

☐ discuss the *importance* of *good record keeping*
☐ list the *common deficiencies* of record keeping
☐ outline the *principles* of good record keeping
☐ outline the *importance of auditing records*
☐ discuss the *legal issues* associated with record keeping

INTRODUCTION
Good record keeping is a fundamental part of nursing (Nursing and Midwifery Council or NMC 2010). An accurate written record detailing all aspects of patient monitoring is important, not only because it forms an integral part of the nursing management of the patient, but also because it can help to protect practitioners if defence of their actions is required. The Clinical Negligence Scheme for Trusts (CNST) also requires its members to maintain high standards of record keeping (Dimond 2005).

The aim of this chapter is to understand the principles of good record keeping, with specific reference to *Guidelines for Records and Record Keeping* (NMC 2010) (Fig. 19.1).

IMPORTANCE OF GOOD RECORD KEEPING
Record keeping is an integral part of nursing, midwifery and health visiting practice. It is a tool of professional practice and one that should

Monitoring the Critically Ill Patient, Third Edition.
Philip Jevon, Beverley Ewens.
© 2012 Blackwell Publishing Ltd. Published 2012 by Blackwell Publishing Ltd.

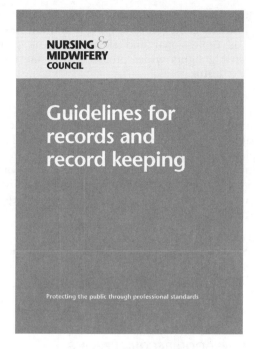

Fig. 19.1 *Guidelines for Records and Record Keeping* (NMC 2010).

help the care process. It is not separate from this process and it is not an optional extra to be fitted in if circumstances allow.

(NMC 2010)

Good record keeping will help to protect the welfare of both the patient and practitioner by promoting:

- high standards of clinical care
- continuity of care
- better communication and dissemination of information between members of the interprofessional health-care team
- the ability to detect problems, such as changes in the patient's condition at an early stage
- an accurate account of treatment and care planning and delivery.

The quality of record keeping is also a reflection of the standard of nursing practice: good record keeping is an indication that the practitioner is professional and skilled whereas poor record keeping often highlights wider problems with the individual's practice (NMC 2010).

COMMON DEFICIENCIES IN RECORD KEEPING

Nearly every report published by the Health Service Commissioner (Health Service Ombudsman) following a complaint identifies examples of poor record keeping that have either hampered the care that the patient has received or have made it difficult for health-care professionals to defend their practice (Dimond 2005).

Common deficiencies in record keeping encountered include (Dimond 2005):

- absence of clarity
- failure to record action taken when a problem has been identified
- missing information
- spelling mistakes
- inaccurate records.

PRINCIPLES OF GOOD RECORD KEEPING

There are a number of factors that underpin good record keeping. The patient's records should:

- be factual, consistent and accurate
- be updated as soon as possible after any recordable event
- provide current information on the care and condition of the patient
- be documented clearly and in such a way that the text cannot be erased
- be consecutive and accurately dated, timed and signed (including a printed signature)
- have any alterations and additions dated, timed and signed; all original entries should be clearly legible
- not include abbreviations, jargon, meaningless phrases, irrelevant speculation and offensive subjective statements
- still be legible if photocopied

- identify any problems identified and most importantly the action taken to rectify them.

It is important to record all aspects of patient monitoring. Some observations will be recorded on the patient's observation charts (e.g. the intensive care unit's [ICU's] observation chart and early warning chart – Fig. 19.2). Dates and times should be clearly visible and standard coloured ink should be used following local protocols. It is also important to ensure that an accurate record is made in the patient's notes. In particular it is important to include interventions and any response to the interventions.

The benefits of good record keeping are (NMC 2010):

- helping to improve accountability
- showing how decisions were made relating to the patient's care
- supporting the delivery of services
- supporting effective clinical judgement
- supporting patient care and communications
- making continuity of care easier
- providing documentary evidence of services delivered
- promoting better communication and sharing of information between members of the multiprofessional team
- helping to identify risks and enabling the early detection of complications
- supporting clinical audit, research, allocation of resources and performance planning
- helping to address complaints or legal processes.

Best practice – record keeping

Records must be:

- factual
- legible
- clear
- concise
- accurate
- signed
- timed
- dated

(Drew et al. 2000)

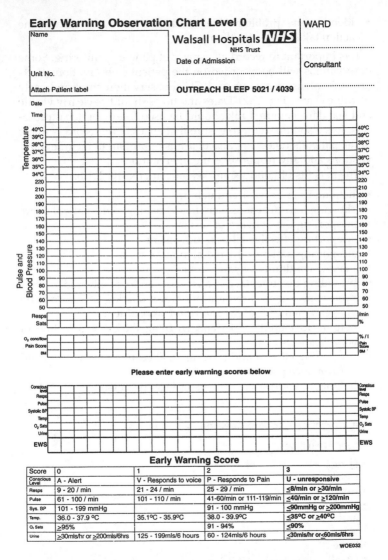

Fig. 19.2 Standard observation chart (Walsall Hospitals NHS Trust).

Notes
- • = Calculate score EVERY time the observations are recorded
- < = less than
- > = greater than
- ≥ = the same or greater than
- ≤ = the same or less than
- • = If the score is three or above inform the nurse in charge who should follow the algorithm
- • = Urine output should be calculated according to body weight i.e. 0.5ml / kg/hr if weight known and from the preceding 6 hours
- • Score 1 - 2 repeat in 1 hour
- • ≥3 follow algorithm
- O_2 record in L / min if Hudson mask, O_2 % if variable mask i.e. venturi

Pain Assessment Tool
1. **Comfortable**
2. **Mild discomfort**
3. **In pain**
4. **In bad pain**
5. **In very bad pain (excruciating pain)**

Fig. 19.2 *Continued* Explanatory notes to standard observation chart.

IMPORTANCE OF AUDITING RECORDS

Audit can play an important role in ensuring quality of health care. In particular it can help to improve the process of record keeping. By auditing records the standard can be evaluated and any areas for improvement and staff development identified. Audit tools should be developed at a local level to monitor the standards of record keeping.

Audit should primarily be aimed at serving the interests of the patient rather than the organisation (NMC 2010). A system of peer review may also be of value. Whatever audit system is used, the confidentiality of patients' information applies to audit just as it does to record keeping.

LEGAL ISSUES ASSOCIATED WITH RECORD KEEPING

The patient's records are occasionally required as evidence before a court of law, by the Health Service Commissioner or in order to investigate a complaint at a local level. Sometimes they may be requested by the NMC's Fitness to Practise committees when investigating complaints related to misconduct. Care plans, diaries and anything that makes reference to the patient's care may be required as evidence (NMC 2010).

What constitutes a legal document is often a cause for concern. Any document requested by the court becomes a legal document (Dimond 1994), e.g. nursing records, medical records, radiographs, laboratory reports, observation charts – in fact any document that may be relevant to the case.

If any of the documents are missing, the writer of the records may be cross-examined as to the circumstances of their disappearance (Dimond 1994). 'Medical records are not proof of the truth of the facts stated in them but the maker of the records may be called to give evidence as to the truth as to what is contained in them' (Dimond 1994).

The approach to record keeping that courts of law adopt tends to be that, if it is not recorded, it has not been undertaken (NMC 2010). Professional judgement is needed when deciding what is relevant and what needs to be recorded, particularly if the patient's clinical condition is apparently unchanging and no record has been made of the care that has been delivered.

A registered nurse has both a professional and a legal duty of care. Consequently when keeping records it is important to be able to demonstrate that:

- a comprehensive nursing assessment of the patient has been undertaken including care that has been planned and provided
- relevant information is included together with any measures that have been taken in response to changes in the patient's condition
- the duty of care owed to the patient has been honoured and that no acts or omissions have compromised the patient's safety
- arrangements have been made for ongoing care of the patient.

The registered nurse is also accountable for any delegation of record keeping to members of the multiprofessional team who are not registered practitioners, e.g. if record keeping is delegated to a pre-registration student nurse or a health-care assistant, competence to perform the task must be ensured and adequate supervision provided. All such entries must be countersigned.

The Access to Health Records Act 1990 gives patients the right of access to their manually maintained health records which were made after 1 November 1991. The Data Protection Act 1998 gives patients the right to access their computer-held records. The Freedom of Information Act 2000 grants the rights to anyone to all information that is not covered by the Data Protection Act 1998 (NMC 2010).

Sometimes it is necessary to withhold information if it could affect the physical or mental wellbeing of the patient or if it would breach another patient confidentiality (NMC 2010). If the decision to withhold information is made, justification for doing so must be clearly recorded in the patient's notes.

CONCLUSION

When monitoring a critically ill patient, it is important to ensure good record keeping. Good record keeping is both the product of good teamwork and an important tool in promoting high-quality health care.

REFERENCES

Dimond, B. (1994) *The Legal Aspects of Midwifery*. Cheshire: Books for Midwives Press.

Dimond, B. (2005) Exploring common deficiencies that occur in record keeping. *British Journal of Nursing*, **14**, 568–570.

Drew, D., Jevon, P., & Raby, M. (2000) *Resuscitation of the Newborn*. Oxford: Butterworth Heinemann.

Nursing and Midwifery Council (2010) *Guidelines for Records and Record Keeping*. London: NMC.

CONCLUSION

REFERENCES

Index

Monitoring the Critically Ill Patient, Third Edition.
Philip Jevon, Beverley Ewens.
© 2012 Blackwell Publishing Ltd. Published 2012 by Blackwell
Publishing Ltd.